Enhancing Human Occupation Through Hippotherapy

Enhancing Human Occupation Through Hippotherapy

A GUIDE FOR OCCUPATIONAL THERAPY

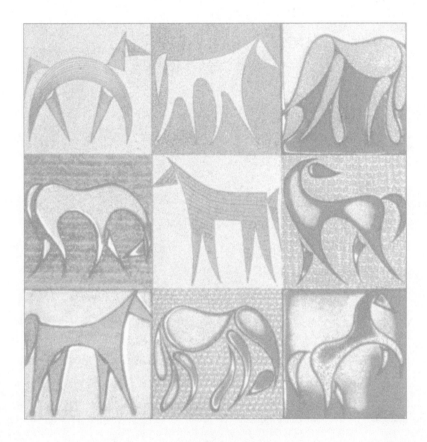

Edited by

Barbara T. Engel, MEd, OTR, and
Joyce R. MacKinnon, PhD, OT(C), OTR

Foreword by Florence Cromwell, MA, OTR, FAOTA

AOTA PRESS

The American
Occupational Therapy
Association, Inc.

Vision Statement
AOTA advances occupational therapy as the pre-eminent profession in promoting the health, productivity, and quality of life of individuals and society through the therapeutic application of occupation.

Mission Statement
The American Occupational Therapy Association advances the quality, availability, use, and support of occupational therapy through standard-setting, advocacy, education, and research on behalf of its members and the public.

AOTA Staff
Frederick P. Somers, *Executive Director*
Christopher M. Bluhm, *Chief Operating Officer*
Audrey Rothstein, *Director, Marketing and Communications*

Chris Davis, *Managing Editor, AOTA Press*
Timothy Sniffin, *Production Editor*
Carrie Mercadante, *Editorial Assistant*

Robert A. Sacheli, *Manager, Creative Services*
Sarah E. Ely, *Book Production Coordinator*

Marge Wasson, *Marketing Manager*
John Prudente, *Marketing Specialist*

The American Occupational Therapy Association, Inc.
4720 Montgomery Lane
Bethesda, MD 20814
Phone: 301-652-AOTA (2682)
TDD: 800-377-8555
Fax: 301-652-7711
www.aota.org
To order: 1-877-404-AOTA (2682)

Disclaimers
This publication is designed to provide accurate and authoritative information in regard to the subject matter covered. It is sold or distributed with the understanding that the publisher is not engaged in rendering legal, accounting, or other professional service. If legal advice or other expert assistance is required, the services of a competent professional person should be sought.
—*From the Declaration of Principles jointly adopted by the American Bar Association and a Committee of Publishers and Associations*

It is the objective of the American Occupational Therapy Association to be a forum for free expression and interchange of ideas. The opinions expressed by the editors of and contributors to this work are their own and not necessarily those of the American Occupational Therapy Association.

ISBN 10: 1-56900-232-0

ISBN 13: 978-1-56900-232-2

Library of Congress Control Number: 2007925092

Design by Sarah E. Ely
Composition by Circle Graphics, Columbia, MD
Printed by Victor Graphics, Baltimore, MD
Cover features an original etching, "Equus," by Jane Lee Ling. The part title pages and chapter heads feature portions of this artwork. Used with permission.

Citation: Engel, B. T., & MacKinnon, J. R. (Eds.). (2007). *Enhancing human occupation through hippotherapy: A guide for occupational therapy.* Bethesda, MD: AOTA Press.

Dedication

This book is dedicated to the occupational therapists who have
devoted their time and effort to forge forward with hippotherapy
strategy in occupational therapy, including those contributors
whose work enriches this text.

To my mentors and teachers, Gayle S. Fidler, A. J. Ayres,
Jennifer J. Thurston, and my daughter, Sandra L. Hubbard,
all who have taught me so much in the fields of occupational
therapy, classical equitation, human interaction,
performance, and the strive to move forward.
—*Barbara T. Engel*

To my parents, Margaret and Robert MacKinnon, who
always encouraged me to follow my dreams; to my uncle,
Gorden MacLeod, who instilled in me his love and passion for
horses; and to the children, parents, staff, and volunteers of the
Special Abilities Riding Institute, who cooperated
with and engaged in my research.
—*Joyce R. MacKinnon*

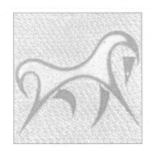

Contents

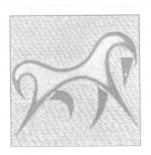

Acknowledgments

We thank Elizabeth Tester for the exceptional job she did in the technical editing of this text in such a short time and Beth LaShell for her hours of computer assistance. We also thank the following people, who gave valuable advice to our contributors and their skill and dedication to this project:

Ann Alman, OTR/L

Stacy Albertson, MS, OTR

Jennifer Almond, MS, OTR/L, CEIS

Rebecca Cook, OTR, HPCS

Marcia A. Cushman, OTR

Ellen Conner Davis, MOT

Roberta S. Devery, MS, OTR/L

Sandra L. Hubbard, PhD, OTR/L, ATP

Christina M. T. Richardson, MS, OTR

Vallery Bisbane Sampson, OTR

Jeannie Seuffert, MS, OTR/L

Kathyrn Splinter-Watkins, MOT, OTR/L, FAOTA, HPCS

About the Editors and Contributors

Editors

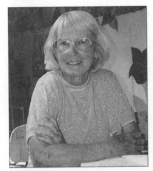

Photo by Seamus T. Millett

Barbara T. Engel, MEd, OTR, is Owner of Barbara Engel Therapy Services, Durango, Colorado, and has written, edited, and published seven books on therapeutic riding and hippotherapy, including *Rehabilitation With the Aid of a Horse* (1997); *Therapeutic Riding II: Strategies for Rehabilitation* (1997); *Therapeutic Riding I: Strategies for Instruction* (1998); and *The Horse, the Handicapped, The Riding Team in a Therapeutic Riding Program: A Volunteer Training Manual* (2nd ed., 1994). Engel practiced occupational therapy for 49 years, working with schools, in-home pediatrics, a rehabilitation center, and a psychoanalytic hospital where she served as the occupational therapy department head and supervisor of clinical training. She has lectured internationally. Engel received the North American Riding for the Handicapped's James Brady Professional Achievement Award.

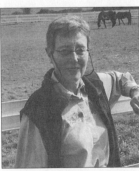

Photo by Barbara T. Engel

Joyce R. MacKinnon, PhD, OT(C), OTR, is Professor Emerita and Former Associate Dean, Faculty of Health Sciences, and Associate Professor, School of Occupational Therapy, The University of Western Ontario, London, Ontario. MacKinnon practiced pediatric occupational therapy in Canada and the United States for 14 years and worked at the University of Western Ontario for 21 years. She has presented papers in England, Greece, Singapore, Australia, and New Zealand.

Contributors

Beatriz C. Abreu, PhD, OTR, FAOTA
Director of Occupational Therapy
Transitional Learning Center at Galveston
Clinical Professor
Department of Occupational Therapy
School of Allied Health Sciences
University of Texas Medical Branch at Galveston
Galveston

Diane E. Allan, MA
PhD Candidate
Research Associate
Centre on Aging
University of Victoria
British Columbia

William L. Bufford, Jr., PhD
Director
Orthopaedics Biomechanics Laboratory
Department of Orthopaedic Surgery and Rehabilitation
University of Texas
Galveston

Dixie L. Carr-Heyn, MPT
Physical Therapist and Clinic Manager
Professional Therapy Services
San Antonio, Texas

Rebecca Cook, OTR, HPCS
AHA Clinical Specialist in Hippotherapy
Right Step Therapy
Grass Lake and Tecumseh, Michigan

Marie Dawson, MA, OTR/L, HPCS
President
Creative Therapy, Inc.
AHA Clinical Specialist in Hippotherapy
Canton, Georgia

Debbie DeTurk-Peloso, CPCU
Equine Insurance Specialist
Markel Insurance Company
Greenville, Florida

Roberta S. Devery, MS, OTR/L
Founder and President
Fun in Motion, LLC
Director of Therapy Services
Riding High Farms
North Princeton Junction, New Jersey

Ashleigh Eccles, OT Reg (Ont)
Canadian Occupational Therapist
Community Association for Riding for the Disabled
Ontario

Linda A. Frease, MHS, OTR/L
Occupational Therapist
Children's Therapy Works
Sarasota, Florida

Rebecca Gewurtz, MSc, OT Reg (Ont)
PhD Candidate
Department of Rehabilitation Science
University of Toronto
Toronto, Ontario

Heather L. Gohmert-Dionne, MOT, OTR/L
Advanced NARHA Instructor
Lake Charles, Louisiana

Patricia Heyn, PhD
Gerontologist Scientist
University of Colorado Health Sciences Center
Denver

Judy Hilburn, OTR/L
Home Health, ADHC
Contract Occupational Therapist
Mastering Abilities Riding Equestrians Program
Bakersfield, California

Christopher Hipsher, MS, COTA/S
Student
Middle Georgia College
Cochran

Paula Hueners, MEd, OTR
School Occupational Therapist
Holman, Wisconsin

Sandra L. Hubbard, PhD, OTR/L, ATP
Post-Doctoral Fellow and Assistant Professor
Occupational Therapy Department
University of Florida
Gainesville

Amy Taylor Johnson, MS, OTR
Private Practice
Owner of Integrated Therapy
Vicksburg, Mississippi

Joanne S. Jones, MS, OTR
Occupational Therapist
TriStar Rehab, Inc.
Gulf Healthcare Center
Galveston, Texas

Nancy King, MS, OTR
Director
A Horse Connection
Anderson Dayhabilitation
Catskill, New York

Deborah Laliberte-Rudman, OT
Former Graduate Student in Occupational Therapy
Department of Occupational Therapy
Elbom College at the University of Western Ontario
London, Ontario

Judith Lariviere, MEd, OTR/L
Assistive Technology Specialist
Skyline College
San Bruno, California

Ann MacPhail, MSc, PT
Physical Therapy Lecturer
Department of Occupational Therapy
Elbom College at the University of Western Ontario
London, Ontario

Brent Masel, MD
President and Medical Director
Transitional Learning Center at Galveston
Galveston, Texas

Cynthia A. Marx, OTR/L
Clinical Specialist
Children's Hospital of Philadelphia
Petersburg, NJ

J. Ashton Moore
Judge
International Equestrian Federation (FEI)
Trainer and Examiner
FEI, U.S. Dressage Federation (USDF), U.S. Equestrian
    Federation, and American Vaulting Association
Faculty Member
USDF Learner Judge Program
San Juan Bautista, California

Samuel Noh, PhD
Epidemiologist/Biostatistician
Associate Professor
Department of Occupational Therapy
Elbom College at the University of Western Ontario
London, Ontario

Karin J. Opacich, PhD, OTR/L, MHPE, FAOTA
Project EXPORT Director
Assistant Director
National Center for Rural Health Professions
University of Illinois–Rockford

Kenneth J. Ottenbacher, PhD, OTR, FAOTA
Director
Division of Rehabilitation Science
University of Texas
Galveston

Rita Patterson, PhD
Deputy Director
Orthopaedics Biomechanics Laboratory
Department of Orthopaedic Surgery and Rehabilitation
University of Texas
Galveston

Timothy A. Reistetter, PhD, OTR
Assistant Professor
East Carolina University
Greenville, North Carolina

Orit Shechtman, PhD, OTR/L
Associate Professor
Department of Occupational Therapy
College of Public Health and Health Professions
University of Florida
Gainesville

Jan Spink, MA
Director and Founder
System of Developmental Riding Therapy
Author of *Developmental Riding Therapy: A Team Approach*
Charlottesville, Virginia

Kathy Splinter-Watkins, MOT, OTR/L, FAOTA, HPCS
AHA Clinical Specialist in Hippotherapy
Associate Professor of Occupational Therapy
Eastern Kentucky University
Richmond

Janine Stoner, MS, OTR/L
Program Director
High View Farm
Killingwood, Connecticut

Melanie M. Tidman, MA, OTR/L
Occupational Therapist—Hippotherapy
Tidman Therapy Services
Albuquerque, New Mexico

Teresa Tisdell, MPH, OTR
Occupational Therapist
MDA Clinic
Integris Southwest Medical Center
Oklahoma City

Ann K. Viviano, MA, MS, OTR, CCC/SLP, HPCS
AHA Clinical Specialist in Hippotherapy
Occupational Therapist
Children's Unit
Good Samaritan Hospital
Puyallup, Washington

Kay Walker, PhD, OTR/L, FAOTA
Occupational Therapy Department
University of Florida
Gainesville

Janet Weisberg, MS, OTR/L
Owner
Hold Your Horses, LLC
Occupational Therapy Hippotherapy Program
Independence, Missouri

Nina Wiger, MA
Vaulting and Riding Instructor
Grue Finnskog, Norway

Colleen M. Zanin, MS, OTR
Public School Staff Therapist
Founder and Therapist
Lift Me Up!
Great Falls, Virginia

Foreword

Disability, regardless of cause, is a cruel partner to anyone seeking to pursue an active life. Whether one has orthopedic, neuromotor, developmental, or psychosocial deficits that make daily life difficult, if not impossible, people with such disabilities will find "mountains to climb" just to manage simple activities of daily living.

For years people attentive to the rehabilitation needs of those with chronic illnesses and developmental disabilities have studied and improvised, seeking solutions to the barriers and opening horizons for participation in everyday occupations. Fortunately, technology and research by rehabilitation specialists now offer multiple solutions or corrections to parents, infants, students, housewives, workers, and people with mild to chronic disabling conditions. Therapists long have been concerned with these efforts, but such developments are not all new. Still, one must search to find!

Among the "solutions" is one strategy that has been well known in Europe and now in the United States. It originated among horseback riders who saw a positive outcome in using the horse as a therapeutic strategy. Called *hippotherapy,* this approach was started by skilled riders in Germany who witnessed positive changes in people with disabilities when they were positioned on horseback to experience the uniquely compatible movement of horses in motion. Soon some occupational therapists in the United States, most well acquainted with horseback riding, saw the approach's potential and became practitioners of hippotherapy, using the horse as a modality.

Now more therapists have added this component to their treatment regimens—or wish to. Hippotherapy is a growing segment for occupational therapy clinical practice.

One important caveat should be noted, however: Anyone targeting a role as practitioners of hippotherapy must not only have expertise in traditional occupational therapy but ideally be skilled horsewomen and men as well.

Because people of all ages and varying disabilities are potential clients, the scope of occupational therapy education provides the ideal base for would-be practitioners of hippotherapy. Universities planning to add preparation for this growing community service option to the curriculum will note the practical content of this volume as ideal for use in a "specialty" class.

As one who has witnessed the gradual growth of interest among occupational therapists, I have noted the successes and increasing publicity such treatment programs attract in community settings. The time is right for more occupational therapy personnel to consider this environment for treatment programs as an ideal place to increase opportunities for balanced human occupation among people with disabilities.

Whether you are a curriculum director planning to add such needed content to your basic studies program or a practitioner of hippotherapy desiring to improve your understanding, this new book will be the right resource for basic information.

I am honored to have been asked to help launch this important professional text. Good reading to all who now are or want to be a practitioner of hippotherapy!

—*Florence Cromwell, MA, OTR, FAOTA*
Claremont, California

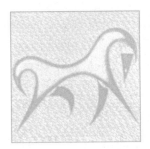

Preface

We expect that there will be five audiences for *Enhancing Human Occupation Through Hippotherapy: A Guide for Occupational Therapy:* (1) undergraduate and graduate students who want to study more about hippotherapy; (2) faculty members who plan to include hippotherapy in their academic curricula; (3) researchers who are studying and documenting hippotherapy; (4) clinicians who are working in hippotherapy or therapeutic horseback riding and want to update their knowledge in research or a particular practice area; and (5) riders or their parents who are interested in the development, application, and benefits of hippotherapy. Although Barbara T. Engel and I hope that this book becomes a text for those studying and working in hippotherapy, we have not targeted the book solely to students, academics, or clinicians. Instead, we focus on making it readable by everyone, although we realize some sections or chapters will appeal to different audiences depending on needs, interests, educational qualifications, and experiential backgrounds.

As far as we can determine, *Enhancing Human Occupation Through Hippotherapy* is the first occupational therapy book detailing the profession's current and potential contribution to hippotherapy. We have not relied on the American Hippotherapy Association's definitions because our book, we believe, has an international perspective written specifically from an occupational therapist's viewpoint.

The organization of this book is divided into five sections, moving from theory to research and from research to practice. Part I starts with a history of hippotherapy and the theory of classical dressage used as the theoretical basis of hippotherapy and the technique's relevance to occupational therapy practice. Next, theoretical concepts and frames of reference from occupational therapy are related to hippotherapy as well as to pertinent literature on hippotherapy. Part II begins with a literature review on research, isolating what we regard as a primary driving force needed in hippotherapy. The chapters move from evidence-based practice to research-based chapters. Part III examines evaluation and treatment planning, providing readers with actual examples of evaluations used in hippotherapy. Part IV offers practice techniques used in hippotherapy, including activity analyses, communication skills facilitation, and treatment of various problems and disabilities ranging from hypotonia to sensory integration. It continues by showing how practitioners of hippotherapy have offered treatment and which interventions appeared to them to be successful. Finally, Part IV examines business management principles and methods, occupational therapy student internships, and insurance.

Differences

Many of the difficulties inherent in writing such a volume are common to any project of this magnitude. Our authors come from varied backgrounds, from hands-on therapists currently practicing in the field to academics involved in research projects. Some authors have had little scientific writing experience but have been ready and willing to learn the basics. Unfortunately, some contributors were lost because of the rigorous demands for which they did not have the time or resources. For this, we are sorry. Thus, readers will find different levels and styles of writing. We tried very hard to maintain a goal of basic rigor in our book.

Other differences arose from essential tensions and contradictions that operate in the field. Many times the politics of meaning came into play as we attempted to navigate our way through turbulent waters. One major issue we were forced to manage was the use of terms, including but not restricted to *hippotherapy* and *therapeutic horseback riding.* So, while most authors have a specific definition of hippotherapy, others do not share that view. We hope this does not confuse our readers. It sometimes is difficult to know how to bridge these differences, and our bridges often were makeshift constructions.

Reading This Book

Were we to write our own critique of this book, we would point to its shortcomings. We have made great efforts to ensure there are theoretical underpinnings and a basic understanding of the research process. We have attempted to include a diverse range of practice techniques and examples, but we realize that many of your favorite areas may be missing.

We do express our own views, which may not fit well with some readers. You, the readers, certainly will have your own reaction to this book, which may highlight issues we do not see. It no doubt will be re-created in future generations of practitioners and researchers of hippotherapy. *Enhancing Human Occupation Through Hippotherapy* is intended not as a final statement but as a starting point for new thought and new work that will sharpen our understanding and provide more insights into hippotherapy's benefits to our riders.

—Joyce R. MacKinnon, PhD, OT(C), OTR
London, Ontario

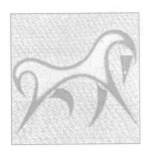

Introduction

Occupational therapists increasingly have shown interest in using the horse as a treatment strategy in their practice, especially those who have had horses in their lives. Some therapists have been Pony Clubbers, have grown up on a ranch or farm, have competed in English or Western riding, or had a trail and companion horse. Some have been introduced to horses through therapeutic riding programs, whereas others always have wished to be involved with horses and now are pursuing this exciting field.

In 1957, I first heard about using the horse in therapy when I read a *Washington Post* article about Joseph Bauer, a Canadian medical doctor who had returned to the saddle after an auto accident injured his back and broke his foot, for which his doctor had no cure in conventional care (Bauer, 1972). It was intriguing to my daughter Sandy and me, because we were recreational riders and enamored by horses. At a psychiatric hospital in the 1960s, I organized a small riding group of patients who also were experienced riders. I was interested in how the horses reacted to certain disorders and how normal behavior occurred in many of the patients while riding. This group was intended to be a social group, involving an activity they had enjoyed in the past. Before therapeutic riding began to be developed in the eastern United States (Butts, 1998), we moved to California and did not think more about it. Then in 1982, I was working with a young teenager with cerebral palsy. His mother asked if I was interested in coming along to a riding program in which the boy was involved. My interest was sparked again and my involvement became serious.

As an occupational therapist, I could see the therapeutic value of the horse in my field. I learned as much about therapeutic riding as was available at that time. Kyne (1980) and Heipertz, Heipertz-Hengst, Kroger, and Kuprian (1984) indicated that the horse provided perpetual sensory excitement through all the receptors in the joints, muscles, tendons, ocular motor systems, and skin. This perpetual stimulation provided an instant feedback that constantly adjusted the movement systems, thus contributing to the maintenance of posture and allowing the client to become a participant involved in purposeful activity. Heipertz and colleagues also stated that the horse was an excellent partner in the treatment of specific disabilities and that space orientation was facilitated through riding while muscle spasms were reduced. They further maintained that various riding skills can be introduced depending on the progress of the client to train motor and behavioral abilities, not to train clients as riders.

I knew from Ayres's (1973) lectures and literature that stimulation and arousal of the vestibular systems are a powerful therapeutic means available to address sensory integration dysfunction. Feldenkrais (1979) stated that the vestibular system is a major system that orients our body in space. The horse provides an ample amount of vestibular stimulation that can be graded and adapted in many ways. Kyne (1980) pointed out an increase in adrenalin is produced by the increase in perceived risk, while an increase in the cardiovascular system appears to improve the muscular reaction beyond what occurs in ordinary therapeutic activity. A graded degree of risk helps the learning process (Rosenthal, 1984). I learned from the German literature that the gait of the average horse resembles that of the human adult. As riders, we know that riding involves and influences the total body's mechanism and all the senses and emotions.

With this limited information on therapeutic riding, I began to use the horse with my private clients. The result of the intervention was astonishing. Not only were occupational therapy theories being applied, but the clients were having a great time—certainly a motivating factor. The children did not take riding as therapy because it was quite different from the conventional methods they had experienced, while the adults were more focused on the horse and being outdoors while learning a new skill.

I was fortunate to be included in a condensed hippotherapy course given under the auspices of the Kürtorium for Therapeütisches Reiten that certified all physiotherapists in Germany. There, we learned the rationale, theory, methods of use, and horse and riding requirements, and we practiced techniques used by the German physicians and physiotherapists. On the way home, I pondered over the information we had received. It was massive and impressive. How does occupational therapy fit into this scheme? I remembered that Gilfoyle, Grady, and Moore (1981) had stated occupational therapy facilitates the adaptation of posture and movement strategies for purposeful activity, which certainly applied to the information we were taught. But they also stressed that the adaptation was for purposeful activity in which an individual was an active participant involved in environment–client–occupational-centered goals.

In 2002, the American Occupational Therapy Association stated that the occupational therapists' domain of concern centers on assisting the client to engage in daily life activities, in this case equestrian activities. Occupational therapy always has focused on the individual as active in meaningful and purposeful activity, while we had learned that the movement of the horse stimulated the client while he or she was passively sitting astride the horse and the client accommodated him- or herself to the movement. There was no active purposeful participation. The client is not actively or purposely involved; therefore, how does occupational therapy fit?

That question led to the development of this book. Occupational therapy uses activities as a strategy for intervention. Therapists help reintroduce activities to those with injuries, diseases, or disabilities to increase their meaningful function and enjoyable life. The horse addresses so many physical and psychological problems clients encounter when they are completely involved with the equine and its environment.

While the initial thoughts about this book were developing, Joyce R. MacKinnon asked me to review a research grant she was proposing at the University of Western Ontario, where she was Associate Dean of Health Science in the School of Occupational Therapy. She had been involved in research in hippotherapy, including writing an article I had read. I asked her if she would be interested in coediting this book with me because she was in academia while I was a practitioner of hippotherapy: This relationship would make a good

fit for this field. We think much alike and have worked well together, and we attracted knowledgeable contributors for this text.

Enhancing Human Occupation Through Hippotherapy: A Guide for Occupational Therapy attempts to cover important issues our contributors feel are significant in their hippotherapy practice. The therapist pursing a practice in hippotherapy, however, must be able to apply skills in areas of neurodevelopment, sensory and perceptual–motor functions, sensory integration, and up-to-date rehabilitation techniques to the equine domain. Additionally, equestrian skills must be acquired to have both knowledge about and a feeling for the qualities of the horse. It is the knowledge of these two areas—one intertwined with the other—that makes hippotherapy an impressive occupational strategy in the treatment of people with many types of dysfunctions.

—*Barbara T. Engel, MEd, OTR*
Durango, Colorado

References

American Occupational Therapy Association. (2002). Occupational therapy practice framework: Domain and process. *American Journal of Occupational Therapy, 47,* 609–639.

Ayres, A. J. (1973). *Sensory integration and learning disorders.* Los Angeles: Western Psychological Services.

Bauer, J. J. (1972). *Riding for rehabilitation: A guide for handicapped riders and their instructors.* Toronto, Ontario: Canadian Stage and Arts.

Butts, E. G. (1998). NARHA—Therapeutic riding in North America: Its first decade, 1970 to 1980. In B. Engel (Ed.), *Therapeutic riding I: Strategies for rehabilitation.* Durango, CO: Barbara Engel Therapy Services.

Feldenkrais, M. (1979). *Body and mature behavior.* New York: International Universities.

Gilfoyle, E. M., Grady, A. P., & Moore, J. C. (1981). *Children adapt.* Thorofare, NJ: Slack.

Heipertz, W., Heipertz-Hengst, C., Kroger A., & Kuprian W. (1984).*Therapeutic riding: Medicine, education, sports.* (M. Takeuchi, Trans.) Ottawa: National Printers.

Kyne, J. P. (1980, June). *Benefit for the physically handicapped through horseback riding.* Paper presented at the 14th World Congress of Rehabilitation International, Winnipeg, Canada.

Rosenthal, S. R. (1984). Research on risk and riding. *NARHA NEWS, 10,* 3–5.

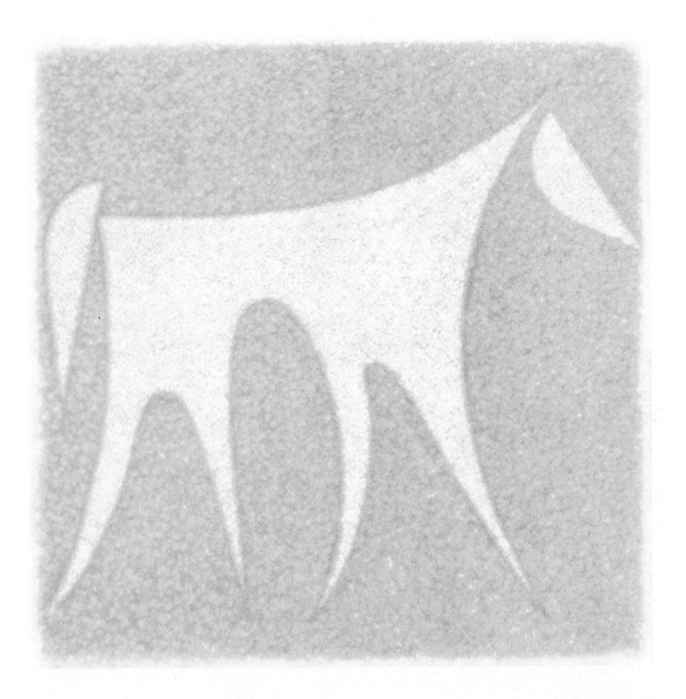

PART I

History, Philosophy, and Theory

I will not change my horse with any that treads but on four pasterns....
When I astride him, I soar, I am a hawk. He trots the air, the earth sings when he touches it, the barest
horn of his hoof is more musical than the pipe of Hermes.
—William Shakespeare, Henry V

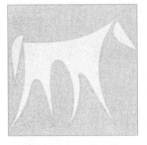

You may bring a horse to the river, but he will drink when and what he pleaseyth.
—George Herbert, 1640

CHAPTER 1

An Introduction to Hippotherapy Terminology and Development

Barbara T. Engel, MEd, OTR

As early as the 1500s, the gentle movement of the horse was felt to be medically beneficial (Riede, 1988). Contemporary use of the horse to treat individuals with disabilities has developed rapidly during the past 45 years throughout the world (Klüwer, 1998) and has been influenced by each country's culture. Initially, English-speaking countries focused on recreational and sports riding. Scandinavian countries were interested in competition, reflecting the impressive accomplishments of Liz Hartel, a woman with post-polio syndrome who rehabilitated herself through riding. Hartel won a silver medal in dressage in the 1952 Olympic Games, the first woman to do so (Klüwer, 1998). Germanic countries based their use of the horse on specialized medical treatment (Klüwer, 1997, personal communication). Today, hippotherapy is practiced in most countries.

In the late 1960s, therapeutic riding was introduced in the United States from Canada and Europe (Butt & North American Riding for the Handicapped Association [NARHA], 1998). The riding model first used by U.S. therapeutic riding centers was adaptive riding or sports riding. These centers were organized under the national NARHA and follow the model of the British Riding for the Disabled centers.

As occupational and physical therapists in North America became involved in therapeutic riding centers, they began incorporating their professional skills of working with both clients and horses (American Hippotherapy Association [AHA], 1992; Gourley, 2002). Barbara Glasow, a physical therapist, began giving clinics that combined her knowledge of physical therapy and the horse as a strategy in treatments in the 1980s (AHA, 1992).

The International Conferences on Therapeutic Riding were held in Paris in 1973; Basel, 1976; Warwick, 1979; Hamburg, 1982; Milan, 1985 (Riede, 1988); Toronto, 1988; Denmark, 1991; New Zealand, 1994; United States, 1997; France, 2000; Hungary, 2003; and Brazil, 2006. The international conferences attracted medical professionals, who have helped move hippotherapy to a scientific arena. These conferences facilitated the exchange of information, making it available internationally. Occupational and physical therapists have incorporated the traditional model in their practice. Thus, clinical application of the use of the horse by U.S. therapists has been modeled on the German–Swiss–Austrian theoretical model.

The term *hippotherapy, hippo* meaning horse, was coined by the Swiss to describe a specialized medical treatment prescribed and monitored by physicians and carried out by physical therapists (called *physiotherapists* in Europe; Klüwer, 1992, personal communication). Strauss (1995), a German neurologist involved with the Deutsches Kuratorium Für Therapeutisches Reiten (the German National Organization for therapeutic riding), has extensive hands-on experience with hippotherapy and defines hippotherapy as follows:

> Hippotherapy is neuro-physiologically based physiotherapy with the help of the horse. The horse at a walk serves as the therapeutic medium by transmitting movement. With the patient in a sitting position, posture reflexes are practiced with the aid of the horse's walk-specific forward movement; as well, delicate coordination responses elicit and exercise balance and equilibrium reactions. Proprioceptive sensorimotor stimulation leads to improved

posture and facilitates the finding and strengthening of the best possible movement patterns of the body, as measured against its hypothetical norm. At the same time this movement correction trains the musculature by dispelling its imbalance and by regulating muscle tone. It also maximizes the possible or remaining range of motion of the joints. (p. 26)

Therapists Jean Tebay, Barbara Glasow, and Jan Spink continued to develop hippotherapy in North America. In 1987, Tebay contacted the German Kurtorium for Hippotherapy, the organization that certifies German physical therapists for practice in this field, and arranged for an intense, 10-day, 10-hour-a-day German hippotherapy course for her and 18 North American therapists. The course covered theory, riding skills, work-in-hand with the horse, and work with clients (AHA, 1992). Subsequently, meetings were held to develop a practice framework. In 1992, the AHA was established, and, their model essentially followed the German–Swiss–Austrian theoretical one. The dimensions of hippotherapy practice in Germany are limited by insurance coverage (Klüwer, 1997, personal interview).

The AHA focuses on physical therapy practice standards, and AHA hippotherapy is similar to the German–Swiss–Austrian model. Riede (1988) stated that the aim of that model "is the client's active and passive adaptation to the undulations of the horse's back" (p. 47). This three-dimensional movement of the horse therapeutically manipulates the client as he or she is placed astride the horse. An instructor trained in the movement of the horse, with knowledge of work in-hand, line-drives a specially trained horse with a quality rhythmic walking gait. The horse also may be led from the side by a lead rope. Based on the client's performance, the therapist, who has been trained in the biomechanical analysis of the horse, advises the instructor to move the horse in various directions and speeds to manipulate the posture of the client (Strauss, 1995). The client's involvement is accommodation to the movement of the horse. The AHA has modified the traditional German–Swiss–Austrian method by adding developmental positions while the horse is moving or standing. Americans refer to the German–Swiss–Austrian model as *classic hippotherapy* and the U.S. model as *American hippotherapy*. In April 1996, the AHA (1996) published a position paper, stating, "Hippotherapy is the overall term used to include a variety of applications of the use of the horse in treatment provided by physical, occupational therapists, and speech and language pathologists."

Hippotherapy generally is accepted internationally as the model for the use of the horse as a treatment strategy, although countries may use different terminology to describe their specific treatments because of language differences. For the purpose of this book, *therapeutic riding* is an umbrella term that encompasses hippotherapy and all other types of riding for individuals with disabilities such as neuromotor and psychosocial disorders. *Hippotherapy* refers to the use of the horse as a "medical treatment strategy" and not as a method to teach riding. Using the term *therapeutic riding* makes it difficult to search the literature to find, for example, literature on hippotherapy. The use of the terms *hippotherapy* and *therapeutic riding* vary throughout the world. In the United States, *therapeutic riding* is the all-inclusive term for all aspects of using the horse with individuals with disabilities. Under the all-inclusive term *equine-assisted activities,* NARHA cites recreational riding, adaptive-sports riding, educational riding, equine-assisted psychotherapy, and hippotherapy (NARHA, 1999).

For the rest of the world, the model of *hippotherapy*—the term referring to treatment with the use of a horse—and the definition of hippotherapy vary dependent on the education and profession of the practitioner and the interpretation of the method of treatment by the country involved (Copeland-Fitzpatrick, 1997). When I attended 2003 Congress of the Federation of Riding for the Disabled International, 15 terms were used in the hippotherapy section to describe a treatment using the horse as a therapy assistant. Terms such as *riding therapy, equestrian rehabilitation therapy, equitherapy,* and *equotherapy* were noted. "Hippotherapy appears to mean many things depending on where [it is done] and who provides the service" (Heine, 2003). Because of the differences in terminology, occupational therapists using the horse as an intervention should make it clear they are practicing occupational therapy within a practice framework, using the horse as a partner or a strategy. For example, occupational therapists would use the term *hippotherapy* in much the same way as they would use the terms *sensory integration* or *neurodevelopmental treatment.*

The purpose of clarifying the professional role (e.g., physical therapist, occupational therapist, other professions) when using the horse in hippotherapy and as a treatment modality is to promote critical research in each profession, which will provide evidence-based interventions such as hippotherapy that are valid. Students and researchers will find relevant information when published articles are clear and consistent. In addition, clarity will assist medical professions and researchers in all countries deciphering the meaning and the treatment protocol.

References

American Hippotherapy Association. (1992, Fall). A brief history. *AHA Newsletter, 2.*

American Hippotherapy Association. (1996, Spring). *AHA Newsletter.*

Butt, E. G., & North American Riding for the Handicapped Association. (1998). Therapeutic riding in North America: Its first decade, 1970 to 1980. In B. Engel (Ed.), *Therapeutic riding I: Strategies for instruction* (p. 1). Durango, CO: Barbara Engel Therapy Services.

Copeland-Fitzpatrick, J. C. (1997, July). *Hippotherapy and therapeutic riding: An international review.* Paper presented at the Ninth International Therapeutic Riding Congress, Denver, CO.

Gourley, M. (2002, April 29). Equine therapy. *OT Practice, 14.*

Heine, B. (2003). *Hippotherapy* (Vol. 12, No. 3). Denver, CO: American Hippotherapy Association.

Klüwer, C. (1998). Federation of Riding for the Disabled International. In B. Engel, (Ed.) *Therapeutic riding I: Strategies for instruction* (pp. 1, 15). Durango, CO: Barbara Engel Therapy Services.

North American Riding for the Handicapped Association. (1999). *NARHA Guide.* Denver, CO: Author.

Riede, D. (1988). *Physiotherapy on the horse.* Riderwood, MD: Therapeutic Riding Service.

Strauss, I. (1995). *Hippotherapy.* Ontario: Ontario Therapeutic Riding Association.

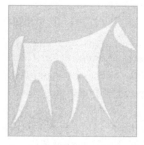

In training horses,
one trains himself.
—Antonio De Pluvinet

CHAPTER 2

Hippotherapy in the Practice of Occupational Therapy

Barbara T. Engel, MEd, OTR

People normally engage in activities that are the essential nature and texture of their everyday lives (Hinojosa & Blount, 2000). Reilly (2005) stated that "man, through the use of his hands as they are energized by mind and will, can influence the state of his [or her] own health" (p. 81). "Purposeful activities have a goal and a meaning and are actively pursued by the individual involved in the task" (Hinojosa & Blount, 2000, p. 4). How occupational therapists employ activities—their extent and their meaning—is the principal core of the occupational therapy profession. When people engage in occupations, they use their motor and memory skills to enhance performance and maintain cognitive and physiological fitness. Occupations require the integration of a person's internal skills to adapt to environmental challenges.

The equestrian environment and the horse provide challenges that are never constant. They offer a nonclinical atmosphere of excitement and new experiences. The love of horses by humans, and of humans by horses, is historical (Podhajsky, 1965; Riede, 1988; Scanlan, 1998). This companionship of horses adds to therapeutic influence and motivation. The horse responds to the individual's mood and gestures, which in turn encourages the individual to respond back. The horse accepts people on their responsive level and does not discriminate against a person's sex, nationality, disability, or form. Some people may need to change their behavior to be accepted by the horse, or the horse may encourage positive interactions with others. The client's activities may vary from session to session, depending on the weather, the horse, and other variables, as well as the individual's goals for the day. All cognizance, memory, motor, and social skills are actively involved in the interaction with the

horse and its environment, as individuals pursue their goal-directed occupations.

Why Hippotherapy?

Hippotherapy as a mode of occupational therapy works on many levels. First, the average-size horse provides the rider with movement that is similar to the walking gait of an adult human (Riede, 1988). This motion provides the adult, who may have difficulty walking, with the feel of a normal gait. In addition, the horse stimulates the spinal system and, in turn, the neuromuscular system (Strauss, 1995). The movement pattern of the horse stimulates the movement of the human pelvis at its center of gravity, a critical point, and enables the person to process the movement impulses of the horse into movement responses and transmit them back to the horse.

Von Dietze (2005) stated that without movement there is no life. Movement is central to the process of adaptation and through movement individuals learn about their environment and how to deal with it (Gilfoyle, Grady, & Moore, 1990). The present inactivity of many in our civilization, especially those individuals with disabilities, threatens the fragile balance of the skeletal muscular system (Riede, 1988). According to Riede, motor inefficiency is at the root of many disabilities and associated problems. The horse and its surroundings provide the basis for functional movement, which is necessary for purposeful activity that is the essence of life.

During occupational therapy sessions in the equestrian environment, the terms used may vary depending on the structure of the session. Therapists may use *hippotherapy* while the client is astride the horse and *equine-assisted occupational therapy* for activities off the horse. How and what terms are used is not as important as describing the intervention during the course of a treatment session. The terminology becomes important for researchers, occupational therapists using evidence-based practice, administrators looking for grants to support occupational therapy, and anyone searching for articles related to specific topics of intervention and practice. Due to the confusion of terminology, a search of past literature may not identify either term, because until recently, the umbrella term *therapeutic riding* or *riding for the handicapped* (Nolt, Brown, Spink, & Tebay, 1994) commonly was used to cover all aspect of riding involving people with disabilities. In keeping with common usage in the field, this book uses the term *hippotherapy* to refer to activities on the horse; related activities are referred to as *equine-assisted occupational therapy.*

The philosophical base of occupational therapy (American Occupational Therapy Association, 2002) states that "engagement in occupation to support participation in context is the focus and targeted end objective of occupational therapy intervention" (p. 611). Henderson, and colleagues (1991) pointed out that the attributes of purposefulness are related to people, not to their activities. The equestrian environment provides many tasks and activities, both on and off the horse, that allow a client to interact with an activity that is *purposeful to them* rather then a randomly selected activity. Baum and Law (1997) stated that occupational performance is "when the person, the environment, and the person's occupation intersect each other to support the tasks, activities, and roles that define who the person is as an individual" (p. 281). The active engagement on and off the horse provides continued challenges and a learning process. The person then receives feedback to support his or her accomplishments as a special person.

The occupational therapist assists individuals' motivation to engage in activities to minimize disability. The therapist also encourages compensatory behaviors and establishes a new repertoire of activities to satisfy basic personal needs and social role essentials (Fidler, 1996). Within the goals established by the individual or parent with the assistance of the therapist, the therapist, through the use of tasks and activity analysis, can develop tasks that are within the person's ability but are still challenging. Occupational therapy's unique contribution is that the therapist creates the opportunity for the person to gain skills and confidence and to accomplish meaningful and productive tasks and activities. In so doing, the individual increases his or her occupa-

tional performance (Baum & Edwards, 1995). The equine setting provides multiple opportunities to gain skills and build confidence in accomplishing meaningful tasks. It also provides the individual with the chance to move beyond the therapy arena to learn skills necessary for job and community opportunities and for riding with a regular riding group and competitors. Reilly stated that occupation promotes a healthy attitude toward life because occupation energizes the mind, body, and motivation (Reilly, 2005).

The treatment sessions using the horse as a partner must follow the occupational therapy frame of references or theoretical models. The physical therapy model, which has been a major focus of hippotherapy in the United States, was developed from the physical therapy model of Europe and does not support the occupational therapy frame of reference. A client-centered practice involves the active participation of the individual and, when possible, choices by the individual that will help him or her achieve chosen goals. In cases in which the client is either too young or incapable of making choices, the parent, caregiver, or therapist makes the choice. The client, however, shows his or her willing involvement by being an active participant. Most treatment session are carried out individually with the therapist. When working with individuals who are physically and cognitively independent while on the horse, a small group of up to 4 persons may be appropriate if they have similar goals. The horse and stable elicit many kinds of interactions that help to improve social skills needed for involvement in school and community. The equine setting allows for participation in a large variety of activities with the horse and its care that help the client achieve goals and skills that carry over to daily life.

In the occupational therapy practice, the horse's movement is of prime importance, as it is for all equestrian activities, both for normal and atypical individuals. The horse's movement can be combined with riding skills, vaulting, and sensorimotor and cognitive development, *as long as the objective is achieving the client goals and not "teaching riding."* Being a living active and sensitive animal, the horse has reactions to both the person and the environment, but it also has special needs that need to be met. This provides individuals, especially children, with the opportunity to care for the horse by feeding, grooming, and nurturing—something many people with disabilities have not experienced. The treatment sessions in occupational therapy may involve sitting astride the horse, therapy off the horse, or both. They may involve active participation by the client on the horse, such as directing the horse by riding aids that facilitate client goals. When off the horse, the client may groom, saddle, or lead it to the mounting block, which facilitates other client goals. For example, grooming provides the client with tactile input, gradation of pressure, range of motion, and spatial relationship; saddling involves cognition skills, strength, and physical coordination; leading facilitates spatial relationship and an acute focus on the horse's reactions.

The American Hippotherapy Association (AHA; AHA, 2004) includes physical therapists and speech pathologists, in addition to occupational therapists, as practitioners of hippotherapy.* Each profession has a different theoretical practice base to which its practitioners must adhere. Many modalities cross the line of occupational therapy, speech pathology, and physical therapy but are used differently according to their theoretical model. The term *hippotherapy* has become familiar to many physicians in the United States and it is internationally accepted as meaning *therapy with the use of the horse*. It should continue to be used when referring to this method of intervention (Hubbard, 2003, personal communication). In 2004, the AHA redefined its definition of hippotherapy as "a physical, occupational, or speech therapy treatment strategy that utilizes equine movement." This definition applies to physical therapy, occupational therapy, and speech therapy, used according to each profession's theoretical models. In occupational therapy, utilizing the movement of the horse while the client is astride it during hippotherapy will be a major factor. Most clients, however, will be actively involved in the riding process, except in the case of vaulting, when they are not involved with directing the horse. Treatment may include off-horse activities with the horse partner. When treating at-risk individuals and individuals with psychosocial problems, one might begin with groundwork with the horse and then mount the horse for additional activities. Bonding is very important and develops as these clients care for *their*

---

*In other countries, occupational therapy education varies a great deal. Therapists who are or intend to be involved in this intensive field of intervention must have a thorough knowledge of theories of occupational therapy, neurology, physiology, development, neurodevelopment, sensory integration, and other intervention techniques. The knowledge of disabilities and types of intervention also are required. In the United States and Canada, occupational therapy curricula continue to be a university-level course. In the United States, it is now a master's degree profession. In addition to university studies, 6 months of internships are required. Also, moderate to high levels of horsemanship skills are required. A degree from a technical school with only 2 or 3 years of training may not provide an occupational therapist with enough knowledge to be involved in hippotherapy.

horse. What part of the equestrian activity is applied during therapy depends on the goals of the client and the skill of the therapist. Activities such as cleaning a stall or wheeling a wagon or wheelbarrow may fall into an occupational task within the occupational therapy session, assisting a person to increase his or her ability to perform purposeful occupations that increase life skills.

The following two examples show how occupational therapy can differ from the traditionally defined hippotherapy model to meet specific goals of these clients and stay within the occupational therapy framework.

Example 1: Girl With Brachial Plexus Birth Injury

An 11-month-old infant, SM had a severe brachial plexus birth injury and was referred for occupational therapy. She was normal in development and intelligence but was not using her right upper extremity. For 1 year, her occupational therapist used many traditional modalities and techniques to address the issue. When nothing seemed to work because SM was convinced she did not need the extremity and was not going to allow someone to pressure her, a joint visit with a physical therapist was arranged to explore modalities, such as muscle stimulation. A muscle stimulation unit was obtained and used during in-home occupational therapy. SM showed improvement in muscle activity but not in function.

At 20 months, SM was put on a pony and given two reins. The goal was for SM to functionally use her right upper extremity. The right rein was reinforced with a strap across the top of the hand. While the horse walked and trotted, the hand was stimulated as the rein moved. Additional activities were introduced to encourage coordination and bilateral hand function. SM eventually began to grasp the rein as she was instructed to turn the pony.

By age 3 years, the right upper extremity was weak, but SM was actively attempting to use it in all activities on the horse and in grooming before riding. Activities always were directed toward her physical and functional goals, even though SM's mind was on learning to ride, because she had no sense of having a disability. One day, SM noticed other children at the riding center had physical problems and asked, "What's wrong with me?" as though she questioned why she was with this group.

During her in-home occupational therapy sessions, SM carried through her horse skills in play activities. She continued occupational therapy and hippotherapy twice a week until age 5, when she moved out of the area. SM continued to ride with a therapeutic sports riding group until she graduated to a higher level. By age 12, she owned her own horse, joined the Pony Club, and progressed through B-ability level. Her doctor told her she had more function than is normally expected for this severe an injury. In October 2003, after completing college, she married and was heading for graduate school. SM said that before she was married, she only had a minimal loss in range of motion but had full function of her right extremity.

Example 2: Boy With Athetoid Cerebral Palsy

A 14-year-old boy, KY, had athetoid cerebral palsy with severe spasms. He had been riding with a recreational group for several years. He was referred for in-home occupational therapy to increase his ability for independent function. After several months, in-home therapy was augmented with hippotherapy once a week.

The initial hippotherapy session was used to evaluate his riding skills and function on the horse. KY's posture was in total flexion and demonstrated continuous associated reactions. KY first sat on a bareback pad and, in his right hand, held the ladder reins (designed for those with less motor control). He needed two sidewalkers (horse leaders) to help him balance. KY said "walk" to start the horse and pulled on the reins to stop and turn the horse. In the second session, a saddle replaced the pad for pelvic and upper body support. The session began with classic hippotherapy methods to inhibit postural reflexes for 10 minutes. KY then was asked to stop the horse by straightening his back and "sitting deep" in the saddle. Facilitation techniques were used to help develop this action. When KY was able to stop the horse consistently, he was given the reins to develop soft finger motions to communicate with the horse's mouth. He was not allowed to pull on the reins.

KY learned to turn the horse by turning his body in addition to using his legs, initially with assistance. He never had used his legs while riding. Facilitation techniques were used to stimulate the legs so that leg aids were slowly added. During this time he was developing body coordination and cognitive skills by learning gymnastic arena figures followed by a dressage test, as well as verbalizing what he was to do, thus adding memory skills. Physically, KY decreased associated reactions, was able to sit tall, and rode with classic riding skills for short periods of time. With increased coordination and verbal skills, KY became verbally more confident and social. After several years of occupational therapy and

hippotherapy, he gave a demonstration at a horse show: doing an introductory Pony Club dressage test at a walk without any assistance. At home, KY learned to roll over and sit up in bed, use the phone, make a sandwich, sit up without flexion, and to carry out a computer accounting job for a nursing home.

Summary

Hippotherapy is a type of treatment strategy used by medical professionals for treating neuromuscular, cognitive, sensory integrative dysfunction, vestibular and proprioceptive, psychosocial, and developmental disabilities. The term—meaning treatment with the help of the horse—is used internationally. Strauss (1995) and von Dietze (2005) both stated that life is movement. When we interact with the horse, whether we are in wheelchairs or on our feet, movement always is involved. On the ground or astride the horse, we move. The horse is a live, large, active and reactive animal and, therefore, provides people with a unique experience.

The horse's size and movement provide both challenges and stress. Rood (1958) believed that the challenge of stress is necessary for growth toward increased development and learning; put differently, stress or misplacement leads to adaptation, increasing a person's ability to function and learn. The riding stable is a unique place with the smell of hay, animals, and farm atmosphere. A mother of a 7-year-old girl, who "awakened" after each ride, stated, "Every time we go to [the stable], there is something new happening. It's like opening a new chapter in a book" (Logan-Carrillo, 2005, p. 15).

Occupational therapy through hippotherapy provides a unique opportunity to gain skills and accomplish meaningful and productive occupations. For example, a child can come home and tell his father that he was responsible for making the horse go and stop. This activity gives him a great deal of confidence.

The two examples demonstrate how traditional hippotherapy, as developed in the Germanic countries, focuses on the influence of the horse's movement on the client. Though movement is a major component, hippotherapy by occupational therapists can be expanded to include the theoretical models of occupational therapy. These models include purposeful and meaningful occupation with full involvement of the client to meet a variety of the client's goals. Learning is stimulated by graded stress. Being on a large animal of which one is not totally in control does provide graded stress for a client.

The equine surroundings provide a rich environment with physical, psychological, and sensory stimulations. They can be adapted to meet the goals of all ages and most disabilities in a nonclinical setting.

When one walks with the horse, the interaction can be immense. In the book *Hippotherapy* (Strauss, 1995), pictures of a horse and a person walking next to the horse and rider portray the similarity of the human movement and the rotation of a person's spine and the rotation of the horse's spine. When one leads the horse, who leads who? Spatial relationship is important, and the bond that often develops comes into focus. Whether the client is on or off the horse, that relationship provides encouragement to move with balance and rhythm. No apparatus that a therapist can use exists to provide movement and interaction in the way a horse does (Riede, 1988). The horse not only provides this movement element but also responds to those who attend to it in a very personal way through its innate nature that, in turn, helps to create motivation and bonding. As Strauss stated, *"the horse is the hippotherapist"* (p. 9). It is the one who responds to our needs and provides the therapy as it is instructed to do by the occupational therapist or the client. The horse is a true cotherapist, our hippotherapy partner.

Within the framework of using the horse in practice, the occupational therapy practitioner must remember that legal boundaries frame the profession and must abide by those boundaries. These issues become more important as practitioners in all disciplines are asked to conform to licensor issues and provide third-party payers with a knowledge-based practice using evidence-based methods (Foto & Collins, 2005). Foto and Collins stated that third-party payers want to see if occupational therapists' knowledge, skills, and judgment really are required and if the patient actually is making progress. Practitioners need to convey the skills, knowledge, expertise, and work that they actually bring to what they do. Denials often are because of the lack of this documentation.

References

American Hippotherapy Association. (2004, Spring). *AHA Newsletter*, pp. 10–11.

American Occupational Therapy Association. (2002). Occupational therapy practice framework: Domain and process. *American Journal of Occupational Therapy, 56,* 609–639.

Baum, C. M., & Edwards, D. (1995). Position Paper—Occupational performance: Occupational therapy's definition of function. *American Journal of Occupational Therapy, 49,* 1019–1020.

Baum, C. M., & Law, M. (1997). Occupational therapy practice: Focus on occupational performance. *American Journal of Occupational Therapy, 51,* 277–288.

Fidler, G. S. (1996). Life-style performance: From profile to conceptual model. *American Journal of Occupational Theory, 50,* 139–147.

Foto, M., & Collins, L. (2005, July 11). Reimbursement perspectives. *OT Practice, 10,* 32.

Gilfoyle, E. M., Grady, A., & Moore, J. C. (1990). *Children adapt: A theory of sensorimotor–sensory development* (2nd ed.). Thorofare, NJ: Slack.

Henderson, A., Cermak, S., Coster, W., Murray, E., Trombly, C., & Tickle-Degnen, L. (1991). The Issue Is—Occupational science is multidimensional. *American Journal of Occupational Therapy, 45,* 370–372.

Hinojosa, J., & Blount, M. L. (2000). *The texture of life: Purposeful activities in occupational therapy.* Bethesda, MD: American Occupational Therapy Association.

Logan-Carrillo, C. (2005, May). One, two, three. Dunny trot! *The Horseman's Voice,* p. 15.

Nolt, B. H., Jr., Brown, O. J., Spink, J., & Tebay, J. (1994, January). *Therapeutic riding as a university curriculum.* Presented at the Eighth International Congress on Therapeutic Riding, Hamilton, New Zealand.

Podhajsky, A. (1965). *My dancing white horses.* (F. Hogarth-Gaute, Trans.). New York: Holt, Rinehart, & Winston, Inc.

Reilly, M. (2005). Occupational therapy can be one of the great ideas of the 20th century. In R. Padilla (Ed.), *A professional legacy: The Eleanor Clarke Slagle Lectures in occupational therapy: 1955–2004* (2nd ed., pp. 80–93) Bethesda, MD: AOTA Press.

Riede, D. (1988). *Physical therapy on the horse.* (A. C. Dusenbury, Trans.). Riderwood, MD: Therapeutic Riding Service. (Original work published in 1986)

Rood, M. S. (1958). Every one counts. 1958 Eleanor Clarke Slagle Lecture. *American Journal of Occupational Therapy, 12,* 326–329.

Scanlan, L. (1998). *Wild about horses: Our timeless passion for the horse.* New York: HarperCollins.

Strauss, I. (1995). *Hippotherapy.* Pickering, ON: Ontario Therapeutic Riding Association.

von Dietze, S. (2005). *Balance in movement: How to achieve the perfect seat.* (C. Hogg, Trans.). North Pomfret, VT: Trafalgar Square.

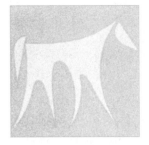

*Where there is an open mind,
there will always be a frontier.*
—Charles E. Kettering

CHAPTER 3

Determining the Goodness of Fit Between Occupational Therapy and Therapeutic Riding

Janet Weisberg, MA, OTR/L

Occupational therapists long have appreciated the quality of life through the lens of activity. From its humanistic origins, the field of occupational therapy recognized that the individual with a physical, psychological, or social disability shares the desire to define a life through action like any other human being. In his 1999 Eleanor Clark Slagle Lecture, Christiansen stated, "When we build our identities through occupations, we provide ourselves with the contexts necessary for creating meaningful lives, and life meaning helps us to be well" (p. 547).

Changes in health care demand that occupational therapy services continue to expand beyond the medical model setting. As inroads continue to develop in community-based programs, day care, home, and recreational environments, occupational therapists must learn to weave their expertise into these settings to facilitate meaningful treatment strategies for clients.

In a profession dedicated to quality-of-life issues, occupational therapists cannot afford to overlook information provided by the individual experience with equine-assisted therapy and activities. Equine-assisted activities, therapeutic riding, and hippotherapy all claim to provide cognitive, physical, and emotional benefit for individuals with chronic illness and disabilities (All, Loving, & Crane, 1999; Casady & Nichols-Larsen, 2004; Heine & Benjamin, 2000). The occupational therapy practitioner brings a unique set of skills and expertise to support the use of the horse as a treatment strategy. Certainly, the philosophy of the profession supports a holistic treatment strategy that can address physical, cognitive, and social skills development.

Although semantics continue to evolve, it should be stated that a clear delineation exists between therapeutic riding and hippotherapy. It is not the mission of this chapter to articulate these differences but rather to inform the occupational therapy practitioner that the setting will dictate his or her role as consultant or a direct service provider. This professional contribution is relevant in regard to medical reimbursement and the creation of a purposeful intervention for the client. In this author's opinion, practitioners with a strong clinical background in sensory processing, neuromotor function, posture, and movement, combined with good understanding of horse behavior and biomechanics, are most likely to be successful with the treatment strategy.

Why the Horse?

As noted earlier in this volume, horseback riding for health is not a new concept. Greco-Roman medicine recommended horseback riding for its physical and spiritual benefits (Bain, 1965; Bracher, 2000). In medical documents dating back to the 16th century, physicians advise equine exercises for the restoration of health, treatment of certain chronic diseases, and relief from the stress of mental illness (Durant, 1878; Swan, 1742). In a more contemporary discussion, Copeland-Fitzpatrick (1997) stated, "We have come to understand in the last half century that the horse has certain unique healing qualities for our bodies and minds. And so, we have recognized those qualities by using the word *therapeutic*" (p. 1).

The American Hippotherapy Association (AHA) recognizes the three-dimensional movement of the horse as a successful intervention to help clients reach functional outcomes. The organization promotes the "use of the movement of the horse as a treatment strategy" and further states that "hippotherapy has been shown to improve muscle tone, balance, posture, coordination, motor development as well as emotional well-being" (AHA, 2005). AHA works with the North American Handicapped Riders Association (NARHA), which states that equine activities "provide opportunities for people with varying ability levels to challenge themselves physically and emotionally and to set goals to improve their quality of life via the horse" (NARHA, 2005).

Both the horse and the environment of the horse offer an opportunity for a nontraditional therapeutic intervention. Health care and wellness practitioners recognize the benefit of treating clients in nontraditional settings. Hinojosa (2003) stated,

> [W]e are agents for change. The goal of all occupational therapists is to assist clients to live more meaningful lives. We create environments and provide interventions that bring about changes in the client's abilities to function in his or her natural world. (p. 226)

The environment of the horse takes the individual away from facilities associated with illness and disability, providing a dynamic treatment medium and an opportunity to experience the natural environment (All et al., 1999; Bracher, 2000). NARHA recognizes more than 650 centers in the United States that offer equine-assisted activities and therapies for individuals with disabilities. According to the *Occupational Therapy Practice Framework,* "understanding the client as an occupational human being for whom access and participation in meaningful and productive activities is central to health and well-being is a perspective that is unique to occupational therapy" (American Occupational Therapy Association, 2002, p. 613).

The challenge to the occupational therapy profession is to combine activities with treatment strategies that are meaningful to the clients and produce purposeful outcomes. This shared understanding of using the natural environment to benefit the individual suggests a theoretical match between therapeutic riding and occupational therapy. As Curtin (2001) wrote,

> Qualitative researchers can reap benefits from involving children as informants, especially when examining childhood occupations (e.g., play), or pediatric occupational therapy practice. This involvement provides an opportunity for the researcher to learn about the children's worlds and perspectives, including the personal meanings children attribute to events and actions. (p. 295)

Method of Analysis

The interview and journal data in this study were analyzed using content analysis (Patton, 1990), "the process of identifying, coding, and categorizing the primary patterns in the data. This means analyzing the content of interviews and observations" (p. 381). Data from both informant groups were categorized and coded (Tables 3.1 and 3.2). Cross-case analysis (Patton, 1990) was used by grouping together answers from each interview of journals to compare answers to common questions. The results were then subject to inductive analysis, in which categories, patterns, and themes were compared and explored as they emerged from the data. Applying the philosophy of health through occupations means first studying the phenomena of occupations that inspire performance. Although the specific phenomena of therapeutic riding will not generalize to other treatment activities, the broader themes of meaning will be relevant to the occupation of children with disabilities.

Therapist Interviews

Occupational therapist informants participated in personal semi-structured interviews. Although each interview covered the same basic content, the interview followed a guide approach, where topics and issues were outlined in advance but the sequence and wording of the questions followed a conversational format that was unique to each interview (Patton, 1990).

Some of the more descriptive excerpts from the interviews and journals follow.

Comments on Perceived Therapeutic Value

All three therapists remarked about the environment and the *sensory integration value.* As an unusual context for treatment, the barn setting provided abundant sensory stimuli to the participant. It also encouraged the participant to continuously integrate the various sensory stimuli while performing the required tasks of the activity, as one therapist described: "They are outside; they get to feel the wind, the sun, the rain occasionally. So you get the environmental, you get the smells, the horse peeing (it smells), emitting gas, they hear all those things, they watch the kitties go by, they hear the horses whinny at each other so you get all the environmental cues."

Although the sensory stimuli frequently provided a positive experience, the therapists acknowledged the important differences in participants who found it disorganizing and displayed defensive behaviors: "Sometimes they [participants] take 15 minutes just to get a

Table 3.1. Summary of Data From Therapist Interviews

Data Category	Data Subcategory
Perception of therapeutic value	• Sensory integration value • Biomechanical value • Psychosocial value
Treatment goals	• Sensory integration • Biomechanics • Cognition
Comparison to traditional treatment settings	• Value of unique qualities of environment
Therapist predisposition for involvement in activity	• Horse enthusiast • Current or previous horse owner • Riding experience • Understanding of the movement and qualities of the horse in relation to disability
Perceived drawbacks of the activity	• Cost • Infrequency of treatment • Limited reimbursement
Professional identity	• Identify impact of occupational therapy's role in activity • Children value activity but don't see it as therapy
Value of availability	• Physical opportunity • Emotional opportunity

Table 3.2. Summary of Data From Children's Journals

Data Category	Data Subcategory
Perception of activity	• Fun • Rode independently • Needed sidewalker or leader • Identified horse's gait • Identified use of equipment • Wrote "I" statements • Identified influence of temperature and weather
Importance of horse	• Identified horse's name • Identified breed • Referred to speed • Drew illustrations of horse • Drew illustrations of self • Identified favorite horse
Expression of positive	• Speed • Independent riding • Love of horses
Expression of negative	• Difficulty holding reins • Unable to ride favorite horse • Giggled too much

helmet on or they are crying and then you have to fight to get the helmet on." The participants with known sensory integration deficits required more preparation prior to participation in the activity: "We spend a lot of time getting these kids ready. . . . We do things prior, whether its getting them on a scooter board, getting them on a swing, you know, having their parents provide a lot of oral input prior to them coming, so they're chewing on licorice or sucking on this to kind of keep their bodies together."

The bounty of sensory information was distinctly valued by the therapists. In contrast to a clinic experience, one therapist remarked, "you don't get the warmth and you don't get the interaction of the horse turning around and sniffing you or the horse sneezing or giving a little shake. The tail coming around (whoosh), batting a fly." In addition, the multidimensional movement of the horse provided a unique *biomechanical value* for the participant to experience:

- "You can get up on a horse and that horse will provide such feedback to you that you can feel exactly what your pelvis is doing."
- "The movement of the horse—you can't simulate a normal movement pattern like the horse has or like we ambulate. We walk, our hips move forward, we get the rotation this way and then we get the rocking back and forth. The horse gives the student that. . . ."

Psychosocial value perceived by the therapists was revealed in some of the following comments:

- "It's a chance for them [the participants] to control something which a lot of these people have very little control over their lives. They get up when somebody gets them up, they get fed when somebody feeds them, they get dressed when somebody dresses them. For them I think it's a window of time that they are in charge of something. Or at least they perceive that they are."
- "This is something they're in control of. This is something that is all theirs. They don't say that I went to a movie and my mom drove me. No, this is, 'I was up on a horse, I was reining that horse.'"

The therapists remarked about the value of participating in an activity that not everyone participates in, able-bodied or otherwise: "I'm doing something that my brother and sister isn't [sic] doing or I'm doing something that I can go to school and show off my ribbons and my trophies that I'm riding a horse and you're not." Another therapist described promoting self-esteem as a primary part of her role in the activity: "It's a place where these kids can go and be successful and feel good about themselves."

In addition, the therapists felt that the participants' relationship with horses was relevant: "The spark that happens between the student and the horse . . . a horse is fun and friendly and not judgmental. It doesn't tease."

Treatment Goals

All three therapists wrote initial evaluations when participants enter the program, which guided the riding instructor in creating lesson plans. The goals formed the following subcategories: sensory integration, biomechanical, and cognitive.

- *Sensory integration treatment goals:* Producing an adaptive response, decreasing gravitational insecurity, decreasing tactile defensiveness, and general sensory integration goals
- *Biomechanical treatment goals:* Developing independence in sitting; increasing trunk control, rotation, and elongation; decreasing tone; improving balance through developmental positional; improving posture; improving coordination; and increasing ability to weight bear through upper extremities
- *Cognitive treatment goals:* Increased verbalization, following direction, attention to task, and improving cognitive awareness.

All of the therapists indicated they used information about the participant from other treating therapists in addition to their own evaluation when formulating therapeutic riding treatment plans. They said, however, that the riding environment often created additional factors to be considered: "Yes, it's great to be able to sit down and look on paper what this child's diagnosis is, what they look like there, but it's a little different when you get them up on a horse." In addition, all three therapists said that their goals for the participants would likely be similar no matter where treatment took place. The use of the horse simply provided an extremely rich opportunity for treatment: "I think that [when] you look at a child and in a clinic or on a horse your goals are the same. You want to make that person as functional as possible. A horse is just a fun way to reach the same goals."

Comparison to Traditional Treatment Settings

Although the therapists said that their treatment goals for a participant would be consistent independent of the setting, they valued how the horse and riding environment contributed to goal achievement: "I said wow, look at this, this is something that there is no way to replicate in a facility."

The importance of the therapeutic riding environment was stressed for several reasons. One said, "They just get a lot more sensory integration, I think, on the horse than they would in the therapy room." The therapist also commented that in addition to facilitating movement, the horse also provides distraction to the child: "I can focus their attention on the horse, they may be stretching their abductors to straddle that horse, but their attention is someplace else, so I can do more."

The therapists validated the importance of the traditional clinic setting for treatment but also advocated for the motivating factors from a nontraditional setting, such as therapeutic riding: "I think you might get more gains more quickly because the participant is more active in the treatment. They are on the horse. It is not that they are not active in a clinic setting but they just may not put as much effort into it because they don't see the value in it as much as say climbing up onto an animal." The same therapist compared the gains of one participant that she saw in both settings: "I can probably see her for an hour and a half in the clinic or in the school and get what I can get in probably 10 to 15 minutes as far as pelvic movement."

In the therapeutic riding setting, therapists perceived their role as providing occupational therapy. They remarked, however, that the participants did not see the activity as therapy: "These people have been to therapy over and over again and it's hard work, it hurts, and they don't like it. When they are riding, they don't even realize that you are a therapist."

Therapist Predisposition for Involvement in the Activity

All three therapists explained their reasons for becoming involved with the activity and what they felt qualified them to facilitate the activity. All identified the importance of an inherent understanding of the activity: "The whole purpose of how you are going to position the rider is to relate to the movement of the horse so you get what you want. So that knowledge is something that is learned. If you have no horse knowledge previously, then you have to come out and you have to observe and you have to learn that."

Perceived Drawbacks of the Activity

In each situation, the therapists interviewed were not the only professionals volunteering for the therapeutic riding program. During the interview, they were questioned about their specific role as an occupational therapist distinct from other professionals facilitating the activity. All were able to identify the effect of their role in the therapeutic riding setting: "I see OT as being a

little bit more important because of the sensory issue. There's no way that if the child's not going to get up on a horse or is gravitationally insecure or has an intolerance to movement that a PT is going to be able to do anything with them. So as far initially, I would say that OT is of utmost importance."

One therapist linked occupational therapy to therapeutic riding through the concept of motivation: "It's what OT goes for. To motivate someone through activity." All of the therapists recognized the importance of meaningful activity and its contribution to client motivation and participation: "I'm not a real traditionalist. I'd rather, if they want to go out doing the skiing or whatever, I'd rather have them try that because first they are interested in it so they are more motivated to participate."

Value of Availability

Therapists also were questioned about the opportunity lost to their clients if the activity was not available. All three identified the participant's interaction with the horse as a primary opportunity provided by the activity. In addition, the therapists indicated a range of physical and emotional opportunities that would be lost. Specific to her clients, one therapist commented,

> I think they would have an increase in joint deformities, they would lose more stability and mobility and lose trunk control. They would probably go back to their sensory defensiveness as far as the vestibular and tactile. . . . I know teachers have said too that when these kids come back to school and they have to write a report, creative imagery comes out of their horseback riding experience.

Another commented, "I think they would lose some of their emotional security and their self-confidence. Some of them would lose the one pleasurable thing they get out of the week. You know, I mean, I hate to say that but for some kids that's the one thing that they would say is really fun."

Journal Excerpts

The categories and subcategories revealed in the writings and drawings of the children often were combined in single comments or drawings. A selection of some of the more articulate entries are shown in Figure 3.1.

Results

Using the inductive, content analysis technique roughly outlined in Patton (1990), a thorough comparison of the

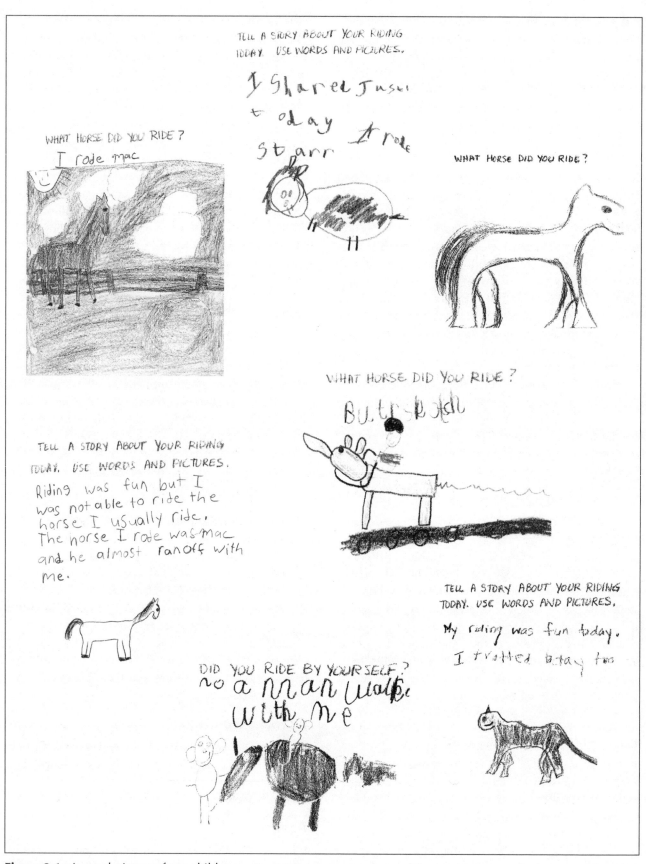

Figure 3.1. Journal pictures from children.

data revealed broad categories and themes. An art therapist provided consultation regarding the journal illustrations. To determine consistency of categories, a second reader who was blind to the previous coding read randomly selected journal and transcribed interviews. Categories and themes are presented in table form. Generalized to other treatment activities, the broader themes of meaning will be relevant to the occupation of children with disabilities.

Discussion: Defining a Meaningful Pattern of Activity

Responding to the difficulty of defining meaningful treatment activities in occupational therapy, this author's research looked toward the individual for information about meaning. The activity, therapeutic riding, represents a popular activity with children and an innovative area of treatment. Exploring the phenomena of the activity provided environmental and motivational clues to performance.

Emerging Themes and Grounded Theory

Qualitative evidence suggested that many categories in both sets of data converged into three dominant themes: autonomy, empowerment, and sensory experience. These themes provide environmental (external) and motivational (internal) clues to the performance of the children participating in the activity. Upon further consideration, a grounded theory evolved:

> Autonomy, empowerment, and sensory experience are meaningful and relevant to the occupation of children with disabilities. The alliance of these elements in therapeutic riding inspired active participation in the therapeutic process. (Weisberg, 1995, p. 78)

Autonomy

The quest for autonomy dominates early childhood and significantly contributes to a child's psychosocial development. Children achieve autonomy by making independent decisions and gaining a sense of control over their environment. Experiencing autonomy is critical to a child's energy, self-esteem, and independence. The experience of autonomy, however, can be elusive to a child with a disability because of physical, social, or emotional barriers to performance. Children may live in environments where the "doing" is done for them. Therapeutic riding offers an important opportunity for "doing."

The horse as a therapeutic strategy provides an opportunity for autonomy. The physical nature of the horse demands certain actions and decisions from a rider. Riding requires mastery of the necessary skills for controlling the horse's movements. Simply interacting with the horse requires appropriate behaviors for safety and respect of the animal's size. These experiences provide a rare opportunity for a child's mind and body to create realistic consequences; the child can assert his or her abilities and then experience the consequences in a supportive and fun environment.

Empowerment

Therapeutic riding and hippotherapy represent an opportunity for a child to participate in a challenge that does not discriminate. Instead of placing a spotlight on children's disabilities, the focus shifts to their ability. This focus on ability creates an opportunity for prestige and a challenge to the individuals' sensory, motor, cognitive, and psychosocial skills in a meaningful format.

In the study, the theme of empowerment also emerged from the relationship between child and horse. Brave drawings in the journals depicted careful consideration of the size and energy of the horse. A smile on the horse's face suggests the child's perception of the horse's willingness to please and be accessible. It is difficult to envision another scenario where a child with a disability could interact and harness the energy of such a powerful living entity. The child's interaction with the animal creates a union where the horse and all of its characteristics become an extension of the child. One child's drawing placed the face and hair of a girl attached to a horse's body. Another drew a horse sticking out its tongue in protest. A 12-year-old girl with Spina Bifida made constant reference in her journal to the speed and movement she experienced. On horseback, this child could experience freedom of movement.

Sensory Integration

The environment of a barn as a treatment facility and the use of a horse as a treatment strategy provide rich opportunity for sensory input and encouragement of adaptive responses. Considering the neurosensory data in the environment, the activity lends itself quite naturally to a sensory integrative frame of reference. Warmth, tactile stimulation, proprioceptive input, and movement of the horse provide valuable information to the participant. According to the therapists, this offered an important opportunity to travel beyond the confines of a clinical setting: "Ultimately we are looking for that functional independence and getting an adaptive response." Drawings and comments in the journals showed sensory awareness. The drawings detailed the movement, size, color, and sounds of the animals.

The feedback of a horse's movement allows the child to determine the effectiveness of his or her performance: "I was trying to get him to canter [sic] but he would not canter so I did not get to canter. I only got to trot." Therapeutic riding involves a challenging combination of gross motor movement and neuro-sensory input essential to child development. To an occupational therapist, this relationship represents an opportunity for achieving sensory integrative, bio-mechanical, and cognitive goals. To a child, it translates as climbing out of a disability and onto the back of a horse.

Implications for Occupational Therapy

With so many challenges facing the profession of occupational therapy (Baum, 2006), practitioners must maintain their broad understanding of quality of life and meaningful treatment strategies (Hasselkus, 2006). The identified themes of autonomy, empowerment, and sensory experience that contribute to experience of children participating in equine therapy need further research for validation. Are these themes relevant to quality of life? Are other therapeutic interventions likely to promote similar outcomes and experiences? Occupational therapists using hippotherapy as a treatment strategy have remarkable stories to tell. How can these stories be measured and used to shape our practice? If they measure only the most narrowly defined outcomes, will they lose their focus on the big picture of human occupation? Ultimately, it is what practitioners learn from their clients that will continue to make professional intervention a valuable contribution to the lives of the people we serve.

References

All, A. C., Loving, G. L., & Crane, L. L. (1999). Animals, horseback riding, and implications for rehabilitation therapy. *Journal of Rehabilitation, 65*(3), 49–57.

American Hippotherapy Association. (2005). *What is hippotherapy?* Retrieved August 15, 2005, from www.american-hippotherapyassociation.org/aha_hpot.htm.

American Occupational Therapy Association. (2002). Occupational therapy practice framework: Domain and process. *American Journal of Occupational Therapy, 56,* 609–639.

Bain, A. M. (1965). Pony riding for the disabled. *Physiotherapy, 51,* 263–265.

Baum, C. (2006). Centennial challenges, millennium opportunities. *American Journal of Occupational Therapy, 60,* 609–616.

Bracher, M. (2000). Therapeutic horse riding: What has this to do with occupational therapists? *British Journal of Occupational Therapy, 63,* 277–282.

Casady, R., & Nichols-Larsen, D. (2004). The effect of hippotherapy on ten children with cerebra palsy. *Pediatric Physical Therapy, 16,* 165–172.

Christiansen, C. (1999). Defining lives: Occupation as identity: An essay on competence, coherence, and the creation of meaning [1999 Eleanor Clark Slagle Lecture]. *American Journal of Occupational Therapy, 53,* 547–558.

Copeland-Fitzpatrick, J. (1997). Hippotherapy and therapeutic riding an international review. *Proceedings of the Ninth International Therapeutic Riding Congress* (pp. 1–12). Denver, CO: North American Riding for the Handicapped Association.

Curtin, C. (2001). Eliciting children's voices in qualitative research. *American Journal of Occupational Therapy, 55,* 295.

Durant, G. (1878). *Horse-back riding: A medical point of view.* New York: Cassell, Peter & Galpin.

Hasselkus, B. R. (2006). The world of everyday occupation: Real people, real lives [2006 Eleanor Clarke Slagle Lecture]. *American Journal of Occupational Therapy, 60,* 627–640.

Heine, B. & Benjamin, J. (2000). Introduction to hippotherapy. *Advances for Physical Therapists and Physical Therapy Assistants, 11*(13), 11–13.

Hinojosa, J. (2003). Therapist or scientist, how do these roles differ? *American Journal of Occupational Therapy, 57,* 225–226.

North American Riding for the Handicapped Association (2005). *About NARHA.* Retrieved August 15, 2005, from www.narha.org.

Patton, M., Q. (1990). *Qualitative evaluation and research methods* (2nd ed.). Newbury Park, CA: Sage.

Swan, J. (1742). *The entire works of Dr. Thomas Sydenham.* London: Printed for Edward Cave at St. John's Gate.

Weisberg, J. (1995). *Exploring meaningful activity: Occupational therapy and therapeutic horseback riding.* Unpublished master's thesis, Rush University, Chicago.

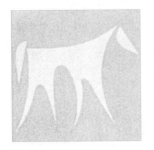

A horse gallops with his lungs, perseveres with his heart, and wins with his character.
—Tesio

CHAPTER 4

Theoretical Frames of Reference Applied to Hippotherapy and Equine-Assisted Occupational Therapy

Barbara T. Engel, MEd, OTR

During my many years as a practitioner of occupational therapy, the profession has moved from the late 1940s and early 1950s, with only one occupational therapy textbook (the first edition of *Willard and Spackman's Occupational Therapy*), to more than 1,300 books on listed on publishers' and book sellers' Web sites (e.g., AOTA Press, Slack, Lippincott or Barnes & Noble, amazon.com). During those early years in meetings, we discussed who we are as occupational therapists. Since that time, the profession has moved to a theoretical basis for occupational therapy and continues a process that is forever undergoing an evolutionary change (Mosey, 1986). From creative, curative treatment projects, the profession has moved to the perspective of meaningful occupation. Occupational therapy's philosophies and basic theories also have slowly developed as the profession has moved into master's-degree and doctorate levels (Serrett, 1985). The original philosophy of work as a curative measure has resurfaced but now with a rationale, depth of meaning, and theoretical reasoning for the profession. Occupation, rehabilitation science, and occupational science have been addressed through numerous theories, but within each concept is the major goal of a holistic approach to improving a person's life within the parameter of his or her functional ability and world (Hopkins & Smith, 1983; Miller, 1993). This remains the aim of the occupational therapy profession (Hopkins & Smith, 1983).

Occupational therapy theorists who have helped spur the profession along are reviewed in this chapter. The process of developing and expanding present concepts, theories, and frames of references are based in part on older theories and models. Theories are dynamic and change to reflect increased knowledge and limitations of theories (Shumway-Cook & Woollacott, 2001).

As an example, we look at Mathiowetz and Bass-Hagen's (1994) review of motor behavior research prior to the contemporary models. Reflex theory of motor control originated from the work of Sherrington, a neurophysiologist, in the early 1900s (Shumway-Cook & Woollacott, 2001). Theories by Bobath and Brunnstrom on neurodevelopmental techniques and Knott, Voss, Kabot, and Rood on proprioceptive neuromuscular facilitation were developed from Sherrington's model in the 1960s. Vibration, inhibiting and facilitation, and neurodevelopmental approaches all were developed from these theories. Further research found many limitations in these models. The hierarchical model followed, which maintains that movement is controlled from the brain, to the brainstem, and down levels of the spinal cord (Giuffrida, 2003). The motor programming theories gave more flexibility over the hierarchical model in that it considers the central nervous system as an action system rather than a reaction system (Shumway-Cook & Woollacott, 2001). This theory did not explain aspects of motor control; thus, Bernstein, a Russian, was responsible for the development of the systems model that came about through research in biology, physics, mathematics, and ecological approaches to perception (Mathiowetz & Bass-Hagen, 1994). The systems model focal point is the interaction of the person and environment (Giuffrida, 2003).

In the mid-1980s, the therapeutic focus shifted from the environment to the individual's ability to increase his or her function with a change or modification within the working setting (McColl et al., 2002). Contemporary theories since have developed a focus on person, environment, occupation, performance, and outcome, with the person in complete collaboration with the practitioner. For example, Dunn's *ecology of human performance framework* centers on the importance of major constructs of the person, environment, occupation, and performance (Dunn, McClain, Brown, & Youngstrom, 2003). *Ecological* refers to the interaction of the motor system with goal-directed behavior and physically exploring the tasks, the environment, and the individual's personal ways to accomplish a task (Giuffrida, 2003).

Although we have not described all theoretical models, I do give one an idea of how theories change as new concepts surface. This chapter reviews the relationship of major theoretical models to hippotherapy and equine-assisted therapy. Furthermore, I show how their clinical application's focal points relate to the treatment practice in using the horse as a therapy partner in occupational therapy.

Physicians, psychiatrists, physical therapists, speech pathologists, psychologists, special education teachers, equine instructors and trainers, and others use the horse to obtain various goals, but the occupational therapy practitioner uses the horse in unique ways to the advantage of the client. How can one differentiate occupational therapy practice from other professions if one does not have a clear perspective of the theoretical base of the profession? How does occupational therapy differ from education, recreational, physical therapy, psychology, or speech pathology in the way the horse is used? If an occupational therapist cannot identify the occupational frames of references in hippotherapy, what is he or she doing—therapeutic riding or physical therapy?

As Strauss (1995) explained, the art of hippotherapy involves much more than putting a client on a horse and moving the horse forward. In the hippotherapy course at the German school discussed in Chapter 1, 18 occupational and physical therapists spent more than 100 hours studying the intricate aspects of hippotherapy, including theory and methods to determine the client's needs, what the horse had to offer, and how to manipulate the horse to gain the desired results, in addition to training requirements of the horse and the therapist. In addition, practitioners must adapt the German theoretical model that addresses physical therapy to the occupational therapy practice model that is used in the United States and Canada. Practice models may vary in other countries where education can vary in university and non-university training and in the number of years needed to obtain an occupational therapy degree. This

difference can vary from a 1- to 2-year course in a technical school to the present 6 years' university training in the United States.

Dunn's (2000) model of best practices fits well for the practice using the horse as a partner. Special skills are needed to work with clients along with large animals. The practitioner not only must be up to date on current occupational therapy practice methods and theories and have a theory base for intervention, but he or she also must have medium-level horsemanship skills that include work-in-hand and understanding training techniques to maneuver the horse to achieve desired results for their client.

The Model Practice Act of the American Occupational Therapy Association (2006) states,

Occupational therapy services are provided for the purpose of promoting health and wellness and to those who have or are at risk for developing an illness, injury, disease, disorder, condition, impairment, disability, activity limitation, or participation restriction. Occupational therapy addresses the physical, cognitive, psychosocial, sensory, and other aspects of performance in a variety of contexts to support engagement in everyday life activities that affect health, well-being, and quality of life. (p. 3)

Occupations encompass all activities that children, adolescents, and adults do during their lives and are at the core and texture of our daily lives (Hinojosa & Blount, 2000). We do both desirable and undesirable activities. The activities we do address the health and welfare of our lives and have a personal meaning, purpose, and goal. Occupation is encompassed in therapy theories, although the construct may be expressed differently by different theorists.

Concepts are ideas that are the understructure of theory (Crepeau & Boyt Schell, 2003). Walker (1993) described a *theory* as "an attempt to explain, predict, or clarify phenomena" (p. 247). Mosey (1986) stated that a theory "is a predicted relationship between circumscribed set of events and phenomena" (p. 376). Reed (1984) defined a theory "as a set of interrelated assumptions, concepts, and definitions that present a systematic view of phenomena by specifying relationships among variables, with the purpose of explaining and predicting the phenomena" (p 677). Kielhofner (2004) stated that when a theory is developed, "researchers who reinterpret, reorganize, and add to interdisciplinary concepts upon which they build are developing new theory" (p. 75).

Relationship of Theory to Practice

To be a researcher in the field of occupational therapy, one would assume that knowledge of theory is very important (Crepeau & Boyt Schell, 2003; Mosey, 1986). A theory may help a practitioner guide the practice technique, predict the course of treatment, and interpret observations or explain how the variables in practice are interrelated (Ottenbacher, 2003). Having a well-understood knowledge of specific theories helps practitioners have scientific support for practice and intertwine the knowledge of theories and practice (Crepeau & Boyt Schell, 2003). For example, practitioners well versed in sensory integration know the importance of understanding the theoretical concept that sensory integration, as developed by Ayres, is intended for children without known neurological disorders (Bundy, Lane, & Murray, 2002). They understand the difference between sensory integration and sensorimotor stimulation or sensory stimulation and what approach to use with a specific child. Without understanding Ayres's theory of sensory integration, it is impossible to use it in practice appropriately.

The following sections summarize the work of occupational therapists whose research has particular relevance to the practice of hippotherapy and equine-assisted occupational therapy.

A. Jean Ayres

Jean Ayres was concerned with the behavior of children with learning disabilities and how it related to sensory processing in the brain (Kielhofner, 2004). Her studies focused on neuromuscular and neurodevelopmental processes and the relationship between sensory processing and behavior (Ayres, 1972).

Ayres's theory was extrapolated from earlier theories by researchers such as Kabat, Rood, Fay, Brunnstrom, and Bobath (Walker, 1993), in addition to her own research in neurology. She developed the sensory integration (SI) test to determine the areas of dysfunction within the learning disability areas, such as communication, behavioral, sensorimotor, and psychological problems (Ayres, 1979). Five major syndromes were identified from the data of the statistical analysis that Ayres gathered, including apraxia, form and position in space, integration of the two sides of the body, visual figure–ground perception, and deficits in tactile perception (Ayres, 2005). Ayres's concern with SI theory and practice was "in children who had no known peripheral or central nervous system deficits" (Walker, 1993, p. 119). She focused on somatosensory, motor, and vestibular processing deficits as indicators of sensory integration dysfunction. SI was focused on processing difficulties in relatively normal children (Ayres, 1972). Sensory integration theory now has provided a base of knowledge that is being reexamined by others (Bundy et al., 2002). Back in 1972, Ayres stated that research is a continuous process dependent on new neurological concepts.

How does hippotherapy fit into the practice of SI? Let us review the five major syndromes Ayres identified as major problems in SI dysfunction (Walker, 1993) and how they relate to hippotherapy.

1. *Apraxia* is the loss of the ability to carry out familiar, purposeful movements in the absence of paralysis or other motor or sensory impairment (Dorland, 1994). This inability to motor plan can be addressed both on and off the horse. Preparing the horse for riding or gymnastic vaulting requires many motor planning activities. Grooming, for instance, requires basic motor movements of the arms and fingers. Astride the horse, stretching exercises, manipulation of the reins, or playing gymkhana games (such as those played on horseback in Pony Club gatherings) also require motor planning. In vaulting, all positions on the horse can be graded from simple movements such as the "seat" to "kneel" to more complicated movements as the "flag" and "stand." All movements require repetition with purposeful and functional meaning that help to improve praxis.

2. Form and position in space are dependent on the *proprioceptors,* the terminals of the sensory nerves in all tendons, muscles, and joint capsules that transmit information pertaining to the force and speed of movement, awareness of body parts, and movements in space (Dorland, 1994; Lane, 2002). The proprioceptive and vestibular systems are believed to address postural responses, balance, and gravitational security (Lane, 2002). Activities on and off the horse address postural responses, balance, and gravitational security. Form and space perception, for example, is addressed in the rider's space relative to the horse's space and position in the arena. This effect is especially true when leading a horse on a lead line. Stimulation can be graded in degrees for proprioception–vestibular input both on and off the horse. While using the reins, the degree and force of movement is critical but can be adjusted for intervention purposes. Where and how the body moves on the horse will affect the movement of the horse. The stimulation of the movement of the horse affects the rider's proprioceptors because the rider's spine is positioned at the center of

gravity of the horse. According to Strauss (1995), "the contact area between the seat bones [of the rider] and the horse's back at its center of gravity is of critical importance. Via this support, the movement impulses of the horse, the primary movements, are transferred to the rider, who receives them, processes them into movement responses and transmits them back to the horse."

3. Integration of the two sides of the body and postural deficits are addressed in all movements and riding positions on the horse. Both riding and gymnastic vaulting skills require separation of the upper and lower body, followed by separation of the right and left side of the body. Leading and grooming the horse assist in rotational and bending movements to encourage segmentation of body parts. Cleaning a stall requires the two sides to coordinate with each other.

4. Deficits in tactile perception and discrimination can be stimulated by touching and petting the horse as well as fingering grain and hay when feeding. Touching and cleaning tack with saddle soap, sponge, and water also are rich in tactile experiences.

5. Visual figure–ground and visual perception are stimulated by the vestibulo-ocular reflex, which helps to stabilize the visual field. The equestrian environment is rich in visual stimulation, including that related to movement as well as colors, figure–ground discrimination, hand–eye coordination, and identification of interesting objects. Many types of games can be added, including placing letters in a mailbox and putting balls in a bucket.

Finally, sensory modulation manifestation, such as gravitational insecurity and lack of tolerance to movement, can be graded easily on the horse by selecting a small horse with a smooth gait that can be increased to faster gaits, then to a larger horse with a smooth and extended gait. Start at walking in straight lines with stops and starts, making turns, and progress to trotting. When a few trot steps are tolerated, more can then be added. Walking over objects or turning in different direction or a simple trail ride adds variety and a change of focus that may help stimulate the sensory system while diverting attention to more interesting areas.

Gymnastic vaulting involves moving in different positions on the back of a moving horse while the horse is being lunged. The individual selects what movements he or she feels capable of, either alone or with another person. All sensory processing mechanisms would be activated, especially anti-gravity, postural responses, and vestibular stimulation.

Gail S. Fidler

Gail Fidler's contributions to the field of occupational therapy were so many that only a few can be focused on in this chapter. She pushed those among her and the field of occupational therapy in general to accomplish all that could be done, and even then pushed more. She strived for a profession that was not subservient to the medical field. Above all, she was a great mentor to many with lasting effects.

Her contributions included the psychodynamic theory (Kielhofner, 2004), and she expressed the value of activities—examining them for a person's healthful and therapeutic benefits and recognizing their importance in the early stage of the formation of the occupational therapy profession. She felt that doing activities or occupations was meaningful and vitally important to a person's life (Elenko, Hinojosa, & Blount, 2000). Fidler was one of the strongest proponents of activity analysis, initially in the field of psychiatry, and helped activity analysis take a prominent role in the occupational field (Wilcox, 1998). She had a strong belief that purposeful activities, well-planned and appropriately timed, were the very core of occupational therapy (Lugwig, 1993). Fidler's theory related to activities addressing the physical, psychological, neurobehavioral, cognitive, and sociocultural aspects of a person and discusses the value of objects and purposeful activity that are in the person's environment and whether they meet the needs of the individual (Miller & Walker, 1993). Fidler focused on the analysis of activities that include motor, sensory integration, cognitive, psychosocial, and interpersonal skills matched to the individual's preparedness to learn (Elenko et al., 2000). Her focus on the aspect of doing always was stressed in her writings and the courses she taught (Fidler, personal communication, July 1969).

Fidler's concepts easily can be adapted to the equestrian environment. Her overall pursuit of occupational therapy should set the stage for practitioners in hippotherapy to be entrenched within the field of research, use occupational frames of reference, and clarify the use of the horse in pursuit of wellness and more productive lives of clients. Fidler's early psychoanalytic thoughts focused on interpersonal relations and symbolic expression of objects and activities (Fidler, personal communication, July 1969). The horse carries great symbolic meaning of power, friendship, and bonding. It allows unique interpersonal relations and expressions without discrimination of appearance or disability, physical or mental (Fletcher & Scanlan, 2005). Fidler's focus on doing was very strong; the application of doing within the equine setting can be directed in caring for the horse, riding the horse, and responding to the feedback that the horse gives to the individual and the behavioral influences it provides.

With individuals with mental disorders, I have experienced many interesting reactions of horses toward riders with different psychiatric problems. The horse's sensitivity can "read" the individual's problems, and the horse can react either by helping or rejecting its rider. Normality can occur on a trail ride with other individuals as the rider is absorbed in the activity and environment. The activity analysis includes the horse and the environment providing a safe and challenging experience. Hippotherapy practitioners must understand every aspect of a horse—its temperament, behaviors, and interaction with the rider—and not just its movements (Strauss, 1995). The practitioner needs to have intermediate skills in horsemanship and safety precautions, including emergency procedures. All activities that the practitioner will use for intervention need to be experienced and analyzed for therapeutic value. An analysis of all activities to be used within this environment needs to be analyzed and experienced.

Fidler strongly believed that *doing* conveys the sense of performing, producing, or causing. It is purposeful action in contrast to random activity in that the action is directed toward the interpersonal (testing a skill), the extrapersonal (clarifying a relationship), or the nonhuman (creating an end product; Fidler & Fidler, 2005). With a live animal and its historic symbolic nature, the horse, its stable, its care, and its companionship provide a unique setting for *doing* in a special purposeful and meaningful occupation.

Mary Reilly

In 1961, Mary Reilly looked back at the profession of occupational therapy to state that its original hypothesis was that "man through the use of his hands, as they are energized by mind and will, can influence the state of his [or her] own health" (2005, p. 80). She felt that, after medical principles, occupational therapy needed to be concerned about the growth and production of humans to grow and be productive and that the power to act creates a need to use the power while failure to use it results in dysfunction and unhappiness (Wilcock, 1998). Her beliefs were based on that of Ayres; she believed that occupation, adaptation, and a balance between work and play were important (Schwartz, 2003). She developed the paradigm of occupational behavior, a signifi-

cant contribution to the evolution of the occupational therapy profession (Law, Baum, & Dunn, 2001). In her view, occupational functioning was the goal of treatment, and the client's task was to integrate motion into total activities to gain work satisfaction and the ability to experience pleasure in what he or she accomplishes (Wilcock, 1998).

Reilly felt that it was extremely important to study and investigate the occupational therapy profession to understand its contribution to science (Elenko et al., 2000). Her Eleanor Clark Slagle Lecture stressed that human productivity provides a person with the most satisfaction and gratification and that occupational therapy is a "profession [that] has as its unique concern the nurturing of the spirit in man for action" (Reilly, 2005, p. 83).

Reilly's belief in the original hypothesis of occupational therapy is reflected in hippotherapy. Within the environment of the horse, the client uses his or her hands and influences his or her health. The client is provided a place to work, to accomplish, and to play. The barn, stalls, and arena provide ample opportunity for the development of work skills. Learning and managing horse care is both interesting and challenging. The interaction with the horse is enjoyable. Learning to communicate with the horse while astride it is a precise skill, and when accomplished, it is enjoyable and motivating and develops self-esteem. Many variables can be addressed to meet individual goals.

Elizabeth J. Yerxa

Elizabeth Yerxa was influenced by Mary Reilly at the University of Southern California (USC). Her premise was that occupational therapy should be aimed at client actualization through choice, self-initiated purposeful activity, reality orientation, and perception of self and the environment (Yerxa, 2005). She developed a doctoral program of occupational science at USC. Yerxa felt that the identification of a scientific base of the human as an occupational being would help support occupational therapy and differentiate it from other professions (Elenko et al., 2000). Occupational therapy and occupational science both focus on occupation, but one focuses on the practice of occupational therapy as a profession, while occupational science is an academic discipline with scholarly inquiry (Larson, Wood, & Clark, 2003).

Yerxa's major factors in occupational therapy are choice, self-initiated and purposeful activity, reality orientation, and reality-orienting influence on the person's perception. Using the horse within a hippotherapy and equine-assisted therapy practice setting brings forth all of Yerxa's features.

Gary Kielhofner

Gary Kielhofner's theoretical concept—Temporal Adaptation: A Conceptual Framework for Occupational Therapy—was later incorporated in the Model of Human Occupation (MOHO; Kielhofner, 1978). Kielhofner stated three assumptions that are the underlying practical application of his model:

1. Man has an innate desire for occupation.
2. Through occupation, a person can shape the health of him- or herself and thus provide a vehicle for health.
3. True occupation must be practiced in occupational therapy with the involvement of purposeful, challenging accomplishment and with satisfaction (Miller, 1993).

The systems panorama states "behavior is dynamic and context dependent, . . . and occupational is essential to self-organization" (Kielhofner, Forsyth, & Barrett, 2003, pp. 213–213). Occupation is how one occupies oneself and, therefore, involves time (Barrett & Kielhofner, 2003).

The intervention of temporal adaptation can be used when a person's life has so changed that his or her past routines and skills must be adapted to account for the life change and to help reestablish someone's occupation and lifestyle. Other persons may have had difficulties establishing priorities in their lives and need to learn how to prioritize time, occupations, activities, and skills (Kielhofner, 2005).

Kielhofner believes strongly that students and practitioners need to know theory and that theory must be an active thinking tool to guide practice (Forsyth & Kielhofner, 2003). He feels that theory is what is going to make practice work.

Occupation is an underlying principle of Kielhofner's model. Occupation is incorporated in all aspects of hippotherapy and equine-assisted therapy. On the ground, horse care has many activity and task components, such as washing and grooming a horse. Learning how to stable, feed, and water a horse is a purposeful task that can support the person's own self-care habits. Being astride the horse encompasses many occupations that are enlightening to the rider, challenging and promoting physical and mental health. Kielhofner points out the need to focus on theory, because theory is the determining force behind treatment in the equestrian environment that determines the meaning of occupational therapy.

Anne Cronin Mosey

Anne Cronin Mosey felt that everyone needs an occupational balance that reaches for equilibrium of potential through purposeful interaction with the environment and needs to be understood within their lifestyles and occupations (Miller & Walker, 1993). She was influenced by Gail Fidler's work in the field of occupational psychiatry. Mosey described seven adaptive skills that are required to reach an equilibrium and maturity:

1. Perceptual motor skills,
2. Cognitive skills,
3. Drive object skills,
4. Dyadic interaction skills,
5. Primary group interaction skills,
6. Self-identity skills, and
7. Sexual identity interaction skills (Miller & Walker, 1993).

Mosey (2003) used the following frame of reference to identify guidelines for practice:

A definition of occupational therapy model of practice: Occupational therapy model of practice provides theory-based guidelines for occupational therapy practice. A model of practice consists of (a) theory describing relationships between occupation and health and (b) theory-based guidelines for therapeutic occupation. (p. 142)

Mosey has been the major player in "addressing the theme of knowledge organization in occupational therapy" (Kielhofner & Forsyth, 1997). Her focus has been on the articulation of frames of reference for occupational therapy (Miller, 1993) that certainly apply to practitioners of equine-assisted therapy and hippotherapy.

Lela A. Llorens

Lela Llorens (2005) developed the Developmental Theory for the Practice of Occupational Therapy, which she explained in her Eleanor Clarke Slagle Lecture. She based her theory on the premise that the human organization develops concurrently in physical, neurophysiological, psychosocial, and psychodynamic areas and continues to grow chronologically through the years. Language, skills of daily living, and sociocultural skills develop at certain periods within periods of development. Mastery of particular skills, abilities, and relationships in each area, developing both horizontally and vertically, is necessary to achieve satisfactory coping, behavioral, and adaptive relationships. That endowment and the stimulation of the family environment work together to provide simultaneous and chronological development. Later, the community, social, and other groups aid in the development. Disruption in growth and development can occur through physical or emotional trauma related to disease, injury, insufficient home environment, and other disturbances, leading to difficulties in coping behavior and adaptive skills (Shortridge & Walker, 1993).

Llorens's principles can be applied to both hippotherapy and equine-assisted therapy. Early developmental skills such as physical, cognitive, sensorimotor, neurobehavioral, and communication skills can be facilitated in this setting both on and off the horse. Later, community, social, and group skills can be developed as the child participates with others in the equestrian environment by riding horses or vaulting with other children.

Winnie Dunn

The Ecology of Human Performance (EHP) framework developed by Winnie Dunn is formed around five major areas: *establish/restore, adapt/modify, alter, prevent*, and *create* (Dunn, Brown, & Youngstrom, 2003, p. 224). The theoretical claim for the EHP framework is that "ecology, or the interaction between person and the context, affects human behavior and task performance" (Dunn et al., 2003, p. 223). The concept of environment is strong within occupational therapy practice. Environment is necessary for humans to perform in a real-life sense with their many tasks.

In addition to Dunn's framework, she also proclaims the difference between the practitioner's standard practice within occupational therapy and what she calls the "best practice" philosophy, which is a way of thinking: "Best practices are a professional's decisions and actions based on knowledge and evidence that reflect the most current and innovative ideas available" (Dunn, 2000, pp. 1–2). The difference is that standard practice is more traditional and routine, while best practice goes beyond the basic principles to obtain and use the latest knowledge in the field and related fields. Dunn also stresses a family-centered care approach (e.g., using first names) and maintenance of the focus on daily-life performance needs that practitioners address, not on the disability.

As mentioned previously, Dunn's best practice would be most appropriate for the equine setting because additional knowledge and skills are required. Additionally, because the field of hippotherapy is relatively new, Dunn's best practice would help a practitioner with research furthering hippotherapy.

Carolyn M. Baum and Charles H. Christiansen

Carolyn M. Baum and Charles H. Christiansen place occupation in the context of sociocultural nature (Elenko et al., 2000). They developed the person–environment–performance–occupation-based framework. This client-centered model aims to improve the performance of individuals in valued occupations (Baum & Christiansen, 2005). They stressed that individuals need "enablers" to overcome obstructions that restrict their participation in tasks and occupations that are important to them. The environment referred to culture, physical, social, and organizational elements. The performance refers to the outcome of the person–environment–occupation. The model focuses on the interaction of the person–environment–occupation or the doing that is meaningful to the person. Baum and Christiansen stated that "to achieve a desired level of participation, people and groups require the support of enablers and must overcome barriers that limit their participation in activities, tasks, and roles that are important and meaningful to them" (p. 244).

In hippotherapy, the practitioner and the horse are the client's enablers that help overcome difficulties. The Baum and Christiansen framework works well in the equestrian environment because environment is a major part of this setting, along with the performance of the person involved. The environment is unique with its many smells and atmosphere. With the horse's help, the practitioner assists the person to develop competence and adapts tasks to overcome barriers.

Mary Law

Mary Law, along with her associates, focused on the client and practitioner relationship that centered on the practitioner working with the client or family (for those too young or impaired to participate) in a partnership to help solve problems rather than the practitioner directing the client to perform specific tasks in the therapy process (Elenko et al., 2000). This approach is referred to as client-centered occupational therapy. Law and her colleagues developed the person–environment–occupation model to incorporate the client, environment, and occupation in the therapy process (Baum & Christiansen, 2005). Law and colleagues (2001) also developed the Canadian Occupational Performance Measure that allows the client to appraise occupational performance. The client-centered occupational therapy approach leads to a similar approach to measurement. This philosophy enables the client to evaluate the outcome of the therapeutic intervention (Law et al., 2001).

The hippotherapy and equine-assisted setting only can be client centers with a partnership with the practitioner. Law and associates' client-centered occupational therapy is fully applied within the equestrian environment and partnership of client–practitioner. The partnership also can include the horse when all work together to resolve problems and develop communication.

Claudia K. Allen

The Cognitive Disability Frame of Reference developed by Claudia Allen is a useful evaluation method for determining the level of adaptive functioning relative to a person's cognitive ability within the field of mental disabilities. One assumption is that "the severity of a mental disorder can be judged by the consequences it has on a person's capacity to think, do, and learn" (Grant, 2003, pp. 261–262). Allen felt that "therapeutic activity compensates for disability by utilizing remaining capabilities to accomplish desirable activities with satisfactory results" (Allen, 2005).

She developed six cognitive levels adapted after Piaget's model. These methods lead to a useful method of treatment. The overall framework for Allen's model is "the pattern of assumptions about what a client can do, will do, and may do…. What a client can do is based on biological factors…. What a client will do is influenced by psychological factors, such as motivation, fears, or the meaningfulness of the activity being performed" (Grant, 2003, pp. 261–262).

Hippotherapy generally helps to motivate an individual to enhance what he or she will do. What a person can do can be adapted to his or her ability. What a person may do can be guided by the practitioner or helpers with the ability of the individual to choose. Therefore, it is easy to see how Allen's framework can be applied to the equine setting for those with mental disabilities or psychosocial dysfunctions.

David Nelson

A conceptual framework of therapeutic occupation developed by David Nelson looks at the term *occupation* in respect to the meaning for occupational therapists and has broken it down into parts; for example, *form* means *object* and *circumstance,* and *performance* is the *doing of occupation* (Elenko et al., 2000). His initial work with children with autism stimulated his interest in meaning, purpose, and the connection among perception, sensorimotor function, symbolic interpretation, language, and social identity (Nelson & Jepson–Thomas, 2003). He looked at the effect of occupation on healthy human beings (Nelson, 2005). Occupation affects a person's productivity and results in being healthy and content. Because occupation refers to whatever someone does, doing can include many enjoyable and fulfilling occupations, including the ability to perform them independently. The contrast of doing would be being idle, which, as one can see in children, is not well-tolerated and can produce helplessness. Occupational therapists base their profession on the use of occupation to enhance the quality of patients' lives and to encourage a healthier state of being (Nelson, 2005). Nelson also felt that a person needs to clearly understand why he or she is asked to do something so that the occupation has a purpose and meaning: "The occupational understands the potentials of various occupational forms and is willing to collaborate in synthesizing occupational forms that are meaningful and purposeful to the person" (p. 115). This collaboration can be adaptive or can enhance normal to near-normal function. Practitioners and students must understand the "critical nature of active doing, how this defines a person and helps him or her develop for the future" (Nelson, 2003, p. 88).

In the equine setting, all of Nelson's principles apply. The semantics Nelson used can help understand and communicate to the team, client, family, occupational therapy assistants, and others important aspects of therapy. The value of each occupation can be easily described and demonstrated. A situation can be developed to produce a cause and effect that helps a person understand how to make the horse go and stop. Off the horse, many activities can demonstrate purpose and therapeutic value. The horse encourages a person to be motivated to do; that, in turn, brings fulfillment of the occupation.

Sally Schultz and Janette Schkade

Occupational adaptation (OA), a theoretical frame of reference, describes two basic occupation therapy concepts: that of occupation and that of adaptation. The success in occupation is dependent on internal and external demands and on a continuous adaptation process throughout life. The demand to "do" happens naturally in the context of person–occupation–environment interaction. When dysfunction or stress is great, the adaptive process demands are the greatest (Schkade & Schultz, 2003). Sally Schultz and Janette Schkade pointed out that occupational therapy always had a holistic nature and that the underpinnings of the profession have involved occupational adaptation. Although a fragmentation in terms of specialization has occurred, as Schultz and Schkade stated, the holistic approach can encamp the total person. Schultz and Schkade (2005), along with their doctoral planning committee at Texas Women's University, stated, "occupation provides the means by which human beings adapt to changing needs and conditions, and the desire to participate in occupation is intrinsic motivational force leading to adaptation" (p. 103). When there is a disability or a developmental delay, a person may need to adapt for occupation to be successful. The equine setting allows for problem-solving of the client and adaptation made by the practitioner to facilitate a successful experience. With the variety of available tasks and with the input of the horse, a person's goals can be addressed in an enjoyable, productive, and purposeful way.

Ann A. Wilcock

Ann Wilcock (1998) developed an occupational theory of human nature: "Its basic concepts of the influence of humans as a result of their biological evolution and enculturation, humans are occupational beings." The central concept of this theory is that people of all kinds initiate complex occupational behavior. Reasons for participation in occupations depend on the need for survival and diverse genetic make-up (Wilcock, 1998). Her recent work focused on the history of occupational therapy and its establishment in the United Kingdom (Kramer, Hinojosa, & Royeen, 2003). She was the founding president of the International Society of Occupational Science and the founding editor of the *Journal of Occupational Science* (Christiansen & Baum, 2005). Her work centered on academic development of the theory of occupational science and applies to theory in the equine field but not to the physical application of hippotherapy.

Summary

This chapter was not intended to exclude occupational therapists who have contributed abundantly to the profession, for there are many, but space limits those I can include. The theorists for occupational therapy always have focused on the individual as a whole being. Although occupational therapy has specialty practices in pediatrics, hand therapy, physical disabilities, psychosocial dysfunction, and assistive technology, to mention a few, occupational performance and environmental areas always must be considered to enhance health and well-being. Furthermore, individuals with disabilities have made it clear that they are people first and then, second, they have a disability, modified behavior characteristics, or environmentally induced disorders (Linton,

1998). Linton points out that this population considers themselves just another group of people among the infants, children, adults, seniors, and nationalities with the same rights as all people. In the equestrian environment, it is easy for the practitioner, the client, and family to be seen as individuals working together to achieve set goals. The horse helps to naturalize the "therapeutic aspect" of the environment, thus making it an occupation performance area where skills and safety factors are developed in a partnership among individuals, clients, family, practitioners, horse, and the environment.

For a practitioner to provide best practice techniques in an environment best suited for intervention and the person's and family's interest, the practitioner must understand the theoretical base of therapy being used. He or she must use evidence-based practice and have the ability to measure outcome. This step is important for the therapy process: to convey to the client that one has the knowledge of one's profession and is able to provide services that support the practice. It is hoped that, in the coming years, occupational therapy practitioners in hippotherapy will strive to produce research to support practice within the occupation theoretical models and the models of classic horsemanship.

References

Allen, C. (2005). Activity: Occupational therapy's treatment method. In R. Padilla (Ed.), *A professional legacy: The Eleanor Clarke Slagle Lectures in occupational therapy* (2nd ed., pp. 395–414). Bethesda, MD: AOTA Press.

American Occupational Therapy Association. (2006). *Model occupational therapy practice act.* Retrieved January 24, 2007, from www.aota.org (membership site).

Ayres, A. J. (1972). *Sensory integration and learning.* Los Angeles: Western Psychological Services.

Ayres, A. J. (1979). *Sensory integration and the child.* Los Angeles: Western Psychological Services.

Ayres, A. J. (2005). The development of perceptual–motor abilities: A theoretical basis for treatment of dysfunction. In R. Padilla (Ed.), *A professional legacy: The Eleanor Clarke Slagle Lectures in occupational therapy* (2nd ed., pp. 108–114). Bethesda, MD: AOTA Press.

Barrett, L., & Kielhofner, G. (2003). Theories derived from occupational therapy perspectives. In E. B. Crepeau, E. S. Cohn, & B. A. Boyt Schell (Eds.), *Willard and Spackman's occupational therapy* (10th ed., pp. 209–212). Philadelphia: Lippincott Williams & Wilkins.

Baum, C., & Christiansen, C. (2005). Person–environment–occupation performance: An occupation-based framework for practice. In C. Christiansen & C. Baum (Eds.), *Occupational therapy: Performance, participation, and well-being* (pp. 242–266). Thorofare, NJ: Slack.

Bundy, A. C., Lane, S. J., & Murray, E. A. (2002) *Sensory integration: Theory and practice.* Philadelphia: F. A. Davis.

Burke, J. P. (2003). Philosophical base of human occupation. In P. Kramer, J. Hinojosa, & C. B. Royeen (Eds.), *Perspectives in human occupation: Participation in life* (pp. 32–44). Philadelphia: Lippincott Williams & Wilkins.

Centola, T. (2005, May). Decoding the written word: New findings on genetic basis of dyslexia. *Advance for Occupational Therapy Practitioners, 21,* 43.

Cottrell, R. P. F. (Ed.). (2005). *Perspectives for occupation therapy-based practice: Foundation and future of occupational therapy* (2nd ed.). Bethesda, MD: AOTA Press

Crepeau, E. B., & Boyt Schell, B. A. (2003). Theory and practice in occupational therapy. In E. B. Crepeau, E. S. Cohn, & B. A. Boyt Schell (Eds.), *Willard and Spackman's occupational therapy* (10th ed., pp. 203–206). Philadelphia: Lippincott Williams & Wilkins.

Dorland, W. A. N. (1994). *Dorland's illustrated medical dictionary* (28th ed.). Philadelphia: W. B. Saunders.

Dunn, W. (2000). *Best practice occupational therapy: In community service with children and families.* Thorofare, NJ: Slack.

Dunn, W., Brown, C., & Youngstrom, M. J. (2003). Ecological model of occupation. In P. Kramer, J. Hinojosa, & C. B. Royeen (Eds.), *Perspectives in human occupation: Participation in life* (pp. 222–263). Philadelphia: Lippincott Williams & Wilkins.

Dunn, W., McClain, L. H., Brown, C., & Youngstrom, M. J. (2003). Ecology of human performance. In E. B. Crepeau, E. S. Cohn, & B. A. Boyt Schell (Eds.), *Willard and Spackman's occupational therapy* (10th ed., pp. 223–224). Philadelphia: Lippincott Williams & Wilkins.

Elenko, B. K., Hinojosa, J., & Blount, M. L. (2000). Perspectives. In J. Hinojosa, & M. L. Blount (Eds.), *The texture of life: Purposeful activities in occupational therapy* (pp. 16–34). Bethesda, MD: American Occupational Therapy Association.

Fidler, G. S., & Fidler, J. W. (2005). Doing and becoming: purposeful action and self-actualization. In R. P. Fleming Cottrell (Ed.), *Perspectives for occupation-based practice: Foundation and future of occupational therapy* (2nd ed., pp. 85–90). Bethesda, MD: AOTA Press.

Fletcher, C., & Scanlan, L. (2005). *Healed by horses.* New York: Atria Books.

Forsyth, K., & Kielhofner, G. (2003). Model of human occupation. In P. Kramer, J. Hinojosa, & C. B. Royeen (Eds.), *Perspectives in human occupation: Participation in life* (pp. 45–86). Philadelphia: Lippincott Williams & Wilkins.

Giuffrida, C. G. (2003). Motor learning: An emerging frame of reference for occupational performance. In E. B. Crepeau,

E. S. Cohn, & B. A. Boyt Schell (Eds.), *Willard and Spackman's occupational therapy* (10th ed., pp. 267–272). Philadelphia: Lippincott Williams & Wilkins.

Grant, S. (2003). Cognitive disability frame of reference. In E. B. Crepeau, E. S. Cohn, & B. A. Boyt Schell (Eds.), *Willard and Spackman's occupational therapy* (10th ed., pp. 261–263). Philadelphia: Lippincott Williams & Wilkins.

Hinojosa, J., & Blount, M. L. (2000). (Eds.). *The texture of life: Purposeful activities in occupational therapy.* Bethesda, MD: American Occupational Therapy Association.

Hopkins, H., & Smith, D. (1983). *Willard and Spackman's occupational therapy* (6th ed.). Philadelphia: Lippincott.

Kielhofner, G. (1978). General systems theory: Implications for theory and action in occupational therapy. *American Journal of Occupational Therapy, 32,* 637–645.

Kielhofner, G. (2004). *Conceptual foundations of occupational therapy* (3rd ed.). Philadelphia: F. A. Davis.

Kielhofner, G. (2005) Temporal adaptation: A conceptual framework for occupational therapy. In R. P. Fleming Cottrell (Ed.), *Perspectives for occupation-based practice: Foundation and future of occupational therapy* (2nd ed., pp. 219–224). Bethesda, MD: AOTA Press.

Kielhofner, G., & Forsyth, K. (1997). The model of human occupation: An overview of current concepts. *British Journal of Occupational Therapy, 60,* 103–110.

Kielhofner, G., Forsyth, K., & Barrett, L. (2003). The model of human occupation. In E. B. Crepeau, E. S. Cohn, & B. A. Boyt Schell (Eds.), *Willard and Spackman's occupational therapy* (10th ed., pp. 212–219). Philadelphia: Lippincott Williams & Wilkins.

Kramer, P., Hinojosa, J., & Royeen, C. B. (2003). *Perspectives in human occupation: Participation in life.* Philadelphia: Lippincott Williams & Wilkins.

Lane, S. L. (2002). Sensory modulation. In A. C. Bundy, S. J. Lane, & E. A. Murray (Eds.) *Sensory integration: Theory and practice* (2nd ed., pp. 101–123). Philadelphia: F. A. Davis.

Larson, E., Wood, W., & Clark, F. (2003). Occupational science: Building the science and practice of occupation through an academic discipline. In E. B. Crepeau, E. S. Cohn, & B. A. Boyt Schell (Eds.), *Willard and Spackman's occupational therapy* (10th ed., pp. 15–16). Philadelphia: Lippincott Williams & Wilkins.

Law, M., Baum, C., & Dunn, W. (2001). *Measuring occupational performance: Supporting best practice in occupational therapy.* Thorofare, NJ: Slack.

Linton, S. (1998). *Claiming disability: Knowledge and identity.* New York: New York University Press.

Llorens, L. A. (2005). Facilitating growth and development: The promise of occupational therapy. In R. Padilla (Ed.), *A professional legacy: The Eleanor Clarke Slagle Lectures in occupational therapy* (2nd ed., pp. 152–164). Bethesda, MD: AOTA Press.

Ludwig, F. M. (1993). Gail Fidler. In R. J. Muller & K. F. Walker (Eds.), *Perspectives on theory for the practice of occupational theory.* Gaithersburg, MD: Aspen.

Mathiowetz, V., & Bass-Hagen, J. (1994). Motor behavior research: Implications for therapeutic approaches to central nervous system dysfunction. *American Journal of Occupational Therapy, 48,* 733–744.

McColl, M., Law, M., Stewart, D., Doubt, L., Pollock, N., & Krupa, T. (2002*). Theoretical basis of occupational therapy* (2nd ed.). Thorofare, NJ: Slack.

Miller, R. J. (1993). Model of human occupation. In R. J. Miller & K. F. Walker (Eds.), *Perspectives on theory for the practice of occupational therapy* (2nd ed., pp. 185–186). Gaithersburg, MD: Aspen.

Miller, R. J., & Walker, K. F. (Eds.) (1993). *Perspectives on theory for the practice of occupational therapy* (2nd ed.). Gaithersburg, MD: Aspen.

Mosey, A. C. (1986). *Psychosocial components of occupational therapy.* New York: Raven Press.

Nelson, D. (1997). Why the profession of occupational therapy will flourish in the 21st century. *American Journal of Occupational Therapy, 51,* 11–24.

Nelson, D. (2005). Why the profession of occupational theory will flourish in the 21st century. In R. P. E. Fleming Cottrell (Ed.), *Perspectives for occupation-based practice: Foundation and future of occupational therapy* (2nd ed., pp. 113–126). Bethesda, MD: AOTA Press.

Nelson, D., & Jepson-Thomas, J. (2003). Occupational form, occupational performance, and a conceptual framework. In P. Kramer, J. Hinojosa, & C. B. Royeen (Eds.), *Perspectives in human occupation: Participation in life* (pp. 87–155). Baltimore: Lippincott, Williams, and Wilkins.

Ottenbacher, K. (2003). Theories provide conceptual scaffolding and show relationships among variables. In E. B. Crepeau, E. S. Cohn, & B. A. Boyt Schell (Eds.), *Willard and Spackman's occupational therapy* (10th ed., p. 205). Philadelphia: Lippincott Williams & Wilkins.

Reed, K. L. (1984). Understanding theory: The first step in learning about research. *American Journal of Occupational Therapy, 38,* 677.

Reilly, M. (2005). Occupational therapy can be one of the great ideas of 20th-century medicine. In R. Padilla (Ed.), *A professional legacy: The Eleanor Clarke Slagle Lectures in occupational therapy* (2nd ed., pp. 80–93). Bethesda, MD: AOTA Press.

Schkade, J. K. & Schultz, S. (2003). Occupational adaptation. In P. Kramer, J. Hinojosa, & C. B. Royeen (Eds.), *Perspectives in human occupation: Participation in life* (pp. 181–221). Philadelphia: Lippincott Williams & Wilkins.

Schkade, J. K., & Schultz, S. (2005). Occupational adoption: A holistic approach for contemporary practice, part 1. In R. P. F. Cottrell (Ed.), *Perspectives for occupation-based practice: Foundation and future of occupational therapy* (2nd ed., pp. 103–112). Bethesda, MD: AOTA Press.

Schultz, K. B. (2003). History of occupation. In P. Kramer, J. Hinojosa, & C. B. Royeen (Eds.), *Perspectives in human occupation: Participation in life* (pp. 18–31). Baltimore: Lippincott, Williams & Wilkins.

Serrett, K. D. (1985). *Philosophical and historical roots of occupational therapy.* New York: Haworth Press.

Shortridge, S. D., & Walker, K. F. (1993). Lela A. Llorens. In R. J. Miller & K. F. Walker (Eds.), *Perspectives on theory for the practice of occupational therapy* (pp. 65–102). Gaithersburg, MD: Aspen.

Shumway-Cook, A., & Woollacott, M. H. (2001). *Motor control theory and practice applications* (2nd ed.). Philadelphia: Lippincott Williams & Wilkins.

Strauss, I. (1995). *Hippotherapy: Neurophysiological therapy on the horse* (M. Takeuchi, Trans.). Toronto: Ontario Therapeutic Riding Association. (Original work published 1991)

Walker, K. F. (1993). A. Jean Ayres. In R. J. Miller & K. F. Walker (Eds.), *Perspectives on theory for the practice of occupational therapy* (pp. 104–154). Gaithersburg, MD: Aspen.

Wilcock, A. A. (1998). *An occupational perspective of health.* Thorofare, NJ: Slack.

Yerxa, E. J. (2005). Authentic occupational therapy. In R. Padilla (Ed.), *A professional legacy: The Eleanor Clarke Slagle Lectures in occupational therapy* (2nd ed., pp. 127–140). Bethesda, MD: AOTA Press.

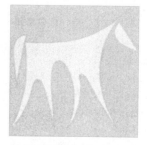

Occupational therapy is a facilitation process which assists the individual in achieving mastery of life tasks and the ability to cope as efficiently as possible with life's expectations....
—Lela Llorens

CHAPTER 5

Relating Hippotherapy to the AOTA *Occupational Therapy Practice Framework*

Kathy Splinter-Watkins, MOT, OTR/L, FAOTA, HPCS

Hippotherapy (American Hippotherapy Association [AHA], 2004) is defined as a "treatment strategy that utilizes equine movement" within the fields of physical therapy, occupational therapy, and speech and language pathology. Each of the practitioners in these professions may choose to use hippotherapy as an effective intervention for their clients. Often this form of intervention looks very similar across disciplines to nontherapists, but in actuality it involves professionally unique approaches, goals, and outcomes. A common saying is that it is all in the perspective of the treating therapist; however, the differences involve not only professional perspective but also theoretical basis and professional scope of practice. For this reason, this chapter will discuss the perspective of the occupational therapy practitioner when using hippotherapy as a treatment strategy by reviewing the occupational base of hippotherapy and its relationship to the *Occupational Therapy Practice Framework: Domain and Process* (American Occupational Therapy Association [AOTA], 2002).

Terminology

Over the years, there has been much discussion and debate as to the terminology and definition of *hippotherapy* and *equine-assisted therapy* (Macauley, 2004). Both terms are appropriate to describe various aspects within an occupational therapy treatment session. Strictly defined, hippotherapy focuses directly on the input from equine movement to effect therapeutic changes in the client. Those therapeutic effects may include, for example, sensory integrative, neurodevelopmental, and perceptual–motor skills changes. Equine-assisted therapy, however, includes activity on or off the horse that may or may not include a moving horse but does

involve the environmental context, performance skills and patterns, activity demands, and client factors.

The sum of both hippotherapy and equine-assisted therapy within an occupational therapy session could be described more clearly as equine-assisted occupational therapy. For practice and reimbursement considerations, this term clearly distinguishes occupational therapy as the discipline in charge of the therapy session and the direction or therapeutic basis from which one is practicing. Additionally, hippotherapy and equine-assisted therapy become specifically oriented treatment strategies to be used within the session. Likewise, each discipline could utilize this structure: equine-assisted physical therapy and equine-assisted speech and language therapy, with hippotherapy being a specified portion of the sessions.

AOTA *Occupational Therapy Practice Framework*

To underscore the connection of hippotherapy with occupation-based practice, it is critical to understand and follow the *Occupational Theraphy Practice Framework* (AOTA, 2002). For occupational therapy, this guide for practice helps to delineate the areas of occupational therapy evaluation, intervention, and outcomes. This document was developed as a revision and replacement for the *Uniform Terminology for Occupational Therapy—Third Edition* (AOTA, 1994) and as a companion to *The Guide to Occupational Therapy Practice* (Moyers, 1999; Moyers & Dale, 2007). The *Framework* offers a structure on which to hang the diverse world of occupational therapy yet focuses on the engagement in occupation and its interaction and relationship with daily life and society. By using the *Framework*, occupational therapists evaluate all areas that may affect performance rather than focus on any one particular area (Holmquist, 2004).

The *Framework* has two purposes: (1) to describe the domain of occupational therapy and (2) to outline the process of occupational therapy practice (AOTA, 2002). With the three main components of evaluation, intervention, and outcomes, the process of occupational therapy is dynamic and interactive. Although evaluation, intervention, and outcomes are not unique to occupational therapy, the domain of occupational therapy is. The domain of practice sets the profession apart from others because it is focused on promoting health and wellness through engagement in meaningful activities or occupations. Thus, the goal of intervention is to facilitate active engagement in occupation within the context of an individual's particular life experience.

Crucial to occupational therapy intervention is an understanding of the occupational needs of the client and the potential benefits to this client as a result of engagement in occupation. Bringing this concept to hippotherapy and equine-assisted therapy, it is critical to assess the occupational needs of the client to determine the potential benefits or contraindications of involvement in equine-assisted occupational therapy.

Evaluation

The evaluation process consists of the occupational profile and an analysis of occupational performance. Often clients come to therapists with standard occupational therapy evaluations and plans of care. The occupational profile assists in gathering information about the client's patterns of activities, roles, interests, values, needs, and functional changes over time. As stated by Roley (2002), "The therapist's analysis of the occupational profile makes our unique focus on occupation central to all other interactions with the client no matter which frames of reference are chosen" (p. 1).

Three areas are considered in the evaluation: client factors, activity demands, and contextual factors. A client's functional abilities are assessed in terms of occupational performance. Performance skills and performance patterns need to be evaluated. What are the client's age, developmental status, and capability? Consider whether additional specific assessments need to be performed to assess sensorimotor, neurodevelopmental, cognitive–behavioral, or psychosocial functioning. What are the client's interests, values, lifestyle, and needs? What are his or her limitations, precautions, or contraindications? For the hippotherapy setting, posture, balance and function are primary considerations for

therapeutic intervention utilizing equine movement. The functional abilities of the client will dictate, for example, what approach to use, which horse to select, length and duration of the session, and ability to address individual goals for that particular client.

The activity demands of being on or around a horse and in that environment must be considered for appropriateness for each particular client. Activity on or around the horse and environment can be used or adapted in a multitude of ways. What are the client's stated goals? What might be the benefits for engagement with this particular activity? What might be the "just-right challenge" in terms of activity demand? How might this particular choice of activity for intervention affect the client's lifestyle or occupational performance? The therapist may adjust or modify the activity as client factors and contexts change or with progression toward goals and objectives.

As evaluation directs treatment, it is especially important to analyze the differences in context between a traditional occupational therapy clinic and a setting for hippotherapy or equine-assisted therapy. What does relating to the horse and equine environment mean for the client? How will this translate to their everyday life, including family, school, societal, or work roles? As practitioners incorporate the occupational profile and occupational performance in evaluations, they increasingly must commit to looking past components and building individualized, context-appropriate, occupation-based activity into their intervention program (Zehr, 2002).

Intervention

Five categories of occupational therapy interventions are listed by the *Occupational Therapy Practice Framework* (AOTA, 2002): (1) therapeutic use of self, (2) therapeutic use of occupations and activities, (3) consultation process, (4) education process, and (5) other. The first category, therapeutic use of self, is critical to equine-assisted occupational therapy in that the therapist must not only understand the goals of occupational therapy practice but also be *knowledgeable and comfortable in the horse environment*. The therapist must thoroughly understand horse behavior, movement, and responses to be effective and safe with clients when involving the horse in therapeutic sessions. Additionally, the confidence of the therapist in that environment imparts feelings of success and safety to the client, which can be critical to motivation and accomplishment of their goals.

The second category includes the *therapeutic use of occupations and activities,* which are selected for specific clients to meet therapeutic goals. Contexts, activity demands, and client factors all should be considered in relation to meeting the client's goals. This category further divides occupations and activities into three groups with different purposes: occupation-based activity, purposeful activity, and preparatory methods. The versatility of the horse and horse environment allows its use in any of these groups depending on the goals and purpose of the intervention.

Strictly defined, hippotherapy can fall into the *preparatory methods* category of intervention for occupational therapy. The client assumes a sitting position, facing forward, on the horse and is passively influenced by the horse's therapist-directed movement. This intervention often can be seen with adult clients where the horse's specifically guided movement influences an adult with physical impairments. The physical multidimensional movement and sensory input of the horse prepares the client for occupational performance.

Hippotherapy, as broadly defined by the AHA (2004), also may be classified under *purposeful activity* because activity on the horse allows the client to engage in goal-directed behaviors or exercises within a therapeutically designed context, leading to occupation or occupations. Thus, for pediatric clients, changing positions from forward sitting to lying supine on the horse, reaching for objects, or stretching the upper extremities to point at different items in the arena as directed by the therapist gives the client purposeful activity within a prescribed context of enjoyable challenges while on the horse. Cognitive or behavioral goals may be reached through questions and answers about the horse and the surrounding environment or responding with verbal cues for the horse to "walk on" and "whoa."

Occupation-based activity is defined by the *Framework* as allowing clients to engage in (1) actual occupations that are part of their (2) own context and that (3) match their goals. Hippotherapy fits with this category because clients may engage in games or purposeful activities while on the horse. An adult client who rode previous to their injury may need to learn to guide a horse again through various patterns in the arena. Alternatively, a pediatric client who needs the vestibular and multimodal sensory input may discover the joy of relating to and riding a horse after a series of developmental steps to increase balance.

Equine-assisted occupational therapy may involve preparing grain or carrots to feed the horse, brushing the horse, leading the horse to the barn, climbing a fence or into the hay loft, tacking or untacking the horse, and carrying the blanket and surcingle back to the tack room. Any of these occupation-based activities should be connected to the client's specific goals and context. For instance, someone who is interested in taking care of their horse should be involved in this aspect of the horse environment as is appropriate to their goals. Brushing the horse may increase both range of motion and strength of upper extremities but also is occupation-based and serves the purpose of readying or caring for the horse. A pediatric client who needs proprioceptive input (or "heavy work") before being able to focus his or her attention may push a weighted wheelbarrow to transport horse feed and then follow up with more fine-motor tasks, such as writing a sentence about the horses. An adult client (previous equestrian) with a brain injury may need to scan the barn environment to locate the horse's brushes, bridle, pad, and saddle before tacking up his or her own horse. This person also may need to learn cues to help remember where equipment should be replaced, learn to space themselves safely while working around the horse, and use proper body mechanics when lifting buckets and equipment.

The third category of *consultation process* is an area in which occupational therapists may be called on to consult with therapeutic riding programs or with clinical or school programs to institute a hippotherapy program. It is imperative that the consulting occupational therapist obtains and maintains his or her own personal and professional training in both therapeutic riding and hippotherapy to effectively consult with programs or individual clients.

The fourth category is the *education process*. One way this category connects with practice is when hippotherapy or equine-assisted occupational therapy is offered within an educational or school system's program as part of their curriculum, special education, or therapy program. This area of practice is becoming more and more viable as programs lend themselves to development in this direction.

In summary, the versatility and flexibility of the horse and equestrian environment lends itself to great adaptability for practice and meeting therapeutic goals within the *Framework* (AOTA, 2002). Critically needed is additional knowledge and research for the evidence-based practice of hippotherapy and equine-assisted occupational therapy.

Outcomes

Without evidence-based practice, neither occupational therapy nor hippotherapy have any standing in the medical arena. It is imperative, therefore, to not only document the evaluation and intervention process but also consistently measure outcomes of practice. Ideally, practitioners all should perform a research study, no matter how small, to add to the body of evidence. Just documenting the changes therapists effect for clients involved in equine-assisted occupational therapy creates a compilation of literature that is critically needed for substantiation of this vital treatment strategy. Of course, as well stated by Roley (2002), the most important outcome of any occupational therapy intervention is to support participation in life through enhanced engagement in occupation. Hippotherapy and equine-assisted therapy can be the just-right meaningful challenge through activity or occupation that enhances the lives of our clients.

References

American Hippotherapy Association. (2004). Statement of practice. *Hippotherapy, 13*(1), 2.

American Occupational Therapy Association. (1994). *The uniform terminology for occupational therapy* (3rd ed.). Bethesda, MD: Author.

American Occupational Therapy Association. (2002). Occupational therapy practice framework: Domain and process. *American Journal of Occupational Therapy, 56,* 609–639.

Holmquist, B. B. (2004, June). Incorporating the occupational therapy practice framework into a mental health practice setting. *Mental Health Special Interest Section Quarterly,* 1–4.

Macauley, B. L. (2004, Spring). Hippotherapy and equine-assisted therapy: Who does what? *Hippotherapy, 13*(1), 10–11.

Moyers, P. A. (1999). The guide to occupational therapy practice. *American Journal of Occupational Therapy, 53,* 247–322.

Moyers, P., & Dale, L. (2007). *The guide to occupational therapy practice* (2nd ed.). Bethesda, MD: AOTA Press.

Roley, S. S. (2002, December). Application of sensory integration using the occupational therapy practice framework. *Sensory integration Special Interest Section Quarterly, 25*(4), 1–4.

Zehr, L. E. (2002). *Linking the* Occupational Therapy Practice Framework *to the therapeutic use of the horse.* Unpublished master's thesis, Eastern Kentucky University, Richmond.

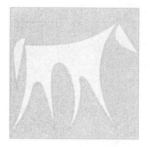

Equestrian art is the perfect understanding between the rider [handler] and his horse. This harmony allows the horse to...carry out all movements with mental and physical enjoyment as well as with suppleness and rhythm. The horse is then a partner, rather than a slave.
—Nuno Oliveira

CHAPTER 6

Classical Dressage as the Underpinning of Hippotherapy

Barbara T. Engel, MEd, OTR

The foundation of hippotherapy is the effect the horse has on its rider (Heipertz, 1981; Riede, 1998). Effective therapy on the horse only can occur when the horse can appropriately balance its own body (Strauss, 1995), a quality that can be obtained through classical dressage. The poor position of a rider generally hampers the horse's movement and balance because of the tension, unwieldiness, or involuntary movement of the rider (Herbermann, 1984). Anyone who rides should understand that a horse is not genetically built to carry a person on its back. The horse, therefore, must strengthen its skeletomuscular system to shift its center of gravity and rebalance to accommodate the additional weight of the rider and tack.

Spink (1993) stated that using a recreational-quality horse with minimal training for therapeutic intervention would be fundamentally incorrect. The therapy horse needs to be athletic and properly trained to be able to accomplish forward–backward–side yielding and other desired movements, as well as to handle changes in tempo and gait. In addition, the horse needs to be trained to focus and be well balanced so the client can receive the full effect of the hippotherapy. When I speak of *focus*, I'm referring to a horse that maintains its focus on the task of what is asked of it and, therefore, is not distracted by factors of the environment nor has a tendency to spook. Many recreational-quality horses have been trained to an introductory level only, which consists of the basic acceptance of being ridden, guided, and controlled at a basic level by the rider. This limited training does not provide the qualities necessary for a therapy horse.

The therapy horse must understand and obey commands by the practitioner or a handler on the ground, requiring a thorough understanding in the communication or cues from the handler, practitioner, or rider, as well as any volunteers. If the horse does not understand what is asked, it cannot accurately respond to a request, a problem that many inexperienced horse people face. Children often will say, "The horse will not listen to me!" How can it when the horse does not understand the child's language? De Pluvinel (1626/1989) insisted on treating the horse with courtesy, sound judgment, and patience. Individuals who have spent a great deal of time with their horses understand their sensitivity and how much a well-trained horse, who has been treated with the respect DePluvinel and Xenophon (430 B.C./1962) expressed, will do to please and perform its job with pleasure and satisfaction.

The Essence of Classical Dressage

Dressage is taken from the French word *dresser*, which means *to train* (*Concise Oxford Dictionary*, 1995), and refers to the gymnastic development of a horse. *Classical* refers to the tradition of time-honored principles (de Kunffy, 2002) that have been developed through centuries. *Gymnastics* refers to exercises involving physical and mental agility, flexibility, coordination, strength, and endurance. The point of classical dressage training is to develop the natural aptitude of the horse by developing its strength, agility, gait, tempo, and natural way of going (i.e., its overall movement pattern) while carrying a person on its back. As the one foundation of classical training of horse and rider that was developed in Europe, dressage can involve many different techniques in teaching to accomplish both the classical goals and many different disciplines in the English and Western variations of riding. It is being rediscovered by some instructors because of its effectiveness. The training originated with Xenophon in 430 B.C. and was developed further by the French. The final theory was put into a theoretical framework by de la Guérinière (1733/1994) in his book *Ecole de Cavalerie (School of Horsemanship).* It is as effective today as it was in the 17th century.

The point of classical training is to develop the natural aptitude of the horse by means of developing its strength, forward impulsion, agility, gait, and tempo while accommodating a rider and performing movements on command (Knopfhart, 1990). One cannot train a rider without first training the horse. Beginning training of the horse is beyond the scope of this book, but one must be able to train the horse to perform to expectations if a readily-trained therapy horse is not available. Throughout this chapter I refer to *classical dressage* as the training and maintenance techniques of the horse to accommodate the rider, not *dressage competition of a rider.*

The Importance of Theory

The importance of theory in practice has been discussed in Chapter 4. Theory in the training and handling of horses provides guidelines, principles, and a systematic approach. Horses respond well to a routine that is kind and consistent. In 1733, de la Guérinière (1733/1994), the great master of equitation, and the father of dressage, stated:

> Practice without true principles is nothing other than routine, the fruit of which is a strained and unsure execution. (p. 75)

> Theory instructs us that we should work from a foundation of sound principles, and these principles, rather then going against nature, must serve to perfect it with the aid of art. Practice gives us facility in the execution of that which theory teaches us. (p.78)

Classical Theory in Hippotherapy Practice

Why should occupational therapists using the horse as a practice strategy be concerned with classical dressage? *It is because classical dressage provides them with a theoretical base that gives a horse the training necessary to become an adequate provider in riding and therapy.* Gymnasticizing a horse can be done only through a proven scheme of proven strategies (de Kunffy, 2002):

> Riders retained only those principles that worked with most horses for most riders, most effectively, most of the time. The classical principles of horsemanship are pragmatic and retain only the best of knowledge, leaving us the task to learn them. Toying with "new" or "innovative" riding methods and "techniques" amounts to a wasteful diversion. (p. ix)

To understand the theoretical base of dressage, how it developed, and why it is still the theoretical base of present-day training in most countries, a review of the work of the old masters and theorists is necessary.

In the field of equitation, theory and practice work together and one is not complete without the other. Theory is the knowledge, practice is the ability (Podhajsky, 1965/1967). This relationship is as true for training horses as it is for the practice of occupational therapy. Practitioners are trained in school to become occupational therapists by steps and develop levels of knowledge and competence, one built upon the other by faculty who are more learned, have researched, or have more experience than students. Therapists live by theory and practice. Education from preschool to a doctoral degree is developed by means of theory (knowledge) and practice (ability). All skilled athletes also are trained by theory. Even baking a cake from scratch is done by knowledge (theory) and ability (practice). Knowledge always must precede practice (Podhajsky, 1965/1967).

Many of the same principles apply to our lives as to equestrian training. Our horses teach us how to be consistent, be in self-control, and understand what goes on in another's mind and the feelings of another creature. These concepts are important precepts for practitioners to know and for clients to learn from the horse and its environment, because in the hippotherapy setting, both practitioner and horse are the enablers and facilitators for the client-centered intervention approach (Baptiste, 2003). With at-risk youths, horses have been used to teach self-control, bonding with another, respect, and caring for another, characteristics that can be applied to the youth's daily life. Podhajsky (1965/1967) felt that only a kind and understanding relationship will bring about desired achievements. That is true with our relationships with each other, with our clients, and with our horses.

De Kunffy (1984) stated that when the practitioner and the client set out to accomplish a specific task, they must have a set goal in mind. In hippotherapy and equine-assisted therapy, the horse is a partner with the client to achieve this set goal. To understand the desired achievements, the practitioner must have the knowledge to judge cause and effect, both in the horse and the rider. The horse acted or performed in a specific way: What was the cause? Was the cue given correctly? Does there need to be change? How can it be corrected, or is it best to avoid it? Practitioners are taught to observe the actions and reactions of their clients. They also must observe and "read the horse" to understand its actions and reactions. The horse may tell much about what is happening with the rider, physically, emotionally, and sensory-wise.

Theory in the training of the horse was developed through the centuries by the acknowledged masters of equestrian training (de Kunffy, 1984). They worked from the knowledge of their predecessors and from observations, experimentation, and years of practice—not so different from how occupational therapy progressed. What works is used and what does not work is discarded (de Kunffy).

The Basis of Classical Dressage

In 430 B.C., a Greek general named Xenophon wrote one of the first books on the gentle training of horses. *The Art of Horsemanship* follows the nature of the horse, which is the foundation of present-day dressage (Xenophon, 430 B.C./1962). Xenophon and his predecessor Simon both maintained that a horse should be considered as a being and not a tool, and must be understood and loved (Oliveira, 1988). Two of the early basic principles were that the horse is trained by understanding, not compulsion, and that training should be by education, not conditioning (Xenophon, 430 B.C./1962). Much of this early theory still is important and applied today.

In the centuries following Xenophon's work, dressage was lost. The 14th century saw the horse used by man as an instrument for his service. In the 16th century, a rediscovery took place in Italy by Frederico Grisone, in the form of equitation (Henriquet, 1991/2004). The methods used then were harsh and not like those used by Xenophon. In the mid-1500s, Antoine de Pluvinel (1555–1620), a Frenchman, revived the training of horse and rider in the gentler style, concentrating on moderation, harmony, and order (Oliveira, 1988). France produced many exceptional practitioners of horsemanship, and riding schools' (*manège*) training went beyond the military schools. That was especially true at the Versailles in France with de la Guérinière (Oliveira, 1988). These master equestrian instructors (*écuyers*) not only produced exceptional students from around the world, but also wrote memoirs and books that have left behind theoretical treatises on equitation.

William Cavendish, the Duke of Newcastle (1596–1676), was another notable horseman who wrote a book delineating his precepts. He was the first Englishman to do so. Cavendish's (1743/2000) work was a turning point in equestrian training, which was considered humane and systematic; his teachings had a long-lasting impact on the development of equestrian skill and horseman-

ship, even though his major focus was on training riders and breeding horses rather than training techniques. Cavendish's education and skill was not limited to equestrian endeavors; he wrote plays and poetry, was knighted in his teens, and became a commander in the British army. Cavendish later was exiled from England and spent the rest of his life in Belgium, where he devoted himself to horses and the equestrian pursuits he truly loved. He stated "that good horses are so rare as not to be valued for money" (Cavendish, 1743/2000, p iii).

One of the notable features that increased the development of equestrian skills in France was the training institutions. École de Cavalerie of Saumur (a school of cavalry) was the major military academy in France and continues as an equestrian *manège* today. Ècole de Versailles, along with the Manège of Versailles (an equestrian school) founded by King Louis XIV and the Manège royal des Tuileries headed by de la Guérinière, concentrates on *haute école* (high school), but de la Guérinière also wrote about the military and what they called "exterior riding" (i.e., hunting, equitation, obstacle jumping, racing) that became popular during the 18th century. Wars disrupted the development of equitation throughout history as it did in France, but helped spread the training to other countries. The wars in France sent many *écuyers* elsewhere in Europe, such as Austria and Germany, where many riding schools were established (L'Hotte, 1997).

In the 18th century, François Robichon de la Guérinière (1688–1751) became an outstanding *écuyer* and is considered the father of today's dressage theory. Using the knowledge of past masters and his own observation and skill, he was the first to develop a true theory. Among the major contributions de la Guérinière gave to dressage were simplifying training with methods to preserve the nature of the horse; developing suppling of the horse by shoulder-in and haunches-in; developing in the rider soft shoulders, hands, and fingers to allow the horse to move forward without resistance; separating upper–lower body for an independent seat; and separating pelvis from legs and arms (de la Guérinière, 1733/1994). His overall aim was to work by a systematic method to develop a riding horse that was obedient, quiet, with pleasant movements, supple, and comfortable to ride. That certainly sounds like a horse that would be suitable to be used in hippotherapy.

François Baucher (1796–1873) was one of the few riding masters who had never been in the military. He trained horses humanely and was an ardent student of the highest level of dressage; his concentration was on training the human to train the horse. He was the first to scientifically analyze the movement of the horse to determine the relationship of the horse's center of gravity to the center of motion, which led to impressive ease and lightness. He was the first to develop unmounted exercises that suppled the horse in 10 to 12 days, an accomplishment that had taken other trainers years to do. He stated that to control the horse, the neck and jaw must be flexible, light, and well-balanced; otherwise the horse could annul all efforts of the rider. He stressed that the horse must seek the hand, not the hand seek the mouth or bit. He also developed mounted suppling on the lunge, which is still used today at the Spanish Riding School of Vienna, Austria (Baucher, 1835/1992). His major goals were suppling to make the horse a docile, subordinate animal that was easy to control and would submit to impulsion (Baucher, 1835/1992). While it was de la Guérinière who is credited with the development of dressage theory, it is Baucher who was able to analyze the how and why of the theory and to develop principles and methods (Baucher, 1835/1992).

Cultural changes were occurring during the time of Count Antoine Cartier d'Aure (1799–1863), who changed his focus as an *écuyer* to outdoor activities such as hunting, racing, steeplechasing, and jumping. Riding now was available to all who could afford it, not just the nobility. D'Aure's schooling consisted of the basics of classical dressage and then extended training in the field to fast-moving riding. He wanted the rider to sit with ease so that the rider's suppleness became united with the horse and that the rider would develop a light and consistent rapport with the horse's mouth through the reins by light pressure of the fingers rather than a clenched fist.

Gustav Steinbrecht (1808–1885), a German *écuyer*, followed the teachings of Xenophon, De Pluvinel, Cavendish, and de la Guérinière, which had become the standard method of practice. He was opposed to Baucher's methods, especially in moving the horse backward, which he felt was unnatural. Steinbrecht (1935/1995) also felt that the English method avoided training the horse to develop its haunches, which caused the horse to weaken its forelegs while its weight was not distributed evenly to account for the additional weight of the rider. In his writings, he was able to describe de la Guérinière's methods in more detail. Steibrecht also included any development of scientific equestrian research that became available during his time and how this applied to or changed training.

Along with Count d'Aure, General Alexis-François L'Hotte (1825–1904) was an *écuyer* at the cavalry school at Saumur, where instruction was permitted only for military officers. L'Hotte, on his own horse and personal time, went beyond the military type of training and pursued the high school education of the horse (Henriquet, 1991/2004). L'Hotte developed the rising trot to be used in outdoor activities such as cross-country and jumping, and he felt these activities were valuable for both horse and rider. He understood the necessity of using classical dressage for the preliminary schooling of the horse before outdoor activities were pursued.

Alois Podhajsky (1965/1967) was the head of the well known Spanish Riding School of Vienna. He spent his life with horses and learned from some of the most knowledgeable trainers of his day. The famous Spanish Riding School then and today follows the teachings of de la Guérinière because they have proven throughout the centuries to work most effectively.

Horse and Practitioner Relationship in Hippotherapy

Russell and Steele (2004) stated, "The horse is a herd animal that seeks a leader. To truly be a team, the horse must accept the trainer [practitioner] as the leader. The trainer [practitioner] builds this relationship through trust, kindness, friendship, and respect" (p. 13). Working directly with both horse and client seems to cement the therapeutic process, because the practitioner is in the horse's direct presence (beside the horse) and the movement of the client cannot be separated from that of the horse. An additional person cuing the horse might confuse it, although the instructor may be involved in a lesser capacity when needed.

Some practitioners may use instructors to work with the horse while the practitioner works with the client. This approach is used in line driving. For instance, my Halflinger horse loves her job. She has been a vaulting horse for 12 years. She knows each child's exercises, recognizes new vaulters, and shows a lot of tolerance when needed. She has endured much from beginners and those who lose their focus, but after so many years, she no longer allows vaulters to kick her on mounting and gives them a reminder warning kick to daunt them, never hurting them. She knows who mounts well and who may not, and she helps to stabilize them during movements on her back. She expects the longeur to know her job, which is to focus on her. If the longeur's attention is on the vaulters, the mare will not maintain her pace well; in other words, *if you don't do your job, I won't do mine.* During demonstrations, however, she performs her best regardless of errors. When younger children warm her up, she will be very patient and lunges well, giving the children great confidence. This mare also had been used for backriding a 2-year-old girl after a near-drowning accident. The mare was able to perceive when the child became tired and would stop moving a second or two before the therapist noted it. She no doubt felt the child's weight drop, which the therapist could not detect.

Many will well understand how much a horse can be a true partner if the handler treats it with respect, acknowledges its sensitivity and abilities, and gives it the training it needs to perform as requested. It is unfair to ask the horse to perform a task for which it has not been conditioned and trained.

Animal professionals, through observation and experiments, are learning more and more about the many abilities of animals, but there is much to learn and the horse's abilities to understand never should be underestimated. Seeing someone pull a horse around like an old wagon certainly is disheartening. In the 17th century literature of the French riding masters, they often say, "*ask the horse to . . . do not demand.*" Russell (2004) stated that in riding, "I often see flagrant misunderstanding between horse and rider. . . . Few trainers have carried the classical knowledge of lightness forward" (p. xii). The horse working with you during a hippotherapy session is the partner whom you ask to perform movements to stimulate the rider. You are the practitioner, he is your assistant, along with an instructor or volunteers; this is the therapy team.

Importance of Balance in the Rider

Hippotherapy during occupational therapy sessions can include numerous goals. Major areas to improve may include the client's symmetrical posture, motor control, and gross and fine coordination to perform desired occupations. The person may have deficits in her or his cognitive abilities, or there may be a need to increase the person's sensory processing and feedback system.

The client's balance with resulting adequate postural control is influenced by the task being performed, the environment, and the individual (Shumway-Cook & Woollacott, 2001). Every activity and its tasks require degrees of postural control; the more motor control one has in postural stability, the easier it is to perform a desired task. This major component of treatment helps occupational therapy practitioners when they help a person achieve occupational independence. Furthermore, Shumway-Cook and Woolacott stated that balance *is* postural stability: "the integration of sensory informa-

tion to assess the position and the motion of the body in space" (p. 165). Von Dietze (2005) stated that one can develop balance only through movement. Practitioners use the horse as a treatment strategy because it provides clients with a natural movement pattern with automatic stimulation rather than an artificial movement pattern, such as being rolled on a therapy ball.

A person is stable when his or her "center of mass is maintained over the base of support" (Shumway-Cook & Woolacott, 2001, p. 164). On a horse, a rider is stable when his or her center of gravity (mass) sits over the pelvis (base of support), which is over the center of gravity (mass) of the horse, allowing the rider to move with the horse and receive the therapeutic influence of the horse's motion. If the rider is sitting in front of the center of gravity (i.e., too far forward) or behind the center of gravity of the horse (i.e., too far back), the rider's position will hamper his or her ability to balance and move with the horse.

For hippotherapy clients dealing with balance or sensory issues, sitting with their center of gravity over the horse's center of gravity is a critical matter. It helps them develop postural stability and a feeling of balance. For an individual who tends to sit flexed forward or who has not inhibited the flexor reaction, such as a person with cerebral palsy, moving with the horse can facilitate a more normalized posture. Swift (2002) recommended that the practitioner help the client at the lower back and in front at the person's center of mass while sitting at the horse's center of gravity. Another approach, which might be an exception to the rule of moving with the horse, is having the person sit slightly behind the horse's movement, which would have the client lean backward until his or her movement reaction becomes more mobile. The method used depends on the client's reaction and therapy techniques.

For a client to develop balance through the horse's influence and use that balance to perform functional tasks effectively, the horse must display fluent movements and balance of its own, qualities that are developed through the principles of classical dressage. Both classical dressage and hippotherapy emphasize that the rider flows with the horse (Schusdziarra & Schusdziarra, 1978/1985). The Schusdziarras further stated that for the horse to move fluently, the rider must remain supple, a primary focal point for intervention. When a person sits at the center of his or her center of gravity and the horse's center of gravity, the movement of the horse will help this person gain an independent sitting posture with initial help from the therapist. The Schusdziarras stated that when riders move with the horse while sitting elastically and staying supple, the spine compensates for the swaying motion of the pelvis to maintain an upright posture.

If the horse is not moving in a balanced way or is moving with inconsistent rhythm or irregular gait or transitions, the client will receive undesirable movement input.

In addition to correcting irregularities in the horse through classical dressage, hippotherapy requires that the horse perform lateral movements like the shoulder-in, shortening and lengthening of strides, and changes of pace to accommodate the different needs of a variety of individuals in their quest for postural stability (Riede, 1998). These movements were developed as an essential part of classical dressage in basic training of the horse to develop the horse's muscles, suppleness, and balance.

Classical dressage theory states that "the two seat bones and the crotch serve as a base for the rider's seat—the full breadth of the seat rests with relaxed muscles on the horse's back. . . ." (Von Dietze, 2005, p. 35). Of course, we understand this for individuals who are trying to become good riders, but what does that have to do with hippotherapy? Balance is needed for all human functions. Balance reactions begin in infancy, and as the infant grows and gains control of his or her balance, functional movements can progress and more difficult tasks can be accomplished. A primary function in hippotherapy is to develop balance at the level an individual is able to function. Infants and small children might begin in a prone position and progress to quadruped, kneeling, and sitting positions on the horse. Balance in all four positions, as in basic vaulting exercises, is advisable for children because kneeling and crawling are useful in activities of daily living.

Some individuals could require adaptations or assistance in the beginning to maintain balance, but the practitioner always needs to work to gain the most normal balance posture as possible, because that is the foundation of all function and a requirement to maintain oneself on the horse. Colangelo (1999) suggested that the child should be given as much support as he or she needs to maintain a correct position to successfully perform a given task *but should not be given more assistance than absolutely needed.* Providing more assistance will deprive the child of developing balance and self-awareness because being held does not allow the body to flow with the horse's movement or find the equilibrium that leads to postural stability. Holding the legs tight

against the horse, as frequently seen in therapeutic activities with individuals with disabilities, does not allow the pelvis to fully flow with the horse's movement and also can hinder the horse's movement by the additional stimulation and erroneous cue.

Von Dietze (2005) stated that movement is life and "*movement* is the expression of the entire personality of an individual"; without movement, there is no balance. To maintain a feeling of security on a horse, suppleness and balance are primary functions, just as they are critical for all human tasks. Balance development begins in the first year of life as the infant begins to control his or her body in space (Case-Smith, 2005).

Von Dietze also felt that the inner self has a great influence on the quality of movement. For example, when people feel good, they are relaxed and show a mental balance with an erect posture. When they feel pressure, stress, chaos, or fear, they react automatically to protective reflexes and stiffness rather than with poise, control, and confidence. Developing a good feeling, therefore, is necessary for the individual when riding a horse.

Riding not only involves balance but teaches one to focus inward to what we feel inside: Where is our center (Swift, 2002)? Are we losing our balance or sitting on our right seat bone? Can we feel our seat bones? What are our limbs doing in space? Are our legs stretching downward or are they flexed? The horse's movement helps us become more aware of our body and helps us to control intrinsic movements and develop coordination, which then can be used while riding using the reins or for other occupations off the horse. Von Dietze (2005) stated that "the 'inner' person has a very decisive influence on the quality of movement," and Strauss (1995) wrote, "if the therapist is unaware of the singular characteristics of his [or her] therapy partner or does not take them into account, the patient will lose out on essential and therapy-enhancing components: not least the joy generated when during treatment on the horse, body, mind and soul are harmonize" (p. 13).

Rider Influence in the Horse

All horses live to move, for that is how they have learned to survive. Foals can run, jump, and gallop within hours of their birth. But as noted by Harris (1993), all horses do not move equally well. Some have great talent while others ramble along, or their movement is hampered because of conformation problems or lack of conditioning. The horse without a rider can perform all gaits in balance, but it must change its balance to accommodate the weight of the rider on its back (Swift, 2002). Harris (1993) mentioned that the horse frequently is asked to perform tasks nature never intended it to do, and that causes it to change its way of going. Not only is the horse asked to carry weight, but it is asked to carry dynamic weight with its own equilibrium and weight distribution (Strauss, 1995). Harris (1993) continued to say that the horse is not free to move as it wishes and may not understand why it should do what is asked by instructors, handlers, and riders who do not always speak *perfect horse language* (cues). The theory of classical dressage can help the horse, practitioner, and instructor learn correct cues and develop the natural way of going. When given correct cues, the horse does what is asked out of generosity and kindness. Practitioners, therefore, must respect the horse and work with it with kindness, caring about its nature, mechanics, and natural movements so that it is comfortable and works with ease and efficiency (Harris, 1993). A horse who shows discomfort, is confused, or shows tension cannot move freely, be supple, or have a balanced body; only when the horse is mentally and physically at ease can it give its best (Swift, 2002). It is an obligation to all that handle the horse to see that it has the best of care.

"Bad movement . . . is hard to ride and uncomfortable, and damaging to the horse" (Harris, 1993, p. 4). Harris further said that a horse cannot achieve its full potential without good movement. Bennett (1988) expressed that a horse should be matched with the required work by physicality, internal functions, heart rate, respiration rate, agility, and strength. Hippotherapy can be demanding for a horse, especially when riders have moderate to severe physical disabilities, poor muscle tone, or increased weight. Some horses are more suited for certain jobs or the way of going than others (Harris, 1993). *The quality of the movement of the horse and the rider's ability (infants to adults) to follow the horse's movement while maintaining postural stability and performing a given task is the heart of the therapy process.*

Classical dressage was developed through the centuries to work in this way, to understand the horse, its abilities and sensitivity, and to develop its agility and strength through the graded gymnastic movements to develop the best the horse has to offer. Classical dressage can be used as a means to improve the abilities of therapy horses as well as a means of better understanding the interaction and biomechanics of movement of the horse and rider.

Connection Between Horse and Rider

The walk of the horse has such great value because the horse's back transfers directly to the rider's body the normal walking pattern that is nearly identical in movement and reactions to human walking (von Dietze, 2005). While the horse walks, the rider is moved up–down, forward–backward, side–side, and rotationally, depending on the quality of the horse and the skills of the practitioner. "Per minute, a full-sized horse at the walk transfers about 110 such multidimensional swinging motions to the rider" (Strauss, 1995, p. 12). If the rider is sitting too far forward or backward, he or she will hinder the horse's movement, and therefore, the influence to the rider's posture will be hampered. The horse's balance becomes more demanding when it is not well balanced itself and carries a problematical rider.

Backriding is a therapeutic technique that is at times used in hippotherapy. It relates strongly to balance with the horse and client and therefore is included here. The goal of backriding is to use facilitation techniques and balance support while the client is being stimulated by the movement of the horse, such as providing head and neck facilitation and balance or inhibiting reflex activity, as in the Bobath technique. The technique requires the practitioner to mount the horse who wears a bareback pad. A client is positioned in front of the practitioner. Sidewalkers are on each side of the horse and pair as safety provides, and a horse handler leads the horse. In this situation, the client sits *before* the motion of the horse and the practitioner sits *behind* the movement of the horse, hindering the horse's movement. Neither the client nor the practitioner, however, is sitting in a stable and secure position because they are not in the center of gravity of the horse. One tends to be moved forward (before the horse's motion) while the other tends backward (behind the horse's motion). Furthermore, the practitioner is sitting on the weakest part of the horse's spine. This practice requires a special horse that is very strong with a short back, exceptionally well conditioned to withstand this procedure without breaking down, and well trained to tolerate this unusual situation.

For the client to move with the horse's motion, the practitioner must move even further back, a risky position, requiring yet another exception—a very well-trained rider with excellent balance. The client must also be a small child who will not unseat the practitioner when he or she makes sudden unbalanced movements. If the sidewalkers hold the child's legs too tight next to the horse to provide extra stability, not only does that interfere with the stimulation given by the practitioner, but it also interferes with the stimulation to the horse. It is a technique that should only be used by hippotherapy practitioners with years of experience in hippotherapy and in neurodevelopment, who are able to question closely the whole situation and understand its value and risks.

Interaction Between Horse and Rider

Systematic schooling in classical dressage teaches the horse how to respond to instant changes in movement, directions, and tempo as requested by the practitioner and instructor, which becomes important when a rider who has a tendency to lean or wobble to regain his or her balance. Strauss (1995) stated that the horse must be given definitive cues by the practitioner or instructor that it must respond to immediately so that balance is not disrupted and the therapy goals can be accomplished. Prodding or pulling the horse by handlers disturbs the movement of the horse, causing faulty balance, and is a disrespectful method of communication. Defective balance in the horse will cause faulty carriage, resulting in poor rhythm and impulsion. This disruption will cause inaccurate sensory input, resulting in faulty movement patterns and balance that then are transmitted to the rider astride the horse (Strauss, 1995; von Dietze, 2005). Additionally, Spink (1993) felt that the horse needs to be attentive, mannerly, and respectful. Simply leading a horse untrained in advanced skills around the arena with a rider astride does not provide that rider with the therapeutic input required for occupational therapy intervention.

In hippotherapy, the horse also must be trained to tolerate certain involuntary movements. Swift (2002) stated that the horse will reflect the posture of the rider, so if the rider is asymmetrical the horse will be asymmetrical. Swift has the rider focus on their body posture for corrections. Von Dietze (2005) stated that a "horse who was stiff on the left side was carrying a student who had stiff, shortened muscles on the left side but conversely, a horse that is stiff on one side can give a rider a sore shoulder when he or she gets off" (p. 210). One must note that the horse and the rider can block each other's movements because the seat of the rider has a close connection to the action of the horse (von Dietze, 2005). Having a skilled rider work with the horse to correct any problems that have occurred because of the client rider's physical disability will help all therapy horses, because von Dietze (2005) felt that most of the horse's problems are transmitted from the rider to the horse.

It is important to develop "feel" in your clients, for this not only will help them respond better to the horse but also learn about their own bodies. The rider's communication with the horse is through the tactile senses, weight aids, pressure aids, vocal aids, and psychological aids, which all riders regardless of age or functional ability will give in some way, "based on the creature's acute perception for things metaphysical: the influence initiated through the rider's thoughts and intentions, colored by personality, mood or emotions, all of which the horses pick up either externally or through sensing the slightest changes that thought power reflects in the rider's body" (Herbermann, 1984, p. 40). Sometimes the horse seems to respond to intentions rather than actions (Herbermann, 1984). Herbermann further wrote that when practitioners lack purpose, they can annoy the horse or, worse, dull it because it does not understand its purpose. This problem can occur when helpers or others are not well trained and have no true connection with the horse and rider.

The Therapy Horse

The quality of the horse is as important as the skill of the therapist and the quality of therapy equipment. What does the practitioner look for when selecting a horse for his or her therapy program? The horse must be cooperative—willing and able to perform prime quality movements with correct rhythm, impulsion, and balance to provide the needed input to the client as requested by the instructor or practitioner. A lame horse, one that is easily distracted or poorly conditioned, or one that will not follow the handler independently will not move with ease and will give inconsistent or disruptive input to the client.

The type of stimulation needed will vary for different people. Therefore, the practitioner needs to have an understanding not only of the horse but also of the child or adult so an appropriate match can be made between horse and rider. For instance, a small child will conform to the movement of a small horse better than to one that is 15 hands or more tall because of stride length and rhythm. Some children need a lot of stimulation and, thus, a horse that will provide them a fast walk or nicely controlled trot. Other children with hyper reaction to stimulation will need a horse with a smooth and rhythmic gait. An adult who is hyper-reactive may not tolerate a horse with a quick, choppy gait, but an adult who is lethargic may need a horse with more spirit to awaken the client's nervous system. Everyone has different needs, goals, and characteristics. The practitioner's responsibility is to match the needs of the client with what a horse has to offer, as well as the task involved. It is somewhat like matching a child receiving sensory integration to the appropriate context.

The horse's stride and rhythm will accommodate the person's movement pattern so that they are in harmony with each other and so the horse can provide the optimal movement stimulation quality to the client (Strauss, 1995). The stride of an average adult equals the stride of a 16-hand horse (Riede, 1998), and this horse would be appropriate for an average adult who needs to regain balance and symmetry through the horse's movement pattern. Beyond the stride length, the degree of sensory stimulation transmitted to the client and the base of support that the horse provides must be taken into account. Mitchell (1997) gave an example of a small horse provided for a 5-year-old boy that would seem appropriate by most standards. The horse was small to compensate for a child who had a fear of heights, and it provided a narrow base of support for a small child to sit astride. A 12-minute ride on this horse, however, resulted in a child who was disorganized and lost his base of support. The following session, he was give a larger horse that provided him with a wide base of support and a movement pattern and organization to which he could adapt. The boy was able to find his own strategy for stability and security.

Characteristics of a Therapy Horse

Because practitioners rarely have a stable full of horses from which to choose, they need to have the skills to adapt a horse to the needs and tasks of several of their clients. That can be achieved by a horse well trained by the systematic steps of classical dressage training principles. The degree of training also will depend on the population with whom the practitioner is working and their needs. Riede (1998) felt that the therapy horse's training needs to be at the basic first or second level of dressage training. These levels of training strive to create a horse with the following characteristics: friendly, submissive, obedient, rhythmic movements, even tempo, smooth transitions, seeks the bit, relaxed forward movement, able to yield to lateral aids, balanced, straight, supple, developed push from the hindquarters, and finally, with weight on the hindquarters and collection. Both Heipertz (1981) and Riede (1998) felt that a therapy horse should have trusting, reliable, and tolerant nature that can accept peculiar behaviors; biomechanics that demonstrate

impulsion, soft active gait, and a comfortable back; and enjoyment of its work.

Strauss (1995) pointed out that while the value of the horse's movement is hippotherapy's primary contribution to therapy, also of great value are remedial education, psychological factors, and sensory motor functions transmitted to the client. The movement of the horse increases activity of the voluntary motor-loop and additional flow of impulses to the tactile, proprioceptive, and vestibular systems through the periphery (Riede, 1998).

Heipertz (1981) stated that while horses are naturally well suited to be used in therapy, they do have natural instincts for flight reactions and may not attend well, have been badly trained, or have developed poor habits. Some horses, therefore, may not be suitable for this type of work.

Sensory Therapy on Horseback

Ayres (1985) described major developmental points that contribute to integration of movement, posture, and function. These points develop from birth to about age 7 in the average child. Through hippotherapy, the horse can assist in stimulating and strengthening weak areas of development that may cause the infant and later the child movement and behavioral problems. Ayres wrote that skills and sensation occur in set steps; if one step is poorly developed, the following steps may be hindered in future integration. At birth the infant can see, hear, and has a sense of self, but these senses are not organized for functional use. The fetus begins to develop touch in the uterus, which is basic to all functions, such as movement (Ayres, 1985).

On the horse, the infant comes in contact with the saddle pad, the mane, coat, and the tail of the horse— rich tactile sources. Touch, vestibular stimulation, gravity reactions, and the movement of the horse provoke integration of movement development in the infant or child. Ayres, as cited in Kimball (1999), stated, "the ability to move against gravity . . . indicates a well-organized nervous system" (p. 127). Gravity input on the horse is a strong therapeutic factor. The vestibular system has a controlling influence on equilibrium and balance that is responsible for the ability to maintain posture (Kimball, 1999). This integration must occur to advance motor function (Ayres, 1985). The horse provides a gentle rocking movement to stimulate vestibular reactions; at the same time, anti-gravity reactions stimulate proprioception of the joints. Moving the horse in different directions, stopping, and starting, causes the infant to make adaptive responses to develop and maintain balance in whichever developmental position they are ready to challenge. Careful monitoring will be necessary to keep the client safe, though one must not intervene in the infant's attempt to maintain or regain his or her balance. Moving the infant or child into a position for which they are not ready would increase his or her instability. For instance, if the movement of the horse is too challenging for the child to control the sitting posture, he or she should be in the presitting stage while on the horse. As Ayres stated previously, if one step is poorly developed, the following steps may be hindered. The selection of a horse that is aware of the infant's ability to balance and able to work to help would be ideal.

Summary

Centered Riding founder Sally Swift depends on the purity of the classical principles in the way she expresses her teachings to reeducate the mind and body for maximum harmony between horse and rider, and to develop greater balance and integration (Swift, 2002). No mystery surrounds the dressage training method, which has been developed through the centuries. It is a systematic training method of natural gymnastic exercises to develop the natural qualities and strength of a horse, whereby it can perform with smoothness in gaits and transitions as requested without injury.

Dressage theory dictates the process of training or retraining a horse. Most horses that occupational therapists use in their practice will have had early training by other individuals. The therapist must obtain as much information about a horse as he or she can, especially regarding the horse's training, the work it has done, and any injuries it experienced. A veterinarian check should be performed, and the horse should be evaluated for conformation, ease of handling, temperament, and rhythm and gait.

Because practitioners work with children and adults with functional and behavioral problems, they need a horse who can be a true cooperative partner in the therapy session, not one who must require special attention to move in the desired way, to focus and not be distracted, or be in tune with its rider. If the rider loses his or her balance, the horse needs to react immediately for the sake of its own and its rider's balance, especially when working with a small child even when the therapist and helpers are assisting.

Classical dressage develops and trains the horse in a way harmonious to the horse's nature and can be fine-tuned to the extent that the horse understands its job and has the ability to be the true therapy partner—the therapy horse. I have experienced numerous situations where the horse has taken its job seriously with great dedication to its rider, both in therapy sessions and vaulting, using its excellent memory uncannily. To allow the horse to be responsible and to give it great praise for his efforts is important; do not treat the horse as something to be pulled around, as a nonentity, or with disrespect. All great masters of equestrian art and those who have fought in battle, whose lives have depended on their horses, understand the unique understanding a horse possesses and the dedication they give to their job and their masters. Horses truly are amazing creatures and a gift to us as helpers in hippotherapy and equine-assisted occupational therapy.

References

Ayres, A. J. (1985). *Sensory integration and the child.* Los Angeles: Western Psychological Services.

Baptiste, S. E. (2003). Client-centered practice: Implications for our professional approach, behavior, and lexicon. In P. Kramer, J., Hinojosa, & C. B. Royeen (Eds.), *Perspectives in human occupation: Participation in life.* Philadelphia: Lippincott Williams & Wilkins.

Baucher, F. (1992). *François Baucher: The man and his methods* (H. Nelson, Trans). London: A. J. Allen. (Original work published 1835)

Bennett, D. (1988). *Principles of conformation analysis* (Vol. 1). Gaithersburg, MD: Fleet Street.

Case-Smith, J. (2005). *Occupational therapy for children* (5th ed.). St. Louis: Elsevier Mosby.

Cavendish, W. (2000). *A general system of horsemanship.* North Pomfret, VT: Trafalgar Square. (Original work published 1743)

Concise Oxford Dictionary. (1995). New York: Oxford University Press.

Colangelo, C. A. (1999). Biomechanical frame of reference. In P. Kramer & J. Hinojosa (Eds.), *Frames of reference for pediatric occupational therapy* (2nd ed.). Baltimore: Lippincott Williams & Wilkins.

de Kunffy, C. (1984). *Creative horsemanship.* New York: Arco.

de Kunffy, C. (2002). *Dressage principles illuminated.* North Pomfret, VT: Trafalgar Square.

de la Guérinière, F. R. (1994). *School of horsemanship.* (T. Boucher, Trans.). London: J. A. Allen. (Original work published 1733)

De Pluvinel, A. (1989). *The maneige royal.* (H. Nelson, Trans.). London: J. A. Allen. (Original work published 1626)

Harris, S. (1993). *Horse gaits, balance and movement: The natural mechanics of movement common to all breeds.* New York: Howell Book House.

Heipertz, W. (1981). *Therapeutic riding: Medicine, education, sports.* (M. Takeuchi, Trans.). Ottawa: Breenbelt Riding Association for the Disabled. (Original work published 1977)

Henriquet, M. (2004). *Henriquet on dressage.* (H. Nelson, Trans.). North Pomfret, VT: Trafalgar Square. (Original work published 1991)

Herbermann, E. F. (1984). *The dressage formula.* London: A. J. Allen.

Kimball, J. G. (1999). Sensory integration frame of reference: Theoretical base, function/dysfunction continua, and guide to evaluation. In P. Kramer & J. Hinojosa (Eds.), *Frames of reference for pediatric occupational therapy* (2nd ed.). Baltimore: Lippincott Williams & Wilkins.

Knopfhart, A. (1990). *Fundamentals of dressage* (N. Bartle, Trans.). London: J. A. Allen. (Original work published 1979)

L'Hotte, A. F. (1997). *Alexis-François L'Hotte: The quest for lightness in equitation.* (H. Nelson, Trans.). North Pomfret, VT: Trafalgar Square. (Original work published 1906)

Mitchell, L. (1997). *Therapeutic riding strategies for rehabilitation.* Durango, CO: Barbara Engel Therapy Services.

Oliveira, N. (1988). *Reflection on equestrian art* (2nd ed., P. Field, Trans.). London: A. J. Allen. (Original work published 1964)

Podhajsky, A. (1967). *The complete training of horse and rider: In the principles of classic horsemanship* (E. Podhajsky & V. D. S. Williams, Trans.). Garden City, NY: Doubleday. (Original work published 1965)

Riede, D. (1998) *Physiotherapy on the horse.* (A. C. Dusenbury, Trans.). Riderwood, MD: Therapeutic Riding SVC. (Original work published 1986)

Russell, M., & Steele, W. (2004). *Lessons in lightness: The art of educating the horse.* Guilford, CT: Lyons Press.

Schusdziarra, H., & Schusdziarra, V. (1985). *An anatomy of riding* (S. Newkirk, Trans.). New York: Breakthrough. (Original work published 1978)

Shumway-Cook, A., & Woollacott, M. H. (2001). *Motor control, theory, and practical application* (2nd ed.). Baltimore: Lippincott Williams & Wilkins.

Spink, J. (1993). *Developmental riding therapy: A team approach to assessment and treatment.* Tucson, AZ: Therapy Skill Builders.

Steinbrecht, G. (1995). *The gymnasium of the horse* (P. Plinzner, Ed., H. K. Gibble, Trans.). Cleveland Heights, OH: Xenophon. (Original work published 1935)

Strauss, I. (1995). *Hippotherapy: Neurophysiological therapy on the horse* (Hippotherapie, Trans.). Ontario: Therapeutic Riding Association. (Original work published 1991)

Swift, S. (2002). *Centered riding 2: Further exploration.* North Pomfret, VT: Trafalgar Square.

Von Dietze, S. (2005). *Balance in movement: How to achieve the perfect seat.* North Pomfret, VT: Trafalgar Square.

Xenophon. (1962). *The art of horsemanship* (M. H. Morgan, Trans.). London: J. A. Allen. (Original work published 430 B.C.)

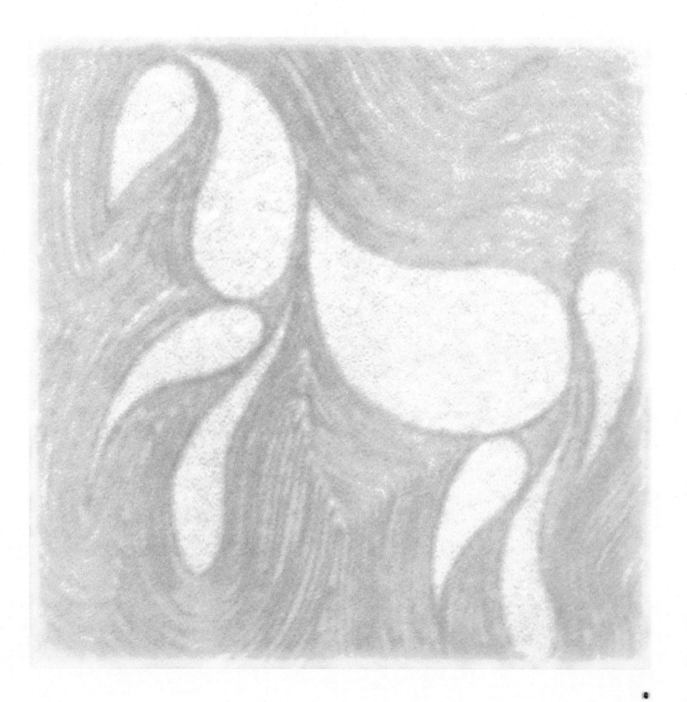

PART II
Research

The sunshine's golden gleam is thrown,
On sorrel, chestnut, bay, and roan;
The horses paw and prance and neigh,
Fillies and colts like kittens play,
And dance and toss their rippled manes,
Shining and soft as silken skeins....
—Oliver Wendell Holmes

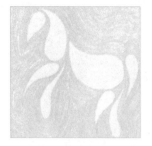

The Horse. Here is nobility without conceit,
Friendship without envy, Beauty without vanity.
A willing servant, yet no slave.
  —Ronald Duncan

CHAPTER 7

A Chronological and Historical Review of Research Related to Hippotherapy

Sandra L. Hubbard, PhD, OTR/L, ATP

Hippotherapy can be defined as neurophysiologically based treatment with the help of the horse. The term comes from *hippos,* the Greek word for horse (Heine, 1997; Heipertz, 1981; Strauss, 1998). Classic hippotherapy has been practiced in Europe since the 1960s, as a method of treating people with cerebral palsy and other neuromuscular impairments. The primary focus of hippotherapy is to use the rhythmic movement of the horse to habilitate and rehabilitate the rider's posture and response control over movement (Heine, 1997). "Movement can only be learned and corrected through movement" (Strauss, 1998, p. 15). Finely tuned trunk coordination only can be developed while walking. Trunk coordination of individuals develops primarily as they learn how to walk and secondarily as a result of atypical gait patterns. According to Strauss, hippotherapy can break this cycle: The rhythmical and three-dimensional movement of the horse facilitates postural corrections that the rider may not be able to achieve on his or her own.

At the Third International Conference on Riding for the Disabled in Poland, Baumann (1974) differentiated the term "hippotherapy," wherein the patient is not asked to guide the horse, from "therapeutic riding," in which horseback riding is used for pedagogical and psychological aims. In a book originally published in German in 1977 and translated to English in 1981, Heipertz (1981) described hippotherapy as "a mainly passive form of therapeutic riding whereby the patient sits on the horse and accommodates himself to the swinging movements of the horse's back" (p. 14). Riede (1988) described hippotherapy as "prescribed and supervised by a physician. . . . the treatment goal is the patient's active and passive adaptation to the undulation of the

horse's back. . . . the patient is therapeutically manipulated by the three-dimensional undulations of the horse's back" (pp. 47–48).

Therapeutic riding is an umbrella term used to denote use of the horse in medicine (hippotherapy) and psychiatry (Riede, 1988). Riede elaborated on the definition of hippotherapy by describing it as a new era in "kinesitherapy" that expands on joint mobilization and muscle strengthening to include modification of sensory feedback (i.e., via the horse). Riede also noted that hippotherapy addresses other unmet needs of people with musculoskeletal disorders: the desire yet decreased ability to move and a need for interesting motor tasks.

This chapter presents research relevant to occupational therapists who practice hippotherapy. To accomplish this task, the chapter presents studies involving hippotherapy as well as those involving therapeutic riding. Because the focus is on research relevant to occupational therapists who practice hippotherapy, studies providing intervention for physical impairment are emphasized. (For example, a study with a sample of people with mental retardation that measured endurance, cardiac function, and oxygen saturation would be included; a study with the same population that focused strictly on behavioral outcomes would not.) The studies presented are not limited to hippotherapy intervention per se because of the inconsistency in use of the terms *hippotherapy, therapeutic riding,* and other various terms. In addition, studies are not restricted on the basis of level of evidence or quality of research design; doing so would have been problematic with older or translated articles and would have ignored potentially good research ideas. In sum, the purpose of this chapter is to describe the wealth of ideas and pilot data that can be gleaned from past research that in turn can be incorporated into future research using current and advanced measurement technology and research design (Table 7.1).

To locate the studies, Medline, PubMed, and Cumulative Index to Nursing & Allied Health Literature (CINAHL) databases using the keywords *hippotherapy, equine, therapeutic riding,* and *horse therapy* were used to search for relevant research literature. Three books on hippotherapy, along with North American Riding for the Handicapped Association and International Therapeutic Riding Congress Conference Proceedings not indexed by the databases, also were included.

Studies Before the 1990s

The medicinal benefits of riding can be traced back to Xenophon and Hippocrates. Chassaigne, in 1870, was perhaps the first to relate riding to improved posture, balance, and muscle control (Bertoti, 1988; Chassaigne, 1870). Therapy riding was recognized in 1951 when Lis Hartel, a Danish riding teacher and an equestrian Olympian with polio, met and established the "Pony-Stable for Disabled Children" in 1953 (Boysen, 1991). Treatment at the Pony-Stable was recommended by physicians and, in 1964, its services became reimbursable by Norwegian health insurance. Also in 1953, the International Polio Fellowship in England began promoting therapeutic horseback riding (Bain, 1965). The First International Congress for Rehabilitation Through Riding convened in 1974 to discuss rehabilitation for people with physical disabilities and mental retardation.

In 1986, Riede published his synthesis of early hippotherapy and therapeutic riding literature in German. The book was translated to English in 1988 (Riede, 1988) and titled *Physiotherapy on the Horse.* Because most of the literature cited in Riede's book is not available in English, this chapter relies on the secondary, translated source. Riede noted that the first German publication on the therapeutic use of the horse was *Gymnastics on the Horse, A Road to Recovery* (Druschky, 1961, cited in Riede, 1988).

Riede (1988) described the effects of hippotherapy as follows:

- Simulation of the human gait through the movement of the horse's back
- Psychological effect of a living exercise apparatus
- Primary atavistic (hard-wired) need to control difficult movements
- Uncontested special relationship between horse and man.

Riede believed that hippotherapy could be used to address the kinesitherapy goal of *coordination training,* defined by Janda (1980, cited in Riede, 1988) as the "treatment of central nervous movement dysfunctions. . . . The three-dimensional undulations of the horse's back are the therapeutic tools promoting stability, normalization of muscle tone, and equilibrium training." Riede described hippotherapy as a medical treatment modality for people with disabilities that is separate from therapeutic riding in psychiatry and riding as a recreational sport, under the direction of a riding teacher. According to Riede (1988), the three-dimensional movement of the horse's back was first described by Quellmalz in 1735. In 1978, both Reisser and Mayberry (cited in Riede) described the relationship between the horse and human gaits; Reisser suggested that the gait of larger horses more closely resembled the human gait.

Mayberry (1978, cited in Riede, 1988) described hippotherapy as unique because it is the only treatment method that provides normal three-dimensional input to the client's pelvis. Mayberry made an important point when he noted that "the gait variations among different horses can be used according to varying therapeutic purposes" (Riede, 1988).

Baumann (1979, cited in Riede, 1988) stated that "the three-dimensional movement of the horse's walk simulates the human gait." Kunzle added that "at the walk, the horse transfers the same movement pattern on to the patient's trunk that two normally functioning legs would create during walking" (as cited in Riede, 1988). The implication is that people unable to walk may experience the sensation of walking by riding a horse because the movement imparted to the rider by the horse at a walk is similar. Gregersen and Lucas (1967, cited in Riede, 1988) performed perhaps the first analysis of the rotation of the human spine when walking. Gottwald (1980, cited in Riede, 1988) achieved similar results as Gregersen and Lucas when he examined the pelvic and lumbar movements of the horse and compared the movement of the horse with the shoulder and pelvic movement of the patient.

In addition to functional effects, physiological effects of hippotherapy have been documented. Findeisen (1974, cited in Riede, 1988) showed that "the straight posture and rhythmic movement during riding facilitate breathing and a beneficial effect on the digestive system." Von Bausenwein (1979, cited in Riede, 1988) suggested that the body warmth of horses, which is 1° warmer than that of humans, promotes muscular relaxation. Note that in his book, Riede (1988) did not

Table 7.1. Intervention Outcome Studies

Author (Date)	N	Intervention	Outcome Measure	Population or Purpose
Findeisen (1974)		Posture, rhythm	Digestive, respiratory systems	Scoliosis
Von Bausenwein (1979)		Horse body temp–rider relaxation relationship		Cerebral palsy (CP)
Gottwald (1981)		Movement of horse ↓	Trunk strength, spinal fixation	Kyphosis
Lindenmann & Mau (1958)			Posture	Scoliosis
Gunther (1968)			To establish limits for safe vibration	
Junghanns (1979)			Spinal movement of rider in mm	Establish safety
Tauffkirchen (1978)	27		Postural tone, equilibrium reactions	Cerebral palsy
Muller (1979)	11	Movement of horse vs. Bobath roll	Lower extremity (LE) spasticity, trunk control (electromyography [EMG])	Cerebral palsy
Meier (1976)		Movement of horse ↓	Coordination, back extensors (EMG)	Cerebral palsy ↓
Raus (1973)			LE spasticity	
Brauer (1971)			Coordination, range of motion (ROM), spasticity	
Hardt (1980)	9		Gait, spasticity (treadmill–videotape)	
Roll (1980)	13		Photometry (photographic images)	
Fox et al. (1984)	19		Balance, coordination, strength, spinal straightness	Cerebral palsy, Spina bifida, learning disabilities, mental retardation ↓
Riede (1988)	291		Movement analysis, muscle testing	Cerebral palsy ↓
Von Bausenwein (1983)	1		Weight distribution: two scales	
Toffola et al. (1988)			Posturographic test, O$_2$ consumption, postural control (EMG)	
Armstrong et al. (1988)	47		Balance, spine mobility, behavior, affect	Mental retardation, Down syndrome
Snir et al. (1988)	4		Strength, gait	Cerebral palsy, minimal brain dysfunction
Brock (1988)	24		Strength, coordination	Traumatic brain injury (TBI), Cerebral palsy, arthritis, visual impairment, epilepsy
MacKinnon et al. (1995)	19		GMFM, posture, activities of daily living, psychosocial behavior	Cerebral palsy
Biery and Kauffman (1989)	8		Balance	Mental retardation
Bertoti (1988)	11		Posture	Cerebral palsy
MacKay-Lyons et al. (1988)	10		Posture, gait, psychological well-being	Multiple sclerosis

(continued)

Table 7.1. Intervention Outcome Studies (*Continued*)

Author (Date)	N	Intervention	Outcome Measure	Population or Purpose
Ricotti et al. (1991)		Movement of horse	Strength (EMG)	Cerebral palsy
Baker (1991)	54		Degree of kyphosis	Kyphosis
Pfofenhauer (1991)	54		Trunk movement	Multiple sclerosis
Selvinen (1997)	6		Gait (video and Ashworth scale)	Multiple sclerosis
Exner et al. (1994)	67		Spasticity, pain sleep, bowel function	Spinal cord injury
Veicsteinas (1994)	36		O_2 consumption, pulmonary ventilation, heart rate	Mental retardation, motor impairment
Weber (1994)	19		Spasticity, gait	Multiple sclerosis
Biery and Kauffman (1996)	8		Balance	Mental retardation
Would (1996)			Pelvic mobility (electronic goniometer)	Cerebral palsy
Kulichova and Zeklova (1996)	13		Vertebrographic measurement	Scoliosis, scoliosis due to Cerebral palsy
Tolson (1997)	2		Echolalia, self-directed behavior	Autism
Stykes et al. (1997)	4		Balance	TBI
Hansen (1997)	5		Gross Motor Function Measure (GMFM; Russell, Rosenbaum, Cadman, Gowland, Hardy, & Jarvis, 1989)	Cerebral palsy
Fox and Peterson (1997)	4		GMFM scores, ROM	
Wasserman (1997)	1		Pediatric Evaluation of Disability Index (PEDI; Haley, Coster, Ludlow, Haltwanger, & Andrellos, 1992) scores	
Wheeler (1997)	1		LE strength	Spina bifida
Cook (1997)	1		ROM	TBI
Sachkov (1997)	93		Electroencephalogram (EEG), pulse, O_2, cardiac activity	Physical, mental disorders
McGibbon et al. (1998)	5		Walking, GMFM scores	Cerebral palsy
Sportwiss et al. (1997)	21		Motor skill, coordination, tone	
MacPhail et al. (1996)	6		Trunk movement, equilibrium	
Haehl et al. (1999)	2		Posture coordination, control, PEDI scores	
Ionatamishvili et al. (2001)	10	Movement of horse vs. Bobath	Muscle tone, memory	Cerebral palsy
Tsverava et al. (2000)	232	Movement of horse	Spine-clinical, X-ray	Spine diseases
Mattila-Rautiainen et al. (2000)	4		Spine mobility, EMG, quality of life, depression	Low back pain
Sahraoui (2000)	29		Posture, equilibrium	Cerebral palsy, diplegia

Table 7.1. Intervention Outcome Studies (*Continued*)

Author (Date)	N	Intervention	Outcome Measure	Population or Purpose
Land et al. (2001)	3	Movement of horse	Sitting posture	Central nervous system, muscle tone disorder
Pasquinelli (2000, 2001)	10		Tone, strength	Dystonia, athetosis
Winchester et al. (2002)	7		GMFM, gait speed	Cerebral palsy, TBI, spina bifida, autism, Down syndrome
Ionatamishvilli (2002)	100		Acquisition of new motor skill, tone	Cerebral palsy
Sterna et al. (2002)	17		WeeFIM (Braun, Msall, & Granger, 1991), GMFM	
Benda et al. (2003)	15		EEG	
Watakabe et al. (2003)	17		Hip adduction contractures	
Lechner et al. (2003)	32		Spasticity	SCI, quadriplegia
Bourgard & Roblin (2003)	16		Balance	TBI, SCI, stroke
Chandler (2003)	12		Canadian Occupational Performance Measure (COPM)	Sensory modulation disorder
Pasquinelli (2004)	4		Strength, motor control, balance, tone	Extrapyramidal disorders, progressive and nonprogressive
Ionatamishvilli et al. (2004)	100			Cerebral palsy

go into detail as to how these effects were measured or the significance of the results.

According to Lippold von Horde and colleagues (1977, cited in Riede, 1988), the "living exercise apparatus demands and maintains concentration and attention" (p. 43). Hippotherapy can be motivational for patients who have become tired of and averse to conventional therapies. Feldcamp (1979, cited in Riede, 1988) wrote that "the air and flair associated with riding is more therapeutic than the riding process" (p. 44). Israel (1984, cited in Riede, 1988) noted the euphoria that can follow physical stress and the liberating and re-energizing effects of sports and physical exercise.

Studies Documenting Three-Dimensional Movement of the Horse

Riede (1988) conducted a study to (1) document and analyze the three-dimensional movement of the horse; (2) measure the forward acceleration and vibration of the horse at the walk, trot, and canter in relation to the strain placed on the human spinal column; (3) document changes in the spinal column length during a rising trot with potential influence on intervertebral disk metabolism; and (4) analyze relationships between acceleration and frequency and horse's height, age, trunk length, sex, and breed. Riede's study was the first to graphically demonstrate the effect of the three-dimensional movement of the horse against the three axes of movement of the rider: up–down, forward–backward, and side-to-side.

Sensors were attached to the saddle of the horse and to the rider (at the sacrum and C7/T1) to measure frequency and acceleration movements of the horse and rider. The measurements were electronically plotted. This information served as a baseline from which to compare horses by age, sex, and height to scientifically substantiate Heipertz (1977, cited in Riede, 1988), who expressed a preference for "rectangular" horses (barrel length greater than height) over "square" horses. The results did not substantiate that rectangular horses were superior to square horses; in fact, the geometry of the horse had no bearing on acceleration or frequency. A minor statistically significant relationship was found between acceleration and the up–down movement of the rider: At the walk, vertical acceleration decreases with the age of the horse. Cold-blood (draft) horses demonstrated increased up–down acceleration compared with warm-blood (recreational) horses, and ponies demonstrated an increased frequency, leading Riede to conclude that only warm bloods were suitable for hippotherapy. Another conclusion was that, although the three-dimensional movement of the horse's movement at the walk simulated human gait at the walk, the horse's trot does not simulate human running.

The International Organization for Standardization (ISO) has established limits for safe vibration upon the spine. Riede (1988) used piezoelectric sensors attached to the saddle to measure the acceleration impulses of the horses (13 warm bloods, 1 cold blood, and 1 pony) to ensure that the vibration to the rider's spine did not exceed the ISO limit. The results indicated that even prolonged exposure to horse acceleration could not damage the rider's spine at the walk, trot, or canter. Studies by Junghanns (1979, cited in Riede, 1988) and Gunther (1968, cited in Riede, 1988) have shown that, while vibration can activate the back musculature, excessive vibration can lead to deceased performance due to fatigue. Consequently, just because the effects of hippotherapy are positive, longer periods of hippotherapy are not necessarily better.

The measurements of the elongation from C7 to S1 taken during the trot showed a variation of 15.7 mm at the sitting trot and 15 mm at the rising trot. This alternating compression and decompression of the intervertebral space at the rising trot suggested that this pumping mechanism could influence the pressure-dependent exchange of fluids in the intervertebral spaces described by Kramer (1978, cited in Riede, 1988).

Research studies comparing the movement of the horse to human gait provided the theories for therapeutic riding and hippotherapy. Subsequentially, European researchers began to apply this theory to document the benefits of this intervention.

Freeman, Wise, Nicodemus, and Osborn (1997) used kinematic motion analysis to quantify and compare the pelvic movement of four horses (a 14.3-hand quarterhorse mare, a 15.3-hand thoroughbred gelding, a 14.1 hand Welsh/quarterhorse cross, and a 17.3-hand Belgium gelding) during hippotherapy when led and long-reined. The investigators found little within-horse difference in pelvic movement when the horses were led versus long-lined; there was a trend of less pelvic movement during long-reining, although the difference was not significant. Because the differences were not significant, the authors concluded that the horse handler should use the method (leading or long-reining) during which the horse was best behaved. Freeman and colleagues also pointed out that the horse should be selected according to the goal of the therapy session. For example, if the goal is to improve lateral trunk lengthening, the Welsh/quarterhorse cross would be the best choice because it demonstrated larger movements than the other horses. Large movement, however, may not be indicated for all therapy sessions (e.g., a client with poor sitting balance and poor head control may benefit more from a horse with shorter and smooth movements).

In their discussion, Freeman and colleagues (1997) compared the horse pelvic-movement values obtained in their study with known pelvic-movement values of humans when walking. They noted 4° of anterior–posterior tilt in the human walk; the mean anterior–posterior tilt of the four horses examined was 3.92° when led and 3.76° when driven. In the human walk, 7° of trunk lengthening occurred; mean trunk lengthening of the horses was 9.08° when led and 7.0° when driven. Finally, the human gait had 10° of anterior–posterior rotation; mean anterior–posterior rotation of the horses was 6.86° when led and 6.16° when driven. One limitation of this discussion is that the nature and source of the human pelvic movement values were not disclosed. Although horse and human pelvic-movement values are comparable, when selecting a horse for a rider with a disability, the therapist should remember that the rider may not be capable of pelvic movement achieved by the average able-bodied rider.

Fleck (1997) compared the pelvic movement in the human walking and horseback riding using the parameters of vertical displacement of center of gravity, lateral pelvic shift, lateral pelvic tilt, and temporal assessment of stride and heart rate. Study participants were 24 able-bodied adolescents grouped according to riding experience. One horse, a 23-year-old Appaloosa mare, was used for all motion analysis data collection. Fleck found significant differences in the vertical displacement of the center of gravity (walking mean = 4.66 cm; riding mean = 3.22 cm), lateral pelvic shift (walking mean = 3.13 cm; riding mean = 5.60 cm), and heart rate (walking mean = 130.66 bpm; riding mean = 105.47 bpm). No significant difference was found in lateral pelvic tilt in walking and riding, and no significant differences were found for experienced and inexperienced riders.

In comparison, Baumann (1974) used film analysis to compare human pelvic movement when walking and riding. Baumann found vertical and lateral displacement of the center of gravity walking and riding equal at 5 cm. Baumann found greater pelvic rotation in riding (8 cm) than in walking (5 cm). While similar to the results obtained by Fleck, variation was noted. Future studies could include a larger number of humans and horses to account for within-subject variation.

Harris, Pulliam, Coffman, Rehkop, and Schroader (1997) used motion analysis to compare trunk kinematics and postural response of 10 able-bodied riders using Grizzle's test for crossover design, *t* tests, and Pearson correlation. The results indicated that walking and riding at the walk exhibit similar trunk movement, according to electromyography [EMG] and muscle activation. The rectus abdominus was significantly more active per stride when participants were riding than when walking. Although not significant, riders in some cases demonstrated greater trunk movement (i.e., in lateral flexion and rotation). Significant indirect correlations were found between stride velocity and trunk flexion and extension in riding and between lateral flexion and stride velocity in riding and walking. The results support the use of hippotherapy to enhance postural muscle endurance and reinforce data on the similarities between the horse's walk and the human gait.

Haehl, Guiliani, and Lewis (1999) used motion analysis to identify parameters that could be used to operationally define postural control and coordination that were sensitive enough to discriminate between levels of riding ability (Phase I). Those parameters could then be used to measure the effect of hippotherapy (Phase II). Measures of stability and orientation were used to define postural control. *Stability* was defined as the maximum excursion of the trunk in the sagittal plane during one stride of the horse's walk. Stability was similar for the novice and experienced rider. *Orientation* was defined as the extent of vertical orientation of the rider's trunk. Novice riders tended to lean forward, whereas experienced riders were more vertical. *Postural coordination* was described by the "temporal phase relationship" between the movements of the horse's back and the movements of the rider's upper and lower trunk. At the walk, as the horse's hindquarters rise, the horse's back moves upward and forward under the child rider; the child's trunk, in response, moves backward. Similarly, when the horse's hindquarters lower, the horse's back moves downward and backward under the child; the child's trunk, in response, moves forward. Thus, in the sagittal plane, the rider's movement is 180° out of phase with the movement of the horse. For experienced riders, muscle activation of the lower trunk preceded that of the upper trunk. That is, as the rider's posture shifted forward and backward with the movement of the horse, the muscles closest to the base of support, the lower trunk muscles, were activated first. That was not the case for novice riders: The novice riders held their lower trunk muscles tight, and their upper trunk reversed direction before the lower trunk.

These parameters describing the interaction between the movements of the horse and rider were then used to document the effect of hippotherapy on two children with cerebral palsy, described in the next section. Table 7.2 summarizes studies on the three-dimensional movements of horse and rider.

Table 7.2. Studies of Movements of Horse and Rider

Author (Date)	Independent Variables	Outcome Measures	Purpose
Riede (1988)	Horse height, age, trunk length, sex, breed	Three-dimensional movement of the horse	Compare horses
Riede (1988)	Acceleration impulses of horse breeds	Vibration in saddle	Rider safety
Freeman et al. (1997)	Gait, breed of horse; method of leading	Pelvic movement of horse and rider	Validate theory, guidelines
Fleck (1997)	Human walk vs. riding Experience of rider	Pelvic movement of rider	
Harris et al. (1997)	Human walk vs. rider	Trunk movement of rider	Compare walking vs. riding
MacPhail et al. (1998)	Cerebral palsy (CP) vs. children without CP	Lateral trunk displacement	Establish normal baseline
Haehl et al. (1999)		Postural control and coordination	Compare CP to baseline

Studies Documenting Benefit to the Rider

Many early hippotherapy studies (1950s–1980s) investigated the benefits of the movements of the horse on spinal disc metabolism. Junghanns (1974, cited in Riede, 1988) coined the phrase "The spine exists through movement" (p. 122). This phrase referred to the benefit of regular loading and unloading of fluid relative to periods of increased and decreased pressure and the negative effect of prolonged maintenance of any position on disk metabolism. Lindemann and Mau wrote in the *Handbuch der Orthopadie* (1958, cited in Riede, 1988) that, from their experience, riding promoted postural training and control for people with scoliosis. Although he provides no scientific evidence, Riede (1988) advocated hippotherapy for the treatment of spinal disorders such as scoliosis. Riede bases his avocation on the assumption that the undulations of the horse's back displace the center of gravity of the rider, thus challenging the rider's equilibrium, which in turn activates the autochthonous back muscles (the deep layers of the long back).

Riede (1988) suggested that the facilitation of automatic proprioceptive and righting responses during riding therapy may be the optimal way to stimulate long-back musculature. Basing his argument on Vaast (1981, cited in Riede, 1988), Riede postulated that, because the trunk musculature has a greater concentration of muscle spindles (sensory organs) per motor unit than the rest of the body, the trunk is less dependent on cortical control than the rest of the body and is more dependent on automatic postural and movement responses. Thus, the externally imposed vibrations and horizontal accelerations on the human spine (i.e., from the movement of the horse) stimulate righting responses through the stretch reflex mechanism. In addition, joint compression affects muscle tone through elongation and activation of surrounding musculature. Heipertz (1977, 1978), Eltze (1978, 1980), and Gottwald (1980, all cited in Riede, 1988) suggest caution when using hippotherapy with clients with fixed spinal segments: Hypermobile and unstable segments adjacent to the fixed segments may become further destabilized.

Von Eltze (1982, cited in Riede, 1988) followed 122 patients with scoliosis with a maximum curvature of 20°. A combination of traditional physical therapy and hippotherapy resulted in improvement in 25% of the participants; 56% of the participants stabilized (i.e., had lack of progression), 9% demonstrated progression, and 9% changed their curvature from a C to an S shape, equaling a success rate of 81%. One problem with this study is that it had no control groups; participants received only physical therapy or no therapy at all. Thus, more information is needed before the 81% success rate can be attributed to hippotherapy.

Von Bausenwein (1983, cited in Riede, 1988) studied lower-extremity adductor spasticity, trunk control, and reciprocal innervations of various muscle groups of 11 children with cerebral palsy, ages 4 to 15, before and after hippotherapy and before and after traditional therapy with a $60'' \times 28''$ roll (simulating a horse's trunk). Adductor spasticity was measured by the patellar reflex because the hip adductors and the knee extensors are innervated through the same spinal segment. EMG measurements of the lumbar back extensors between L2 and L4 during ambulation were used to measure trunk control. Co-contraction of peripheral muscle groups also was recorded, although the method of recording was not mentioned (or perhaps was lost in the translation). The authors concluded that hippotherapy normalizes muscle tone, improves coordination, and reduces reflex activity when compared to traditional physical therapy treatment of exercises using a roll or ball. No statistical results were provided. Muller (1979, cited in Riede, 1988) achieved the same results as Von Bausenwein, noting that the roll permitted only two-dimensional movement. Muller used the Wilcoxon test ($N = 11$) to determine that spasticity was significantly reduced, although p values and other data were not available.

Meier (1976, cited in Riede, 1988) used telemetric EMG tests to document improved coordination of movement sequences, more rhythmic and economizing innervation, and increased stimulation of the back extensors with hippotherapy. However, "success" was not defined, and methods and statistical results were not provided.

Raus (1973, cited in Riede, 1988) found an increase in lower-extremity abduction of 10% to 30% during sitting and standing following hippotherapy. Although a 10% to 30% gain in range of motion is impressive, no control group received traditional therapy techniques; thus, more information is needed before this gain can be attributed to hippotherapy.

Brauer (1971, cited in Riede, 1988) evaluated children with cerebral palsy (N unknown) before and after 25 therapeutic riding sessions over an 8-week period. Brauer's evaluation included 10 exercises that tested coordination. Brauer found improvement in relaxation and psychosomatic function; coordination; balance; and range of motion and efficiency of hip abductors and knee flexors and extensors. Again, statistical significance was not provided. Hardt (1980, cited in Riede, 1988) videotaped 9 participants with cerebral palsy walking on a treadmill before and after their riding sessions. Subjective, visual evaluation of the videotapes revealed reduction in adductor spasticity and improved postural control.

Roll (1980, cited in Riede, 1988) experimented with the use of photometry, comparisons of photographic images of the body outline taken before and after hippotherapy sessions, as a method of objective documentation of treatment results. Photometry proved an unsatisfactory method of measurement, however, because it did not control for age-related changes and the children (3 with cerebral palsy and 10 with mental retardation) tended to be uncooperative.

Between 1969 and 1983, Riede (1988) incorporated hippotherapy into the treatment program of more than 600 clients. The most frequent diagnoses were functional and postural deficits, scoliosis, neuromotor dysfunction, bilateral osteoarthritis of the hips, and coordinative dysfunction related to trauma. The children reported preferring hippotherapy to swimming, group exercises, vocational therapy, and remedial sports. Riede devised a test of postural dysfunction that included movement analysis, muscle testing, a dual-scale test whereby the participants stood with each of their legs on one of two scales, a forward flexion of arms test, a measurement of thoracic kyphosis, and measure of thoracic and lumbar curves. Twenty-nine children with cerebral palsy ages 10 to 15 were administered this test of postural dysfunction before and after weekly therapeutic riding sessions. Improved coordination and a more erect posture in the sagittal plane was observed and measured in 90% of the participants.

In summary, Riede (1988) described therapeutic riding as "the youngest shoot on the tree of physiotherapy," with improvement in coordination as the primary goal. He stated that therapeutic riding is the only treatment that provides vibration to the spine of the rider, generated by the movement impulses of the horse, which in turn improves postural stability, normalizes muscle tone, and increases balance and coordination. Also special about therapeutic riding is the contact with another living being and the harmony of movement of the horse and rider. Psychological and physiological benefits in addition to musculoskeletal benefits occur.

Studies Not Appearing in Riede (1988)

Several studies of hippotherapy from the 1970s to the 1980s are not described in Riede (1988). Tauffkirchen (1978) performed a study in Austria; only the abstract has been translated into English. Tauffkirchen concluded that "improvement in postural tone, inhibition of pathological movement patterns, facilitation of normal automatical [*sic*] reactions, and the promotion of sensorimotor perceptions is achieved. By adjustment to the swaying movement of the horse, the child feels how to retain straightening alignment, symmetry, and balance" (p. 405). Tauffkirchen based these conclusions on a study of 27 children with cerebral palsy. The methods, however, are not included in the English translation of the abstract.

VanLiet (1995) compared the balance and posture of two groups of children with spina bifida; both groups received traditional physiotherapy, swimming, and remedial gymnastics. The test groups also received therapeutic riding once a week for 30 minutes for a period of 1 year. Sheepskin was used in lieu of a saddle. Exercises were performed at a walk and trot. The Functional Activities Scoring System was used to measure the functional status of locomotion. Equilibrium was tested by laterally tilting the participants while on a therapy ball or roll. Spinal curve was measured using the Cobb technique. Results indicated that sitting posture improved in 5 out of 7 participants; those who improved could balance on the horse without external support or without holding on. The two participants whose sitting balance did not improve also were the only participants with spinal or hip deformities (i.e., hip dysplasia and fixed hip flexion with 32° of scoliosis). The one child in the test groups with scoliosis experienced a 2° reduction in the spinal curve, whereas the only child in the control group with scoliosis experienced a 12° gain in spinal curve. The investigators concluded that (1) the movement of the horse facilitated righting and equilibrium reactions and strengthening of the trunk and (2) perception of space of movement is enlarged through proprioceptive experiences benefiting the mental development of the child.

A copy of Gottwald and Biewald (1981), a study mentioned in Riede (1988), was obtained through PubMed, but only the abstract has been translated in English. The study supported the use of hippotherapy in the treatment of Scheuermann's disease (kyphosis); the abstract stated that riding therapy strengthened the musculature of the trunk and reduced segmental fixation of the spinal column as confirmed by clinical examinations and x-rays. These conclusions should be interpreted with caution, however, because the entire study was not available in English, and it is logical that the movement of the horse could adversely affect a fixed spinal segment.

At the Department of Aerospace Engineering Sciences at the University of Colorado–Boulder, Fox, Lawler, and Luttges (1984) designed and built an apparatus that used automated data collection to objectively test balance and coordination (stability and accuracy) and changes in strength. The device was piloted with 19 participants with cerebral palsy, spina bifida, learning disabilities, and mental retardation. Testing was administered before and after each 2-hour riding session. In addition, spinal curve measurements were taken to monitor straightness. Balance accuracy improved by 19%, with practice effects accounting for no more than 4% of the improvement (according to earlier pilot studies). Balance and coordination stability improved by 7% and were considered immune to practice effects. Arm strength increased by 8% and leg strength increased by 14%. An 18% improvement toward more normal spinal curvature also occurred. Unfortunately, no other studies appear to have used this device.

Armstrong, Sandilands, Myco, and Miller (1988) examined balance, spinal and joint mobility, behavior, and affect to test the hypothesis that horseback riding would benefit physically and mentally handicapped adults. Forty-seven participants over age 18 were divided into two groups. One group rode 3 times per week for 6 weeks, followed by a 2-week break and another 6-week session. The control group rode for a 6-week period, then ceased riding for the duration of the study. Western saddles were used. Of interest is the study's physical assessment parameter. Mobility standards developed by the Committee for the Study of Joint Motion of the American Academy of Orthopedic surgeons were used to measure change in spine and joint mobility. When comparing the intervention and control groups, significant changes in left shoulder rotation ($p = .03$), right ankle flexion ($p = .01$), left ankle flexion ($p = .008$), right knee flexion ($p = .005$), right hip flexion ($p = .02$), left knee flexion ($p = .02$), and left hip flexion ($p = .000$) were found. An uncontrolled confounder in this study was the variation in diagnoses: For example, 16 participants had mental handicap, 4 had Down syndrome, 5 had cerebral palsy, 2 had multiple sclerosis, and 1 had had a stroke.

Snir, Dlin, Ayalon, Yazdi, and Inbar (1988) studied the effects of horseback riding as a form of therapy on biomechanical, physiological, and psychomotor factors in four children ages 13 to 15. Three participants were diagnosed with minimal brain dysfunction, and 1 had mild cerebral palsy. Participants rode twice a week for 60 minutes. Strength was tested on a Cybex II isokinetic machine. Ground reaction forces in gait were evaluated with a Kistler force plate. A posturographic test was performed using four plates that measured the vertical ground reaction forces for the heel and forefoot of both legs. Psychomotor variables included eye–hand coordination, balance, reaction time, kinesthesia, manipulation, and weight distribution. Physiological measures included cardiorespiratory testing and walking efficiency with the following parameters: O_2 consumption, anaerobic threshold, maximal ventilation, maximal mechanical power, maximal heart rate, and mechanical efficiency. Improvement in walking efficiency was noted in all participants, although statistical results were not provided. Significant improvement occurred on two of the psychomotor parameters: body movement imitation ($p = .05$) and the kinesthesia test for the right hand ($p = .047$).

Toffola, Bar, Petrucci, Pfazza, and Ricotti (1988) compared 10 youths with cerebral palsy, ages 4 to 19, with 10 control group participants without, ages 9 to 14, all of whom were participating in a riding program. Baseline data were gathered 3 months after the riding program had been suspended for summer break. Data were collected after 6 months of riding: once per week for 30 minutes of actual riding time. According to the results, participants with cerebral palsy demonstrated increased EMG activity compared with the controls. The EMG activity of the paravertebral muscles at the cervical, dorsal, and lumbar levels (evaluated using a biofeedback DUAL EMG SATEM device, a type of electrogram used in Europe) of participants with cerebral palsy decreased following the hippotherapy intervention. Although consistent changes for participants with cerebral palsy were noted at the individual level, in reflex activity following stimulation of the Achilles tendon and the tibialis posterior nerve at the popliteal fossa, the changes before and after intervention were not significant when tested as a group.

Brock (1988) performed two studies of the efficacy of therapeutic riding for improving strength and coordination for adults with physical disabilities. The participants' ages ranged from 19 to 41; diagnoses included head trauma, visual impairment, arthritis, cerebral palsy, and epilepsy. Study I used a pretest–posttest design. Study II compared the posttest results of 24 adults with physical disabilities randomly assigned to a riding or nonriding group. For both studies, the intervention consisted of horseback riding twice a week for 8 weeks. The midweek class was 60 minutes long, and the weekend class lasted 90 to 120 minutes. Sessions included stretching and centering exercises, walking, trotting, posting, turns, and circles. Barrels, bean bags, poles, and buckets also were used. Psychomotor measurements of arm and leg strength and coordination were taken using the Strength and Coordination Instrument (Fox et al., 1984). The results indicated significant changes in arm and leg coordination ($p = .01$) for Study I and significant changes in arm coordination ($p = .01$) for Study II.

Bertoti (1988) measured change in the posture following a therapeutic riding intervention of 11 children ages 2 to 9 who had spastic diplegia or quadriplegia cerebral palsy. A repeated-measures design was used. A postural scale developed by the author was administered by three blinded pediatric physical therapists; interrater reliability was 0.82. Data were collected at baseline, following a 10-week period of no riding, and again after a 10-week therapeutic riding program in which participants rode in groups of three twice a week for 1-hour sessions. The intervention consisted of the horses led at a walk with two side-walkers positioning and stabilizing the participant as necessary. Each participant rode on a sheepskin in prone, side-lying, and sitting positions. Soft saddles with stirrups were introduced toward the end of the study and were alternated with the sheepskin, and work in squat and standing was introduced. Results of a Friedman's test showed significant improvement in posture ($p = .05$).

MacKay-Lyons, Conway, and Roberts (1988) studied the effects of a therapeutic riding intervention on postural sway; gait; neurological status, function, and neurological impairment; and psychological well-being of 10 participants with multiple sclerosis. The intervention consisted of two 45-minute therapeutic riding sessions per week for 9 weeks. A series of exercises in circles and serpentines was performed to elicit equilibrium reactions. Gaits included the walk and the trot. Postural sway was measured using a computerized force platform, gait analysis with a microprocessor-controlled walkway, neurological status and function with the Minimal Record of Disability, neurological impairment with the Kurtzke Expanded Disability Status Scale, and psychological well-being with the SCL-90-R. Data were collected at baseline and following the intervention. Gait analysis revealed significant increases in the relative speed of free speed walking ($p = .029$) and stride length ($p = .008$). In addition, the walking of three participants improved such that they were able to walk without their ambulation devices following the intervention. Depression also was significantly reduced ($p = .03$).

Biery and Kauffman (1989) looked at the effect of therapeutic riding on balance of 8 individuals with mental retardation. Balance was measured using 10 balance tasks developed by Cratty (1967). Data were collected at baseline, after 6 months of no intervention, and after 6 months of intervention. The intervention consisted of 20-minute riding sessions once per week for 24 weeks. Wilcoxon matched-pairs signed-rank test and paired t-test results found significant changes ($p = .013$) in balance after the 6 months of intervention; no significant changes were found after the 6 months of no intervention.

Studies During the 1990s

In a study of 5 patients with infantile brain damage (spastic tetraplegia), Ricotti and colleagues (1991) found that hippotherapy improved muscle performance as measured by EMG signals. Significant changes were found in H_{MAX}/M_{MAX} and T_{MAX}/M_{MAX} values were attributed to a reduction in alfa and gamma motoneuronal excitability, resulting in better activity of tibialis anterior muscle because of reduced spastic hypertonia of antagonist counterparts (triceps surae) and better recruiting of paretic muscles (foot dorsiflexors).

On the basis of a mathematical relationship between acceleration, speed, and change of location, Pfotenhauer and colleagues (1991) devised and tested an acceleration transducer positioned between the third and forth lumbar vertebrae to measure movement of the human walking and riding. Twelve adults with and 42 without multiple sclerosis participated. The investigators found this method of evaluation to be an appropriate measure of the effect of hippotherapy: Graphs were produced that allowed comparison of human acceleration in three planes (right–left, up–down, and forward–backward). Thus, trunk movement at the walk and when riding could be compared. This preliminary data suggested hippotherapy improved the walking gait of individuals with multiple sclerosis.

Baker (1991) studied the effect of hippotherapy on flexible kyphosis of four adults with developmental disabilities. A single-subject, alternating-treatment design with participants serving as their own controls was used. Kyphosis was measured before and after hippotherapy sessions with a device fabricated for the study. During the nontreatment sessions, participants sat on a bolster in an approximation of the mounted position for 15 minutes; kyphosis was measured before and after. Three of the four participants demonstrated decreased kyphosis following hippotherapy and a tendency toward increased kyphosis with no intervention. The client who did not show improvement had a less flexible kyphosis.

Veicsteinas, Melorio, Turner, Belleri, and Sarchi (1991) monitored heart rate as an outcome of therapeutic riding. Their study involved two groups: Group A included 15 people with mental impairment, and Group B involved 15 participants with physical impairment ($N = 30$). Measurement of heart rate was ongoing throughout the riding session. The session consisted of 10 minutes of riding at the walk followed by 20 to 30 minutes of exercises while on the horse. The results indicated that riders with physical impairment exerted more effort than riders with mental impairment. When both motor and mental impairment were present, however, heart rates remained similar to that of people with only mental impairment. The authors concluded that "[heart rate] increase depends more on the mental condition than on the muscular control of the subject" (Veicsteinas et al., 1991, p. 112). The results were presented as graphs for 9 of the participants. The study did not address confounding factors, such as degree of impairment and experience with riding.

Exner, Engelmann, Lange, and Wenck (1994) published in German a study of 67 patients with paraplegia and quadriplegia who received hippotherapy (only the abstract was translated into English). They reported statistically significant effects on the reduction of spasticity, pain, and impaired joint mobility. Associated positive effects included easier catheterization, more rhythmical bowel function, more balanced mood, improved sleep, and improved motivation. Veicsteinas, Melorio, and Sarchi (1994) studied the energy expenditure in a typical therapeutic horse riding session ($N = 36$, 20 in the intervention group and 16 in the control group). Oxygen consumption (VO_2), pulmonary ventilation (VE), and heart rate (HR) were monitored in people with mental retardation (Group 1), motor impairment (Group 2), and a control group. All participants were between the ages of 15 and 37. Baseline VO_2, VE, and HR measures were taken following exercise in the laboratory. VO_2, VE, and HR measures were taken again following riding the horse at a walk and after a series of exercises on the walking horse. The results indicated that the cardio-respiratory stress imposed during riding was higher than the stress resulting from exercise in the laboratory, perhaps because of the muscle tone required to balance on the horse and emotional factors associated with being on the horse. The increased values were not severe enough to represent a risk to the health of the rider. The

energy expenditure was greatest for Group 2, followed by Group 1 and the control group.

EMG (to measure changes in muscle activation) and acceleration (to measure change in the center of gravity of the body) data were found to be valuable methods to monitor qualitative changes of movement and coordination during hippotherapy (Webster et al., 1994) in 9 participants with and 10 without multiple sclerosis. EMG and acceleration measurements were taken before and after the hippotherapy session. Improvement was noted in 6 of the 9 participants: Post-hippotherapy, the mean values of the participants with multiple sclerosis were similar to the values of the participants without multiple sclerosis. Changes noted in participants with multiple sclerosis included a decrease in adductor spasticity, improved gait quality, and reports that walking was easier following hippotherapy. P values were not reported.

Hoff (1994) investigated two methods of using the reins by individuals with cerebral palsy when riding: an opening rein and an opposition direct rein. (The article was written in French, with a somewhat cumbersome translation to English.) Hoff developed an extensive prehension assessment that included factors related to prehension, such as vision, trunk control, and coordination. Hoff found that some participants were successful at using an opening rein (which required upper-extremity [UE] abduction, forearm extension [external rotation], and hand supination), whereas others were successful with an opposition direct rein (UE adduction, forearm extension [internal rotation], and hand pronation). Hoff validated the effects of the two types of reining with the horse's hoof prints to make sure the horse was indeed moving in correspondence with the driving rein. Although this study provides only indirect evidence for the efficacy of hippotherapy, it does provide support for theories that postulate that people with disabilities develop movement patterns that are successful, even though they may not be considered developmentally normal.

MacKinnon, Noh, Lariviete, MacPhail, and Allan (1995) randomized 19 children with spastic cerebral palsy (who could sit independently in a chair for 2 minutes) into a group who received therapeutic riding and a group who went on a waiting list. The study controlled for degree of impairment by stratifying the sample into mildly and moderately involved levels of cerebral palsy. Participants in the mild group focused on the development of functional riding skills, and participants in the moderate group rode on pads with surcingles. Participants rode for 1 hour per week for 6 months. The people who administered pretests and posttests were blinded. Analysis of covariance (ANCOVA) was used to compare change in the treatment group to change in the control group, controlling for pretest score. Outcomes included a postural scale (Bertotto, 1988) and scores on the Gross Motor Function Measure (GMFM; Russell et al., 1989), Peabody Developmental Motor Scale (PDMS; Folio & Fewell, 1983), Bruininks-Oseretsky Test of Motor Proficiency (Bruininks, 1978), Vineland Adaptive Behavior Scales (Sparrow, Balla, & Cicchetti, 1984), Harter Self-Perception Scale (Harter, 1985), and the Child Behavior Checklist (Achenbach & Edelbrock, 1983). Grasp improved significantly, but perceived self-adequacy diminished. Grasp is an important skill that is especially difficult for children with cerebral palsy. Of concern is why self-adequacy diminished; the measure was completed by parents, and the authors proposed that the parent reporters may have inflated the pretest abilities to ensure that the child was selected for the study.

Biery and Kauffman (1996) found a significant difference ($p = .01$) in the balance scores of 8 study participants with mental retardation ages 12 to 22, 7 of whom were diagnosed with Down syndrome. Balance (measured by tests by Cratty, 1967) was measured initially, then again after 6 months of no riding intervention, and finally after a 6-month intervention of riding once per week for 20 minutes. The intervention consisted of a 5-minute warm-up, during which riders rode without holding on and were asked to follow the horse's motion. Next was a 10-minute period of intensive activity, followed by a 5-minute cool-down period, during which participants rode with their shoulders protracted and arms externally rotated with arms hanging loosely at their sides, palms facing forward.

Would (1996) used a Penny and Giles electronic goniometer fastened to the rider's back (*N* unknown) to measure the pelvic angle relative to the lumbar spine and pelvic movements. This movement was then graphed to compare riders with and without cerebral palsy. This method then was used to monitor changes in stability, asymmetry, and balance over time. More recently, Would (2000) investigated changes in walking patterns and reduction in energy expenditure after hippotherapy.

Kulichova and Zenklova (1996) demonstrated the benefits of hippotherapy for 13 individuals with scoliosis ages 12 to 20. Diagnoses included hemiplegia due to cerebral palsy, idiopathic juvenile scoliosis, and dis-

orders of the pelvis. Vertebrographic measurements were taken prior to the intervention, after riding twice per week in 40-minute sessions, and again after riding once every 2 weeks for 6 months. Harmony of the horse and rider movements was emphasized during the riding intervention. According to paired *t* tests, significant changes in deviation in the frontal axis occurred between the first and second measurement time points ($p = .0008$) and the second and third measurements ($p = .006$). The curvature of the spine was significantly reduced after 6 months of riding twice per week (mean = 18.2° [13.0°]). The preintervention mean was 22.1° (19.5°). After less intensive riding (once every 2 weeks), the curvature worsened slightly (mean = 20.8° [14.3°]).

Selvinen (1997) investigated the effect of a single riding therapy session on the walk and the active and passive leg movements of 6 people with multiple sclerosis ages 25 to 54 and the effects of riding therapy on their daily activities. Participants were included if they could walk independently with or without walking aides, reported problems with paraparesis and extension, and had no prior experience with riding therapy. Participants rode three times with 2 days between sessions. The same horse was used for all sessions and participants: a cold-blood horse with a brisk gait. Assessment of walk (via videotape), walk time, step height and length, and spasticity (Ashworth Scale) were performed before each session and 30 minutes following the session. An interview was administered immediately after the session, and questionnaires were completed in the evening following the riding sessions. Results were reported using median values. The most distinctive changes were an increase in step height (median increase from 72 to 94.5 cm), followed by a decrease in spasticity. Participants reported feeling "looser" and reported "better balance."

Using a single-subject design with 2 children with autism, Tolson (1997) collected data on echolalia, self-directed behavior, and other-directed behavior for 15 weeks in the classroom. During approximately Weeks 7 to 9, the intervention—eight 1-hour therapeutic riding sessions—took place. The intervention then was withdrawn for the remaining weeks. Echolalic and self-directed behaviors decreased for both participants during the intervention and returned to baseline following the intervention. Other-directed behavior increased for both participants during the return-to-baseline phase. Data were not serially dependent.

Several case studies have documented the positive effects of hippotherapy. Using a multiple single-case design with 4 study participants with brain injury, Stykes and colleagues (1997) found that hippotherapy improved functional balance as measured by computerized balanced platform and videotaped analysis of gait. Participants rode once per week for 16 weeks. Each session was individualized based on an initial physical therapy evaluation. Hansen (1997) used a case study approach to document the effect of hippotherapy on five children ages 8 to 11 with mild to severe spastic cerebral palsy. Effect was measured by change in GMFM scores (Russell et al., 1989). Participants rode for 16 individual, once-a-week, 30-minute sessions. Five participants used a surcingle, and 3 used an English saddle. The GMFM is scored as a percentage of task completed; higher percentages indicate less impairment. The baseline GMFM scores ranged from 25.74% to 74.10%. The mean change in GMFM score before and after intervention was 5.41%, with a range of 0.30% to 7.02%. The participant with the least change demonstrated the most severe impairment. Change most often was seen in balance and graded trunk and extremity control.

Fox and Peterson (1997) reported on a multiple-case design that used the GMFM as well as goniometry to assess changes in hip range of motion (ROM) and sitting ability in 4 children with mild to moderate spastic diplegic or quadriplegic cerebral palsy. Participants received hippotherapy for one 30-minute session per week for 6 weeks. None of the participants demonstrated improvement in GMFM sitting dimension scores. A paired t test revealed significant changes ($p = .016$) in right hip abduction but not left hip abduction ($p = .139$). Type II error due to small sample size could have been a factor in the lack of significance in change in left hip abduction. Examination of raw data, however, does show more change in right hip abduction across all 4 participants: Change in left hip abduction ranged from $-1°$ to $14°$, and change in right hip abduction ranged from $9°$ to $20°$. The same horse was used for all sessions per client, but whether the same horse was used for all clients was not mentioned. All participants rode on bareback pads.

Using a single-case design, Wheeler (1997) documented an increase in hip and knee strength and progression from a walker to independent household ambulation in a 7-year-old child with L4 myelomengingocele after 28 weekly sessions of hippotherapy. Martin and Stormont-Smith (1997) documented improvement in static and dynamic balance and broad jump abilities of a 6-year-old child with spastic cerebral palsy who rode once weekly for 45-minute sessions for 6 weeks. Wasserman and Keeney (1997) used a single-case design to document the effects of hippotherapy (20-minute sessions, once weekly for 8 weeks) on an 8-year-old child with spastic quadriplegic cerebral palsy and cortical blindness and who had had a dorsal rhizotomy at age 6. The child rode the horse prone because of limited pelvic mobility. Only postintervention lower-extremity ROM measures were provided, so a comparison with preintervention scores could not be made. On the Pediatric Evaluation of Disability Index (PEDI; Haley, Coster, Ludlow, Haltwanger, & Andrellos, 1992), the score on the social function/caregiver assistance domain increased from 0 to 39.6 points. If this change reflected an increase in standard score, it would mean a nearly 4 standard deviation increase (mean = 50, standard deviation = 10) because the maximum raw score obtainable in this domain is 25. Other PEDI scores remained unchanged. Anecdotal reports described change in head control, especially active extension, and increased ROM in elbow extension, forearm supination, and hip extension.

Cook (1997) also used a single-case design to document an increase in active ROM in a 22-year-old woman who received 3 years of riding therapy that began 4 years following traumatic brain injury (TBI). The woman, who used a wheelchair, had been discharged from traditional therapies due to lack of progress. Increased left upper-extremity ROM was documented in shoulder flexion and hyperextension ($+30°$), abduction–adduction ($+25°$), elbow flexion–extension and forearm supination ($+25°$), wrist dorsiflexion ($+50°$), and thumb and digits ($+20°$ to $+30°$). Increase in ROM could be attributed to a decrease in spasticity and, ultimately, an increase in functional movement. In addition, according to the Scorable Self-Care Evaluation, a 30% increase in self-care tasks was noted.

At the Ninth International Therapeutic Riding Congress in Denver, Colorado, in 1997, research ideas from around the world were presented. In Russia (Harris et al., 1997), a group of researchers were focusing on using objective measurement; they examined 93 institutionalized adults who had diagnoses including autism, cerebral palsy, Down syndrome, and schizophrenia using measures of physical change including pulse, blood oxygen saturation, electroencephalogram, cardiac activity, and pletismogram (heart rate). German investigators (Sportwiss, Heipertz-Hengst, & Wohlschlegel, 1997) were in the midst of a randomized control trial. At the time of the conference, 21 participants had completed the trial. Although the analyses had not been performed, the hippotherapy group appeared to be performing better in sitting, standing, walking, balance, coordination, flexibility, and muscle tone.

McGibbon, Andrade, Widerer, and Cintas (1998) used a repeated-measures design to investigate the effects of an 8-week hippotherapy program for 5 children with cerebral palsy who walked independently with or without assistive devices; the study took two baseline measures 8 weeks apart, then provided an 8-week intervention. Outcome variables were energy expenditure walking, stride length, velocity, cadence during walking, and GMFM scores. The intervention consisted of 16 30-minute sessions. Equipment included fleece and surcingle, bridle and reins, halter, and lead line. Data were collected at each session. According to the results of Wilcoxon signed-rank tests, Friedman analysis of variance (ANOVA), and multiple comparisons tests, significant changes were noted in the energy expenditure index ($p < .05$) and the GMFM Dimension E (walking, running, and jumping; $p < .05$). The results suggest that hippotherapy reduces energy expenditure, increases efficiency in walking, and improves gait-related motor function for children with cerebral palsy.

The early motion analysis studies compared the movement of the horse and human movement at the walk. Later studies (Haehl et al., 1999; MacPhail et al., 1998) went a step further by looking at the interaction between the movement of the rider and the horse. MacPhail and colleagues used motion analysis to compare the trunk movements of children with cerebral palsy ($n = 6$) and without cerebral palsy ($n = 7$) to determine whether normal equilibrium reactions were being elicited during therapeutic riding. All participants rode the same horse. The mean lateral trunk movement of the children without cerebral palsy was half the magnitude of the horse's pelvic movement. The mean lateral trunk movement of the children with cerebral palsy was close to the magnitude of the horse's pelvic movement and significantly different ($p < .01$) from that of the children without. The children without cerebral palsy demonstrated postural movements that followed the movement of the horse. The children with diplegic cerebral palsy demonstrated postural movements that were similar to the movement of the horse but with time delays 65% to 75% of the time. The postural movements of children with quadriplegic cerebral palsy followed the movement of the horse only 10% to 35% of the time. The mean trunk displacement of the children without cerebral palsy was 5.8°, compared with 10.2° for the children with.

Note that this study did not look at change in postural reactions over time but rather analyzed the horse–rider interaction during three trials (i.e., 1 stride near the beginning and 1 stride near the end of each trial, for a total of 6 strides). The article did not mention the timing of the trials. Trials were not compared to each other, as in a time-series or repeated-measures design, but rather mean trunk displacement of the children without cerebral palsy was compared to mean trunk displacement of the children with cerebral palsy. Thus, although MacPhail and colleagues concluded that hippotherapy did not elicit normal equilibrium reactions for children with cerebral palsy, especially those with quadriplegia, the study did not address the question of how the equilibrium reaction could change over the duration of intervention.

Haehl and colleagues (1999) examined the effect of hippotherapy on postural control, postural coordination, and functional performance over time (12 weekly sessions). A collective case study design was used ($N = 2$). The same horse was used for all sessions. Participants sat on a pad with surcingle or a saddle. The sessions lasted 20 minutes for Participant 1 and 40 minutes for Participant 2. Over the 12 sessions, postural control and stability increased for both participants. The postural coordination of Participant 2 progressed from being inconsistent and out of synchronization with the movement of the horse's back to that of an experienced rider. The trunk movement of Participant 1 followed the movement of the horse's back throughout the study; however, the lag time of the rider adjusting to the horse's movement decreased from 5% to 0.5%. In summary, both participants progressed to postural coordination sequencing similar to that of the experienced rider in Phase I (see Studies Documenting Three-Dimensional Movement of the Horse). Change in functional skills was measured with the PEDI. The PEDI-scaled scores of the functional skills domain increased for both participants, although the change was only significant for Participant 2.

Studies During the 2000s

In the country of Georgia, Tsverava, Rukhadze, and Loria (2000) studied the use of hippotherapy to treat 232 adults with osteochondrosis of the spine (neck, thorax, and waist) who were ages 19 to 52. A treatment group received remedial exercises, massage, and riding therapy, and the control group received only remedial exercises and massage. Outcomes included clinical, x-ray, and functional investigations, along with studies of the degree of the clinical picture, frequency and duration of exacerbations. The reported therapeutic effect after treatment was 97% in the treatment group and

89% in the control group. The treatment group demonstrated a significant ($p < .001$) decrease in exacerbation and a significant ($p < .001$) increase in "clinical picture," which was not defined. The investigators concluded that the frequency and amplitude of vibrations from the horse's back positively affect the nervous and endocrine systems and metabolic processes and that this proprioceptive excitation from the horse facilitates new motor stereotypes. They also concluded that the rider's body mechanisms that are affected include centering of the decentered nuclei of the spine, improved metabolism in the intervertebral discus and surrounding tissue, decompression of the nerve trunk and blood vessels, isotonic and isometric strengthening of muscles, and a decrease in the dystrophic process that accompanies osteochondrosis of the spine. Note that little detail was provided on the clinical data that supported these conclusions.

In Finland, Mattila-Rautiainen, Korhonen, Nyman, and Tossavainen (2000) studied hippotherapy as an intervention for 4 patients with marked, chronic low-back pain. Magnetic resonance imaging (MRI) revealed degeneration but no prolapse or disc protrusion. Three of the 4 participants had associated sleep disorders. Measures of depression (Beck Depression Inventory), quality of life, spine mobility, balance and electronic response from low-back muscles (using the muscle tester ME3000), and tiring of low-back muscles and muscle activity in forward–backward bending (measured with EMG) also were recorded. The EMG was connected to video and computer for analysis. Reported pain decreased between preintervention and postintervention and continued to decrease at 5 months' postintervention. Mean depression scores decreased from 21.5 (moderate to difficult) to 14.8 (mild to moderate). Quality of life improved, and falling asleep became easier. Low-back muscle strength improved by 30%. Video EMG analysis showed increased balance between back muscles on the left and right sides, and the tiring test showed that the muscles had more durability. Patients reported a warm feeling in lower extremities and decline of nerve pain. Raw data and levels of significance were not provided. One could question whether this intervention could be considered hippotherapy and tapping some of the same mechanisms evaluated in the early hippotherapy studies examining spinal disc metabolism (Mattila-Rautiainen et al., 2000).

Sahraoui (2000) measured the effects of hippotherapy on upright posture of 29 children ages 5 to 17 who had spastic diplegia cerebral palsy. A force platform created in Wroclaw, Poland, detected the vertical component of force applied horizontally and thereby measured the dynamics of postural sway (force vs. time in the sagittal and frontal planes) before and after hippotherapy. Participants rode for 30 minutes 4 times per week for 12 months. The results were presented in frequency polygons that were rather difficult to interpret. Sahraoui, however, reported improvement in 25 of the 29 participants.

Mattila-Rautiainen (2000) used motion analysis to analyze riders' movement before, during, and after hippotherapy. The intervention consisted of 3 riding sessions per week for 8 weeks. Mann–Whitney U' tests were used to determine whether the lumbar movements that occurred in each rider–horse combination were significantly different at the free and the collected walks. A limitation of this publication was that little information was available about how the movements were different, as well as confusion between the assessment of differences in the horses' movements versus the rider's movements at the free and collected walks. The implications were that the gait of the horse should be chosen on the basis of the desired degree of movement in the rider's spine and pelvis.

Land, Errington-Povalac, and Paul (2001) also used motion analysis to measure the effects of the movement of the horse on sitting posture. Three participants, ages 10 to 40 with documented disturbance in muscle tone because of central nervous system damage, were videotaped two times on two separate days and then received the intervention. The intervention consisted of a 1-hour riding session, once per week for 8 weeks. All participants used a saddle and reins. Participants were tested again on two separate days, post-intervention. Repeated measures ANOVA indicated significant changes ($p \leq .05$) in 4 of the 8 measurements of sitting posture.

Ionatamishvili, Tsverava, Loria, and Avaliani (2001) studied the effects of riding therapy on 30 children with cerebral palsy and 10 children without between ages 6 and 12. The children were divided into three groups: one received riding therapy, the second received traditional therapy using a Bobath approach, and the third was a control group of children without cerebral palsy who were riding amateurs. Group 1 rode 6 times per week for 90–120 minutes, in 5–6-minute turns with breaks. Group 2 participated in gymnastic exercises 6 times per week for 90 minutes. Group 3 engaged in off-horse activities that involved perceiving the environment. The dependent variables were intensity of hyperkinesia, memory abilities, and knowledge of the horse. Although significant changes occurred in all three groups ($p < .001$) for all three variables, the greatest change was found in Group 1, and the least change in Group 2. Moreover, the positive results in the riding groups were achieved more quickly than in the other group.

Pasquinelli, Allori, Raupach, and Caterion (2003) studied 10 people with nonprogressive extrapyramidal disorders (ED) that included dystonia and athetosis with or without spasticity. Participants were ages 10 to 57. Participants rode twice a week for 1 year in 50-minute sessions using an English saddle, reins, and stirrups. The mean intervention duration was 2 years, 5 months. The more severely affected participants used a special handle attached to the saddle in addition to or in place of the reins. Each session consisted of a program designed specifically for each participant. Assessments included the Dystonia Movement Scale (Burke, Fahn, & Marsden, 1985), the ED Assessment Scale Results (Papini, Pasquinelli, Allori, & Biagini, 1995), videotaping, and direct observation. Improvement in muscle tone and strength was noted in 100% of the participants; 55% demonstrated improved balance reactions, 67% demonstrated a decrease in involuntary movement, and 60% experienced improved motor planning and coordination. The improvements translated to improvement in sitting for 50% of the participants and improvement in standing and walking for 50% of the participants. The investigators found that, in the majority of participants, improvement was generalized to neuromotor competencies on the ground after 6 to 12 months.

Winchester, Kendall, Peters, Sears, and Winkley (2002) studied 7 children ages 4 to 8 who had diagnoses of cerebral palsy, spina bifida, Down syndrome, autism, and TBI. Inclusion criteria included the ability to sit unassisted for a minimum of 2 minutes and sufficient hip abduction to sit astride a horse. Exclusion criteria included uncontrolled seizure disorder, allergies to animals, atlanto–axial instability as determined by a physician, body weight exceeding 200 pounds, uncontrolled hypertension, open skin areas on weight-bearing surfaces, and a scoliotic curve of greater than 30°. The study was carried out at a therapeutic riding center. Prior to the intervention, baseline measures were gathered over two testing periods to determine a single pretest value. For the baseline measure, participants were assessed by a physical therapist using the GMFM and, if ambulatory, gait speed during a timed 10-meter walk.

The intervention was described as a 1-hour, once-weekly riding session for a period of 7 weeks. Appropriate horse and tack were selected at the beginning of the study by a certified riding instructor. Participants wore approved helmets. The horse, trained horse-handler, and sidewalkers remained consistent throughout the 7-week intervention for each participant. Each treatment session emphasized muscle relaxation and stretching, symmetrical postural alignment, independent sitting and standing balance, dynamic weight shift to facilitate automatic righting and equilibrium reactions, and following commands from the instructor. Posttreatment measures were taken both at 1 week and 7 weeks after the intervention ended. A repeated-measures, one-way ANOVA blocked by subject, $\alpha \leq .05$, was used to analyze the results, followed by Tukey multiple comparisons to test pairwise differences. Significant differences in GMFM scores ($p < .01$) were found in the omnibus test (ANOVA); pretest scores had a mean of 60.2% + 24.1%, and posttest scores had a mean of 71.0% + 20.1%. Post hoc testing revealed a significant difference between the pretest and Posttest 1 and the pretest and Posttest 2. No significant difference was found between Posttests 1 and 2, indicating that the effect of the intervention did not subside 8 weeks after the intervention. No significant changes were found in gait speed.

Ionatamishvili and associates (2002) conducted what appears to be a randomized control trial involving 100 participants; the study was published in Russian with only the abstract translated to English. Ionatamishvili and colleagues (2001) found the therapeutic riding intervention to be significantly ($p < .0001$) more beneficial than the Bobath therapeutic gymnastics intervention given to the control group. Therapeutic riding benefits included acquisition of new movement skills, reduction in spasticity and hyperkinesis, and mobilization of compensatory abilities.

Sterna, Rogers, France, and Vokes (2002) examined the effect of "recreational riding" on the gross motor function of 17 children with mild to severe cerebral palsy. This study is interesting because the investigators (two physicians, an occupational therapist, and a physical therapist) reported using a recreational riding intervention, not a hippotherapy intervention, although they used the terms *recreational therapy* and *therapeutic riding* interchangeably. The intervention consisted of 1-hour sessions, once per week for 18 weeks. The objectives of the sessions were to develop sensorimotor and perceptual–motor skills based on the Developmental Riding Therapy methods of Spink (1993). The WeeFIM (Braun, Msall, & Granger, 1991) and GMFM were administered 6 weeks in advance of and again immediately prior to the intervention; no significant change was noted. Significant changes ($p < .02$) on the GMFM Dimension E (walking, running, and jumping) were noted after 12 weeks of intervention; the scores remained elevated at 6 weeks' postintervention. The results are similar to the results obtained by McGibbon and colleagues (1998), who provided a hippotherapy intervention.

Lechner and colleagues (2003) hypothesized that a "rhythmical side flexion and extension of the patient's trunk combined with trunk torsion have a beneficial effect on spasticity" (p. 502). Their rationale was that the inhibition of spasticity would be achieved (1) while in saddle position—that is, hip flexion, abduction, and external rotation; (2) through the rhythmical and three-dimensional movements of the horse; and (3) via psychosomatic effects. The study took place between 1996 and 2001 and involved 4 women and 28 men, ages 16 to 72 (mean age = 37), with spinal cord injury between C4 and T12. The total number of sessions per participant ranged from 5 to 24 and each session lasted 25 to 30 minutes. A measurement of spasticity using the Ashworth Scale with the participant in prone was taken before and after each hippotherapy session.

Seven physiotherapists, all trained by the same person, participated in the testing; the same physiotherapist performed the participant's pretest and posttest. The physiotherapists met regularly to discuss experiences and check inter- and intrarater reliability. During the intervention phase of the study, participants sat on sheepskin (no saddle), while the horse (Icelander) was led at a walk by a trained equestrian. A physiotherapist walked beside the horse and rider facilitating postural changes and repositioning if necessary. Some patients with high lesions were backridden. The Wilcoxon signed-rank test was used to analyze the data; α was set at $p = .05$. The results indicated a significant change ($p < .001$) in Ashworth values. The decrease in spasticity of the lower extremities was most pronounced in participants with high spasticity. Individual mean Ashworth values were 17.6 to 53.3 before the intervention and 16.6 to 42.0 postintervention. The effects were immediate; there was no longitudinal effect or decreasing trend. This study provided evidence of the short-term effect of hippotherapy on spasticity of people with spinal cord injury. This research team plans to investigate the duration of the effect in future studies.

Benda, McGibbon, and Grant (2003) used a pretest–posttest design with a control group design to examine the effect of hippotherapy on the symmetry of muscle activity in children with cerebral palsy. Muscle activity

was measured using a remote telemetered surface EMG. The objectives were to determine whether changes in muscle activity after a short hippotherapy session occurred and to compare the effects of symmetrical sitting on a barrel to symmetrical sitting on a rhythmically moving horse. Inclusion criteria included the ability to sit independently without back support; to stand and walk independently, with or without an assistive device; and to cooperate and follow directions as well as adequate hip adduction to sit astride a horse or barrel. Exclusion criteria included dorsal rhizotomy, uncontrolled grand mal seizures, surgical procedures, casting, or botulinum toxin injection within 12 months prior to testing; moderate to severe mental retardation; and hearing loss. Fifteen children with cerebral palsy ages 4 to 12 were randomized (using sealed envelopes) to either the hippotherapy intervention or the barrel intervention.

The test protocol consisted of a 10-second EMG recording of all muscle groups while participants sat quietly on a bench, a 10-second EMG recording of all muscle groups while participants stood still, and an EMG recording during two 10-foot walking sessions. The test protocol was administered before and after the intervention. The hippotherapy intervention was performed on a trained therapy horse, tacked with a fleece pad and surcingle. A horse handler led the horse on a designated track at a steady walk for 4 minutes clockwise and 4 minutes counterclockwise. A physical therapist and an assistant walked on either side of the horse and rider for safety but provided no postural support. The control group sat on a barrel and watched a video for 8 minutes to encourage attention and quiet sitting. A t test was used to analyze the data. The mean change in symmetry scores for the experimental group was 55.5 (82.5) and 11.9 (29.9) for the control group ($p = .24$). The mean change in percentage improvement from pretest to posttest was 64.6% (28.3) for the experimental group and −12.8% (88.8) for the control group ($p = .051$). The greatest improvement was noted in muscle groups displaying the highest asymmetry prior to hippotherapy.

In France, Bougard and Roblin (2003) used a computerized posture analysis platform to measure the change in balance before and after hippotherapy intervention with 16 participants. Diagnoses ranged from TBI to stroke to multiple sclerosis. All participants were able to maintain a standing position. The hippotherapy sessions lasted 20 to 25 minutes; the study did not mention how many sessions were provided. The authors reported improvement in balance but did not provide raw data or results of statistical analyses.

In Japan, Watakabe and colleagues (2003) studied the effect of hippotherapy on the contractures of hip adductors in children with cerebral palsy ages 5 to 14 ($N = 17$). All participants had never been on a horse. Riders rode on saddle pads with surcingles, once a month for 3 months, for 15–20-minute sessions. Hip abduction was measured when the resistance for rapid hip abduction occurred (F-ROM). Hip abduction was also measured by slowly abducting the hips (S-ROM). In general, S-ROM becomes smaller when soft tissues surrounding a joint (tendons, ligaments, and muscles) become shorter or stiffer. F-ROM represents the degree of spasticity in cerebral palsy. Measurements were taken by an orthopedic surgeon and two physical therapists; one of the therapists restrained pelvic movement by holding the participant's pelvis firmly, and the other therapist moved the lower limbs. The surgeon evaluated the ROM values. The mean differences before and after riding at the third riding session were analyzed. S-ROM increased by 7.2° in the right hip and 8.6° in the left hip, meaning the hip adduction contracture improved. The F-ROM also increased by 7° in the right hip and 7.6° in the left hip.

A second objective of Watakabe and colleagues (2003) was to explore accelerometry as a means of quantitative measurement of the interaction between rider and horse during riding. The rider–horse interaction of 3 experts without cerebral palsy and 3 beginners who had no riding experience was compared over the course of 1 year using two triaxial miniature accelerometer sensors, one applied to each rider and one applied to each horse. The results found no difference between beginners and experts while the horse walked. However, a distinct difference between beginners and experts was found in forward and backward acceleration at the trot. The beginner movements were uncoordinated, but the experts synchronized their movements with the horse's up-and-down movement. The beginners actually moved in a direction opposite of the horse. The investigators concluded that accelerometry provides useful information relating to the movement of both rider and horse.

Chandler (2003) examined the effect of summer camp at a therapeutic riding facility; although the study did not involve classic hippotherapy, its findings are nevertheless important to the occupational therapy profession. Participants included 4 girls and 8 boys ages 5 to 13 who were diagnosed with sensory modulation disorder by an occupational therapist. Two to 4 weeks prior to camp, the therapist administered a modified

interview format of the Canadian Occupational Performance Measure at the child's home. Families were then asked to identify three goals to be addressed at summer camp. The results of the Wilcoxon signed-rank test indicated that the change between precamp and postcamp ratings was statistically significant for performance and satisfaction ($p = .0001$), indicating overall positive change in the children's behavior. A limitation of the study was that, although it took place in a therapeutic riding facility and riding and horse care were included activities, there was no mention of a therapeutic riding intervention or related outcomes.

Pasquinelli and colleagues (2003) examined the effect of *therapeutic riding* (using the term interchangeably with *hippotherapy*) on extrapyramidal disorder. All 4 participants were male, ranging in age from 3 to 14. According to the Gross Motor Function Measure (Palisano, Rosenbaum, Walter, Wood, & Galuppi, 1997), 2 of the participants were at Level V (no independent mobility), 1 was at Level II (ambulatory indoors on level surfaces), and 1 was at Level IV (independent mobility with power wheelchair). Participants received ongoing 50-minute therapeutic riding using an English saddle. Sessions were videotaped every 3 months for the first year, then yearly thereafter. Video then is played in slow motion, and the following factors are analyzed: torsion dystonia, opisthotonus, stiffness, segmentary inconsistency, involuntary movement, functional competency, tone, strength, and timing. The time needed to maintain the positive effects achieved while riding, on the ground, was calculated. Results were presented per participant, thus a case series design. The authors concluded that a reduction in involuntary movement and dystonic postural patterns was observed during the initial therapeutic riding session. As riding progressed, a decrease in reflexes such as the startle, decrease in spasticity, and improvements in tone and timing allowed for the development of riding skills in some of the participants, meaning that the intervention facilitated the development of a functional skill.

Ionatamishvili, Tsverava, Loria, Avaliani, and Rukhadze (2004) studied an intervention group of 50 children with cerebral palsy (30 dystonic, 20 spastic) and a control group of 50 children who received therapy using Bobath techniques. Unfortunately, the control group is not described. Ride therapy sessions occurred 3 to 5 times per week for 90 to 120 minutes for 2 to 4 months; participants took turns riding for 3 to 5 minutes, then would take a break and ride again. A point system was devised to measure spasticity, dystonia, and the motor activity of the horse. Prior to intervention, the groups had no significant difference in points. A significant difference ($p < .001$) was found postintervention, however. The authors noted that ride therapy involves more active participation than Bobath therapy, resulting in an improved sense of self-control and increased motivation.

Debuse (2003) found that physiotherapists in England and Germany rated the benefit of hippotherapy to children with cerebral palsy as 8 or higher on a scale of 1 to 10. Regulation of muscle tone was rated as the most important effect of hippotherapy, followed by coordination and sensory input, then psychological benefit. One conclusion of the study was that physiotherapists are not really sure about what they should be measuring and how.

Conclusion

The evidence for hippotherapy has evolved internationally over the past 40 years. Many countries are engaged in research related to hippotherapy and therapeutic riding, perhaps because people with disabilities, along with horses, ponies, mules, or donkeys, are in all countries of the world (Lavric, Burja, & Zadnikar, 2000). It could be speculated that therapeutic riding is more available in medically underserved countries than in those that have modern, state-of-the-art rehabilitation facilities. Perhaps the countries with more developed rehabilitation—that do not consider hippotherapy or therapeutic riding a medically indicated intervention—could lend their science to the less-developed countries that are providing rehabilitation with available resources: horses.

Hippotherapy requires specialized training of a therapist or physiotherapist and thus is likely to be less available and less understood than therapeutic riding. For example, a therapeutic riding program in Slovenia that began in 1992 with two donated, 3-year-old, untrained horses has as its goal recognition of hippotherapy and organization of hippotherapy seminars (Lavric et al., 2000). Although the quality of the available studies vary from region to region, the ideas under investigation are plentiful and worthy of further study.

This chapter reviewed 75 research studies ranging from randomized control trials to single case studies. Movement of the horse was the independent variable for the majority of the studies; four of the studies compare hippotherapy with more traditional neurodevelopmental treatments. Outcome measures have varied from digestive, cardiac, and respiratory function to spinal health, posture, muscle tone, gait, balance, and range of motion. Initially, in the 1970s, hippotherapy was investigated as an intervention for scoliosis, kyphosis, and cerebral palsy. More recent studies have included individuals with autism, brain injury, multiple sclerosis and spinal cord injury.

Although the evidence for hippotherapy and therapeutic riding presented in this chapter is not conclusive, many interesting study designs and intervention effects have been explored. Hippotherapy researchers are an international community. Terminology varies across cultures and translations and, indeed, within publications. In fact, the field of occupational therapy is not recognized internationally. The underlying theme, however, is that evidence from around the world suggest that the horse is being used successfully in medically based interventions.

References

Achenbach, T. M., & Edelbrock, C. (1983). *Child Behavior Checklist and Revised Child Behavior Profile.* Burlington: University of Vermont.

Armstrong, C. A., Sandilands, M. L., Myco, F. M., & Miller, D. (1988). *Validation of horse riding as a therapy for physically and mentally handicapped adults.* Paper presented at the 6th International Therapeutic Riding Congress, Toronto.

Bain, A. (1965). Pony riding for the disabled. *Physiotherapy, 51,* 263–265.

Baker, E. A. (1991). *A comparison of change in flexible kyphosis of the trunk pre- and post-hippotherapy.* Paper presented at the 7th International Therapeutic Riding Congress, Aarhus, Denmark.

Baumann, J. U. (1974). *Therapeutic exercise on horseback for children with neurogenic disorders of movement.* Paper presented at the 3rd International Conference on Riding for the Disabled, Warwick, England.

Benda, W., McGibbon, N. H., & Grant, K. L. (2003). Improvements in muscle symmetry in children with cerebral palsy after equine-assisted therapy (hippotherapy). *Journal of Alternative and Complementary Medicine, 9,* 817–825.

Bertoti, D. (1988). Effect of therapeutic horseback riding on posture in children with cerebral palsy. *Physical Therapy, 68,* 1505–1512.

Bertotto, D. B. (1988). Therapeutic riding conferences—Positive progress. *Proceedings of the 6th International Therapeutic Riding Congress.* Toronto, Ontario: International Therapeutic Riding Congress.

Biery, M. J., & Kauffman, N. (1989). The effects of therapeutic horseback riding on balance. *Adapted Physical Activity Quarterly, 6,* 221–229.

Biery, M. J., & Kauffman, N. (1996). The effects of therapeutic horseback riding on balance. *Scientific and Educational Journal of Therapeutic Riding.*

Bougard, P. M., & Roblin, M. (2003). *Re-education of the postural stability of the trunk with equestrian therapy—Evaluation of the efficacy of the technique for improving the postural tonus using an analytical platform.* Paper presented at the 11th International Congress: The Complex Influence of Therapeutic Horse Riding, Budapest.

Boysen, T. (1991). *The education system for therapeutic riding in Norway.* Paper presented at the 7th International Therapeutic Riding Congress, Aarhus, Denmark.

Braun, S., Msall, M. E., & Granger, C. V. (1991). *Manual for the Functional Independence Measure for children (WeeFIM) Version 1.4.* Buffalo: State University of New York, Center for Functional Assessment Research.

Brock, B. J. (1988). *Therapy on horseback: Psychomotor and psychological change in disabled adults.* Paper presented at the 6th International Therapeutic Riding Congress, Toronto.

Bruininks, R. H. (1978). *Bruininks–Oseretsky Test of Motor Proficiency: Examiner's manual.* Circle Pines, MN: American Guidance Services.

Burke, R. E., Fahn, S., & Marsden, C. D. (1985). Validity and reliability of a rating scale for the primary torsion dystonia. *Neurology, 35,* 73–77.

Chandler, C. (2003). Sensory integration and therapeutic riding at summer camp: Occupational performance outcomes. *Physical and Occupational Therapy in Pediatrics, 23,* 51–65.

Chassaigne, R. (1870). *Physiologie de l'equitation, se son application a l'hygiene et a la therapeutique.* Paris: University of Paris.

Cook, R. (1997). Remedial ridging therapy: A study of a traumatic brain injured adult. In B. T. Engel (Ed.), *Rehabilitation with the aid of a horse* (pp. 249–272). Durango, CO: Barbara Engel Therapy Services.

Cratty, B. J. (1967). *Development sequences of perceptual–motor tasks: Movement activities for neurologically handicapped and retarded children and youth.* Palo Alto, CA: Peek.

Debuse, D. (2003). *An exploration of German and UK physiotherapists' views of the effects of hippotherapy on patients with cerebral palsy and the measurement of these effects.* Paper presented at the 11th International Congress: The Complex Influence of Therapeutic Horse Riding, Budapest, Hungary.

Exner, G., Engelmann, A., Lange, K., & Wenck, B. (1994). Basic principles and effects of hippotherapy within the comprehensive treatment of paraplegic patients. *Rehabilitation, 33,* 39–43.

Fleck, E. (1997). Hippotherapy: Mechanics of human walking and horseback riding. In B. T. Engel (Ed.), *Rehabilitation with the aid of a horse* (pp. 153–173). Durango, CO: Barbara Engel Therapy Services.

Folio, M. R., & Fewell, R. R. (1983). *Peabody Developmental Motor Scales Manual.* Allen, TX: DLM Teaching Resources.

Fox, J., & Peterson, B. (1997). Enduring effects of hippotherapy on passive hip abduction in children with spastic cerebral palsy. In B. T. Engel (Ed.), *Rehabilitation with the aid of a horse* (pp. 277–296). Durango, CO: Barbara Engel Therapy Services.

Fox, V. M., Lawlor, V. A., & Luttges, M. W. (1984). Pilot study of novel test instrumentation to evaluate therapeutic horseback riding. *Adapted Physical Activity Quarterly, 1,* 30–36.

Freeman, G., Wise, D., Nicodemus, C., & Osborn, D. K. (1997). A comparative instrumented kinematic analysis of the pelvic movement of four horses trained for hippotherapy. In B. T. Engel (Ed.), *Rehabilitation with the aid of a horse.* Durango, CO: Barbara Engel Therapy Services.

Gottwald, A., & Biewald, N. (1981). New aspects in the treatment of Scheuermann's disease with hippotherapy. *Zeitschrift für Orthopädie, 119,* 351–355.

Haehl, V., Guiliani, C., & Lewis, C. (1999). Influence of hippotherapy on the kinematics and functional performance of two children with cerebral palsy. *Pediatric Physical Therapy, 11,* 89–101.

Haley, S. M., Coster, W. J., Ludlow, L. H., Haltiwanger, J. T., & Andrellos, P. J. (1992). *Pediatric evaluation of disability inventory (PEDI). Version 1.0.* Boston: New England Medical Center Hospitals.

Hansen, K. (1997). A group case study: Hippotherapy as a means of improving gross motor function in children with cerebral palsy. In B. T. Engel (Ed.), *Rehabilitation with the aid of a horse* (pp. 233–240). Durango, CO: Barbara Engel Therapy Services.

Harris, A., Pulliam, R., Coffman, C., Rehkop, M., & Schroader, D. (1997). *Comparison of postural trunk response in human walking vs. horseback riding using EMG and 3-D kinematic analysis.* Paper presented at the 9th International Therapeutic Riding Congress, Denver, CO.

Harter, S. (1985). *Manual for the Self-Perception Profile for Children.* Denver: University of Denver.

Heine, B. (1997). An introduction to hippotherapy. *NARHA STRIDES, 3*(2), 10–13.

Heipertz, W. (1981). *Therapeutic riding. Medicine, education, sports.* Ottawa: National Printers. (Original work published 1977)

Hoff, J. P. (1994). *Analysis of manual gripping during therapeutic riding in a rehabilitation's project.* Paper presented at the 8th International Therapeutic Riding Congress, Hamilton, New Zealand.

Ionatamishvili, N., Tsverava, D., Loria, M., & Avaliani, L. A. (2001). Riding therapy rehabilitation methods of child cerebral palsy. *Federation of Riding for the Disabled International Scientific Journal, 7,* 51–57.

Ionatamishvili, N., Tsverava, D., Loria, M., & Avaliani, L. A. (2002). The advantages of ride therapy in different forms of infantile cerebral palsy (therapeutic riding). *Zh Nevrol Psikhiatr Im SS Korsakoval, 103*(2), 25–27.

Ionatamishvili, N., Tsverava, D., Loria, M., Avaliani, L., & Rukhadze, M. (2004). Ride therapy—Method of teaching and development of movement habit among the children with cerebral palsy. *Scientific and Educational Journal of Therapeutic Riding, 10,* 45–50.

Kulichova, J., & Zenklova, J. (1996). The influence of horseback riding under the supervision of a sports medicine doctor on the posture of children and young adults. *Scientific and Educational Journal of Therapeutic Riding.*

Kuprian, W. (1981). Hippotherapy and riding therapy as physiotherapeutic treatment methods. In K. Heipertz (Ed.), *Therapeutic riding—Medicine, education, sports* (pp. 14–15). Ottawa, ON: National Printers.

Land, G., Errington-Povalac, E., & Paul, S. (2001). The effects of therapeutic riding on sitting posture in individuals with disabilities. *Occupational Therapy in Health Care, 14,* 1–12.

Lavric, A., Burja, C., & Zadnikar, M. (2000). *Therapeutic riding in Slovenia.* Paper presented at the 10th International Therapeutic Riding Conference, Anger-Saumur, France.

Lechner, H. E., Feldhaus, S., Gudmundsen, L., Hegemann, D., Michel, D., Zach, G. A., et al. (2003). The short-term effect of hippotherapy on spasticity in patients with spinal cord injury. *Spinal Cord, 41,* 502–505.

MacKay-Lyons, M., Conway, C., & Roberts, W. (1988). Effects of therapeutic riding on patients with multiple sclerosis: A preliminary trial. *Physiotherapy Canada, 40,* 104–109.

MacKinnon, J. R., Noh, S., Lariviere, J., MacPhail, A., Allan, D. E., Laliberte, D. (1995). A study of therapeutic effects of horseback riding for children with. *Physical and Occupational Therapy in Pediatrics, 15,* 17–34.

MacPhail, H. E. A., Edwards, J., Golding, J., Miller, K., Mosier, C., & Zwiers, T. (1998). Trunk postural reactions in children with and without cerebral palsy during therapeutic horseback riding. *Pediatric Physical Therapy, 10,* 143–147.

Martin, K. S., & Stormont-Smith, J. (1997). T.H.E. C.H.A.P.S. hippotherapy pilot project: A case study. In B. T. Engel (Ed.), *Rehabilitation with the aid of a horse* (pp. 227–231). Durango, CO: Barbara Engel Therapy Services.

Mattila-Rautiainen, S. (2000). Biomechanical aspects to study riders' lumbar and spinal area movements in therapeutic riding. *Federation of Riding for the Disabled International Scientific Journal.*

Mattila-Rautiainen, S., Korhonen, T., Nyman, M., & Tossavainen, S. (2000). *An experimental study of the effects of riding with chronic low back pain patients.* Paper presented at the 10th International Therapeutic Riding Conference, Anger-Saumur, France.

McGibbon, N., Andrade, C. K., Widerer, G., & Cintas, H. L. (1998). Effect of equine-movement therapy program on gait, energy expenditure, and motor function in children with spastic cerebral palsy: A pilot study. *Developmental Medicine and Child Neurology, 40,* 754–762.

Palisano, R., Rosenbaum, P., Walter, S., Wood, E., & Galuppi, B. (1997). Gross motor function classification system for cerebral palsy. *Developmental Medicine and Child Neurology, 39,* 214–223.

Papini, M., Pasquinelli, A., Allori, P., & Biagini, B. (1995). *Treatment of extrapyramidal disorders in children with sulpiride: Preliminary report.* Paper presented at the 7th Annual Meeting European Academy of Childhood Disability, Intern Sven Jerring Symposium, Stockholm.

Pfotenhauer, M., Leyerer, U., David, E., Schemm, S., Larsson-Pfotenhauer, E., Rimpau, W., et al. (1991). *Hippotherapy—Scientific programme in Herdecke. An example. Registration of hippotherapeutic effects by evaluating acceleration with walking patients suffering from multiple sclerosis.* Paper presented at the 7th International Therapeutic Riding Congress, Aarhus, Denmark.

Ricotti, S., Citterio, D. N., Alfonsi, E., Bilucaglia, E., Carenzio, G., & DallaToffola, E. (1991). *Horse riding therapy: Neuro–motor rehabilitation.* Paper presented at the 7th International Therapeutic Riding Congress, Aarhus, Denmark.

Riede, D. (1988). *Physiotherapy on the horse* (P. A. Dusenbury, Trans.). Riderwood, MD: Therapeutic Riding Services. (Original work published 1986)

Russell, D. J., Rosenbaum, P. L., Cadman, D. T., Gowland, C., Hardy, C., & Jarvis, S. (1989). The Gross Motor Functional Measure: A means to evaluate the effects of physical therapy. *Developmental Medicine and Child Neurology, 31,* 241–352.

Sachkov, R. (1997). *Objectification of hippotherapy efficiency.* Paper presented at the 9th International Therapeutic Riding Congress, Denver, CO.

Sahraoui, R. (2000). *Influence of riding therapy on postural steadiness in children with cerebral palsy.* Paper presented at the 10th International Therapeutic Riding Conference, Anger-Saumur, France.

Selvinen, S. S. (1997). The effect of riding therapy on the walk and leg movement of patients with multiple sclerosis. In B. T. Engel (Ed.), *Rehabilitation with the aid of a horse* (pp. 3–14). Durango, CO: Barbara Engel Therapy Services.

Snir, D., Dlin, R., Ayalon, A., Yazdi, O., & Inbar, O. (1988). *Effects of therapeutic riding on disabled children.* Paper presented at the 6th International Therapeutic Riding Congress, Toronto.

Sparrow, S., Balla, D., & Cicchetti, D. (1984). *Vineland Adaptive Behavior Scales: Survey form manual.* Circle Pines, MN: American Guidance Service.

Spink, J. (1993). *Developmental riding therapy: A team approach to assessment and treatment.* Tucson, AZ: Therapy Skill Builders.

Sportwiss, Heipertz-Hengst, C., & Wohlschlegel, A. (1997). *Evaluation of outcome in hippotherapy.* Paper presented at the 9th International Therapeutic Riding Congress, Denver, CO.

Sterna, J. A., Rogers, B., France, A. P., & Vokes, D. A. (2002). Horseback riding in children with cerebral palsy: Effect on gross motor function. *Developmental Medicine and Child Neurology, 44,* 301–308.

Strauss, I. (1995). *Hippotherapy* (M. Takeuchi, Trans.). Pickering, ON: Ontario Therapeutic Riding Association.

Strauss, I. (1998). Hippotherapy—Its unique position within physiotherapy. In Deutsches Kuratorium für Therapeutisches Reiten e.V. (Ed.), *Therapeutic riding in Germany* (pp. 15–17). Warendorf, Germany.

Stykes, M., Gouge, D., Newstead, A., Freeman, G., Tomberlin, J. A., & Mossberg, K. (1997). The effects of therapeutic horseback riding on balance in persons with brain injury. In B. T. Engel (Ed.), *Rehabilitation with the aid of a horse* (pp. 127–135). Durango, CO: Barbara Engel Therapy Services.

Tauffkirchen, E. (1978). [Hippotherapy: A supplementary treatment for motion disturbance caused by cerebral palsy.] *Padiatr Padol, 13,* 405–411.

Toffola, E. D., Bar, D., Petrucci, L., Pfazza, F., & Ricotti, S. (1988). *Clinical and instrumental evaluation in patients suffering from infantile brain damage and undergoing hippotherapy.* Paper presented at the 6th International Therapeutic Riding Congress, Toronto.

Tolson, P. (Ed.). (1997). *Therapeutic horseback riding and behavior change in children with autism: A single subject study.* Durango, CO: Barbara Engel Therapy Services.

Tsverava, D., Rukhadze, M., & Loria, M. (2000). *Integration of hippotherapy in the system of physical rehabilitation of spine diseases (osteochondrosis, scoliosis).* Paper presented at the 10th International Therapeutic Riding Conference, Anger-Saumur, France.

VanLeit, B. (1995). Using the case base method to develop clinical reasoning skills in problem based learning. *American Journal of Occupational Therapy, 49,* 349–353.

Veicsteinas, A., Melorio, G., Turner, J., Belleri, M., & Sarchi, P. (1991). *Heart rate as an index of cardiovascular stress during therapeutic horse riding.* Paper presented at the 7th International Therapeutic Riding Congress, Aarhus, Denmark.

Veicsteinas, A., Melorio, G., & Sarchi, P. (1994). Energy requirement and cardiorespiratory readjustment during therapeutic horse riding in disabled. *Scientific and Educational Journal of Therapeutic Riding,* 23–31.

Wasserman, R., & Keeney, A. M. (1997). Hippotherapy for the child with cerebral palsy. In B. T. Engel (Ed.), *Rehabilitation with the aid of a horse* (pp. 241–248). Durango, CO: Barbara Engel Therapy Services.

Watakabe, M., Mita, K., Akataki, K., Ito, K., Oki, T., Kaneko, M., et al. (2003). *Biomechanical analysis of therapeutic effects of horseback riding.* Paper presented at the 11th International Congress: The Complex Influence of Therapeutic Horse Riding, Budapest, Hungary.

Webster, A., Pfotenhauer, M., David, E., Leyerer, U., Rimpau, W., Aldridge, D., et al. (1994). *Registration and evaluation of effects of hippotherapy with patients suffering from multiple sclerosis by means of electromyography and acceleration measurement.* Paper presented at the 8th International Therapeutic Riding Congress, Hamilton, New Zealand.

Wheeler, A. (1997). A case study of a boy diagnosed with spina bifida. In B. T. Engel (Ed.), *Rehabilitation with the aid of a horse* (pp. 221–226). Durango, CO: Barbara Engel Therapy Services.

Winchester, P., Kendall, K., Peters, H., Sears, N., & Winkley, T. (2002). The effect of therapeutic horseback riding on gross motor function and gait speed in children who are developmentally delayed. *Physical and Occupational Therapy in Pediatrics, 22*(3/4), 37–51.

Would, J. (1996). Study on posture and the development of balance in disabled riders. *Scientific and Educational Journal of Therapeutic Riding.*

Would, J. (2000). *Research into the effects of hippotherapy on walking ability of children with cerebral palsy.* Paper presented at the 10th International Therapeutic Riding Conference, Anger-Saumur, France.

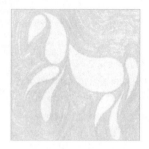

Far back,
far back in our dark soul
the horse prances.
—D. H. Lawrence

CHAPTER 8

Hippotherapy and Evidence-Based Practice

Beatriz C. Abreu, PhD, OTR, FAOTA; Joanne S. Jones, MS, OTR;
and Karin J. Opacich, PhD, OTR/L, MHPE, FAOTA

One way to become competent in the use of hippo-therapy in occupational therapy is to become knowledge-able in the process of evidence-based practice (EBP). Clinicians use EBP in their decision-making to develop and support effective clinical programs as well as main-tain efficient assessment and intervention procedures (Tickle-Degnen, 2002). Today, every occupational therapy practitioner is responsible for the validation of his or her occupational therapy services; institutions' providers, clients, and payers expect and demand support for the services provided (Holm, 2000; Ottenbacher & Hinderer, 2001). Practitioners, however, face the chal-lenge of searching through and sorting out a dramatic explosion of information, which includes impressive research advances. In addition, the evidence is used on a limited basis to support clinical practice.

This chapter introduces EBP as it applies to the practice of hippotherapy. The chapter also contains a review of the evidence-based literature that supports and guides the practice of hippotherapy for a variety of con-ditions. After describing the five steps involved in the process of implementing EBP, the chapter identifies examples, strengths, and limitations of the practice. It concludes with research and education implications for hippotherapy using EBP.

Evidence-Based Practice: Definition and Relation to Hippotherapy

Evidence-based practice is the formal gathering and synthesis of information from research studies by using a systematic research review to determine and conduct best clinical practice. This method is derived from evidence-based medicine (Law, 2002; Sackett, Straus, Richardson, Rosenberg, & Haynes, 2000). Clinical prac-tice should provide sufficient evidence to establish the

effect of occupational therapy services on health out-comes, and the benefits of the outcomes should show that occupational therapy interventions are effective, beneficial, and cost-effective (Abreu, 1998; Foto, 1996). Evidence-based practice is an evolving process. It had its roots in medical outcomes, was transformed to evidence-based medicine, expanded into evidence-based practice, and more recently further expanded to the broad area of evidence-based health care (Ottenbacher, 2002). The distinctions among these concepts are not clear and continue to develop.

For this chapter, the authors determined the studies for hippotherapy in a broad-ranging search that included the keywords *hippotherapy, horseback riding,* and *horses and rehabilitation.* Computer-aided searches were conducted using the following databases: PubMed, Medline, Cumulative Index to Nursing & Allied Health Literature (CINAHL), PsycINFO, Cochrane Register, and Occupational Therapy Bibliographic System. An extensive manual search and cross-referencing from review and original articles also were performed. Articles not written in English were excluded. Numerous studies, however, were reported in the German literature. The results are shown in Table 8.1.

The inclusion criteria for this summary of evidence are as follows: (1) studies that involved use of horses as a rehabilitation tool or (2) studies that involved use of horses for leisure and recreation. Studies were not included in the summary if they were anecdotal or pro-motional material for programs.

Five Steps to Follow in Evidence-Based Practice

A complete description of the EBP process for managers is beyond the scope of this chapter. Nevertheless, it is

Table 8.1. Results of Database Searches for Hippotherapy-Related Publications

Database	Time Frame	Search Term	No. of Articles
PubMed		Hippotherapy	17
		Horseback riding	50
		Rehabilitation and horses	63
Medline	1966–November Week 1, 2003	Hippotherapy	17
		Horseback riding	78
		Rehabilitation and horses	44
CINAHL	1982–November Week 1, 2003	Hippotherapy	13
		Horseback riding	77
		Rehabilitation and horses	4
PsycINFO		Hippotherapy	5
		Horseback riding	0
		Rehabilitation and horses	5
Cochrane Register		Hippotherapy	3
		Horseback riding	3
		Rehabilitation and horses	1
Occupational Therapy Bibliographic System		Hippotherapy	25
		Horseback riding	16
		Horses and rehabilitation	1

possible to describe some highlights of the five steps for using EBP in clinical reasoning and problem solving: (1) set the question, (2) search and sort the evidence, (3) critically appraise the evidence, (4) apply to practice (reject or accept), and (5) self-assess.

1. Set the Question

The first step is to turn the clinical problem into the form of a question. The question must be framed within the structure of the evidence-based process. Therefore, the questions are categorized from a medical literature perspective: (1) therapy and prevention, (2) etiology and harm, (3) prognosis, (4) diagnosis, and (5) economic analysis (Sackett et al., 2000). Additionally, knowledge gaps in hippotherapy practice, as well as specific client needs, may guide the formulation of questions.

The best research outcomes provide the best evidence for hippotherapy practice. EBP provides therapists with opportunities for better client care, optimal program evaluation, and quality improvement systems. The therapist can frame evidence-based searching related to client care questions in many ways.

For example, two types of treatment questions within the categories deal with effectiveness and efficacy. Effectiveness studies answer the questions, Did clients receiving hippotherapy improve? How much did they improve? Evidence on treatment efficacy in hippotherapy, however, is difficult to obtain. This type of evidence

examines the relation of the intervention to outcome measures under controlled or optimal conditions (Ottenbacher & Hinderer, 2001) and can answer the question, Which hippotherapy treatment made the clients better?

Controlled experiments have two or more groups of participants; one group receives the treatment under investigation, and a second group of study participants receive a standard treatment or a placebo intervention (a treatment with no known therapeutic value). Efficacy evidence requires the use of the most rigorous experimental research designs: *randomized controlled trials (RCTs),* which allocate participants to treatment or control groups in an unsystematic, or random, fashion that guarantees no selection bias. RCTs are valued as having the most powerful experimental design and evidence for evaluating the effectiveness of a treatment.

Blinding is another way of enhancing quality and eliminating bias in research. In single-blind studies, participants do not know which type of intervention they are receiving; in double-blind studies, neither participants nor the investigators know which treatment (experimental or control) they are receiving.

2. Search for and Sort the Evidence

The second step is a systematic and explicit search to identify, select, and summarize evidence. It is a complex and labor-intensive task. The EBP process does not include searching traditional textbooks as sources of evidence because they are not updated yearly, are lightly referenced, and many times do not provide evidence in support of the statements made in the book (Sackett et al., 2000). EBP is best conducted through the use of scientific databases. Access to certain databases requires user codes, which are readily available to college students and faculty but are less accessible to therapists. One free public access database is PubMed (www.ncbi.nlm.nih.gov/PubMed/), which, in addition to citations, links to other related Web resources. Other useful databases are listed in Table 8.1.

Regardless of the database used, searches for evidence can be conducted using two major categories of sources: primary and secondary. *Primary research* or *primary publications* are studies that report original analytical investigations; they can be experimental or observational. *Secondary studies* are those that summarize and draw conclusions from primary research or previously published or unpublished studies (McKibbon, 1999). Secondary studies include meta-analyses; systematic reviews; nonsystematic reviews; and other documents, such as editorials and practice guidelines. EBP only draws from meta-analyses and systematic reviews. A meta-analysis is a quantitative analysis of data from published scientific papers that estimates treatment effects of a particular intervention. A systematic review attempts to summarize published and unpublished material; the review uses objective and orderly methods to avoid bias in the report and synthesis of the research studies (Egger & Smith, 1997).

A useful resource for locating high-quality evidence from primary and secondary publications is the Cochrane Library database. The Cochrane Library is an electronic-format collection of information, available from university libraries on the Internet and in CD-ROM format, developed by the Cochrane Collaboration Group to help people make informed decisions about health care.

3. Critically Appraise and Formally Evaluate the Evidence

The third step is critical appraisal and formal evaluation of the evidence to determine its soundness, magnitude, and usefulness to the practice question. Guidelines for grading evidence vary and reflect the complexity of the research design used during the investigation (Geyman, Deyo & Ramsey, 2000; McKibbon, 1999; Sackett et al., 2000). The level of evidence in primary research originally was ranked by Sackett using numerical indexes

from I to V or letter indexes from A to D, where I or A represents the greatest level of rigor and control. The ranking is based on the characteristics of the research design, the number of study participants, and the level of *external* and *internal validity*. External validity represents the extent to which the findings of the study are relevant to participants and settings beyond those in the study. Internal validity is the extent to which the results of a study can be attributed to the intervention rather than to the flaws in the research design. Readers are referred to the Center for Evidence-Based Medicine at http://cebm.jr2.ox.ac.uk for more detailed appraisal criteria for interventions.

4. Apply Scientific Research Findings to Practice

The fourth step is the outcome of the search process. The systematic integration of the evidence with client factors, institution factors, and staff expertise results in either rejection or integration of the research findings into clinical practice. Clinical decisions using EBP are based largely on the quality of quantitative research design (e.g., the power of the study and the use of randomization techniques in treatment studies).

5. Evaluate the Process

This step involves appraisal of the procedures undertaken in the preceding four steps and reflection on the way in which the clinician formulated the question, tracked down the evidence, critically evaluated the evidence, and integrated the evidence into practice (McKibbon, 1999; Sackett et al., 2000). This necessary step determines the value of using this process within the occupational therapy workplace.

Review of the Evidence on Hippotherapy

For people who share an affinity for horses, learning to ride can be a satisfying and awesome endeavor. Success in riding an animal whose size and athleticism so far exceed human capabilities hinges on physics, communication, and collaboration. *Horse-mediated therapy* (also known as *equine-assisted therapy, therapeutic riding,* or *hippotherapy,* depending on the researcher and the focus of the research) is a multidimensional intervention that appeals to people across the life span as well as across a spectrum of abilities and disabilities. The potential for manipulation of the dimensions of this approach to therapy is nearly limitless, especially for those skilled with horses who understand the intricacies of therapy. The variables inherent in horse, rider, context, equipment, and approach make horse-mediated therapy ideal for scientific inquiry. Moreover, horse-mediated therapy lends itself to quantitative, qualitative, and triangulated investigative strategies. Limited studies, however, support the efficacy or effectiveness of hippotherapy.

Horseback riding has been used therapeutically for centuries. Health professionals frequently use horses as a tool in rehabilitation. Many physical and psychological benefits of therapeutic horseback riding have been reported (All, Loving, & Crane, 1999; MacKinnon, Noh, Laliberte, Lariviere, & Allan, 1995), including recreational, psychosocial, and physical benefits (Platford, 1999). Physical benefits include improved strength and agility, muscle tone, and weight-bearing ability (Bertoti, 1988); improved standing ability (MacKinnon et al., 1995); and enhanced self-esteem, self-image, and interpersonal skills (Bliss, 1997). Although the desired outcome of horse-mediated therapy may be different for each group of riders, understanding its many dimensions and phenomena can enlighten and support those who want to use horses as therapeutic agents.

Horse-mediated therapy uses the multidimensional movement of the horse to improve posture, balance, and function (Engel, 1997). The rider's body smoothly and rhythmically moves with the horse in a manner similar to the human gait, promoting normal movement. Clinicians argue that the displacement of the riders' center of pressure produced during horseback riding can facilitate righting and equilibrium responses (MacPhail et al., 1998). This type of treatment is considered an occupational therapy approach; however, it is also considered under other disciplines that provide rehabilitation, leisure, and recreation services (Bracher, 2000; DePauw, 1986; Heine, 1997; Whalley, 1980). Occupational therapists may analyze and perceive the challenges of riding differently, because riding is subtle and is not as easy as it appears.

The benefits of horse-mediated therapy differ among populations. If the goals of riding are largely physical, then evidence pertaining to its effects on balance, strength, and coordination ought to be gathered to support therapeutic decisions. If the goals are psychosocial, social outcomes need to be clearly articulated and tracked. For example, horse-mediated riding for autistic children might entail studying improvement in following a sequence of activities related to riding. In yet another situation, the desired outcome might be to enhance neurosensory processing to improve tolerance to tactile stimuli (e.g., grooming and touching the horse) or tolerance of movement (e.g., changing pace while riding). Understanding the interplay between physical demands and psychosocial phenomena will best illustrate the unique value of horse-mediated therapies.

Although minimal research about hippotherapy is available in the literature, a few descriptive studies report benefits in people with disability. The systematic review performed for this chapter did not find any RCTs. Most of the studies' sample sizes were small; the highest *N* was 29 (Cawley, Cawley & Retter, 1994). The populations studied were primarily children with cerebral palsy and mixed physical and other disabilities. The effectiveness of hippotherapy has been measured mostly at the impairment level, with subjective outcome measures. Subjective quality-of-movement assessments included muscle tone, coordination, and postural control. The length of the programs ranged from 5 to 24 weeks, and follow-up was minimal. In general, the studies reviewed described subjective positive effects; however, given the limitations of the research design of the studies, the review of the literature did not provide sufficient evidence about the efficacy of hippotherapy. The studies reviewed are summarized here and in Table 8.2:

- Bertoti (1988) reported on an observational postural assessment tool used with children with cerebral palsy before and after participation in a 10-week therapeutic riding program; the children benefited at the impairment level in areas of muscle tone, posture, and balance, and their functional skills improved as well.
- Biery and Kauffman (1989) reported improvement in postural alignment in quadruped positions in children and young adults with the diagnosis of Down syndrome as the result of a 6-month therapeutic riding program.
- Cawley, Cawley, and Retter (1994), in an 8-week study of 29 students ages 11 to 17 who had educational needs, reported a small increase in self-concept as measured by the Piers Harris Children's Concept Scale.
- MacPhail and colleagues (1998) studied the kinematics analysis of horse and rider in 13 children (6 children with cerebral palsy and 7 children without disability). They found that the children with cerebral palsy displaced the trunk almost twice as much and responded with less frequent equilibrium reactions than the children without disability.
- Haehl, Giuliani, and Lewis (1999) studied 2 children with cerebral palsy for more than 12 weeks and reported positive subjective effects in postural control and coordination that did not generalize to functional performance in the Pediatric Evaluation of Disability Inventory (PEDI).
- Land, Errington-Povalac, and Paul (2001) reported positive benefits in selected sitting postures in 3 children who participated in an 8-week therapeutic riding program.
- More recently, Sterba, Rogers, France, and Vokes (2002) demonstrated improved gross motor function

Table 8.2. Summary of Studies Reviewed

Study	Population	Condition	Length of Study	Outcome
Bertoti (1988)	Pediatric	Cerebral palsy	10 wks.	Improvements in muscle tone, posture, balance, and functional skills
Biery & Kauffman (1989)	Pediatric and young adults	Down syndrome	6 mos.	Improvements in postural alignment in quadruped positions
Cawley et al. (1993)	Pediatric, ages 11–17	Educational needs	8 wks.	Increase in self-concept (Piers Harris Children's Concept Scale)
MacPhail et al. (1998)	Pediatric	Cerebral palsy		Kinematics analysis demonstrating increased trunk displacement and less frequent equilibrium reactions
Haehl et al. (1999)	Pediatric	Cerebral palsy	12 wks.	Subjective improvements in postural control and coordination but no improvement in functional performance (PEDI)
Land et al. (2001)	Pediatric		8 wks.	Selected seated posture improvements
Sterba et al. (2002)	Pediatric	Cerebral palsy	18 wks.	Improved overall gross motor function (Gross Motor Function Measure & WeeFIM)
Blinde & McClung (1997)	Adults	Mixed physical disabilities		Improved sense of control in physical and social lives
Sykes et al. (1997)	Adults		20 wks.	Improved functional standing balance

in 17 children with cerebral palsy following 18 weeks of hippotherapy. Outcome measures used included the Gross Motor Function Measure and the WeeFIM (Sterba et al., 2002).

- Blinde and McClung (1997) reported positive, subjective benefits in sense of control in the physical and social lives of 23 adults with mixed physical disabilities after a program of hippotherapy.
- Sykes and colleagues (1997) described positive results in functional standing balance after a maximum of 20 weeks of hippotherapy intervention in 4 adults ages 18 and older.

Direct Care, Research, and Reflections on Education

Although EBP is being promoted in occupational therapy practice, not all the areas have been systematically investigated or their effectiveness supported. Hippotherapy is a specialty in occupational therapy practice that requires the following activities to improve its research base:

- Better outcome measures at all levels—impairment, disability, and participation
- More systematic qualitative and quantitative investigation
- Improved research designs.

EBP advocates quantitative research. Multiple methods of inquiry, however, can expand the understanding of the therapeutic relationship, cultural differences, and institutional philosophies and visions. Qualitative research and philosophical reflections on

hippotherapy also can expand our understanding of this specialty practice. A broad-based inquiry beyond EBP is needed to integrate the art and science of occupational therapy practice.

The process of imparting and acquiring knowledge about EBP in occupational therapy practice is in its early stages. Many organizations lack both a research culture and time for research as a result of their heavy direct care commitments in the clinic or teaching responsibilities. In addition, a limited number of role models are available for teaching and applying EBP. As a result, the attention to investigating and disseminating evidence of relevant studies is diminished. As increasing numbers of occupational therapists pursue postgraduate work, clinical research will become more integrated with educational institutions.

The responsibility of applying EBP needs to be accepted cautiously. Although occupational therapists are expected to incorporate research findings into their practice and be accountable to their clients and institutions, they often lack the research knowledge and workplace support to carry out EBP approaches. In addition, qualitative research that investigates the subjective and meaningful perceptions of clients', families', and caretakers' feelings and satisfaction during and after hippotherapy is essential.

References

Abreu, B. C. (1998). Additional uses for data. In J. Hinojosa & P. Kramer (Eds.), *Occupational therapy evaluation: Obtaining and interpreting data* (pp. 213–234). Bethesda, MD: American Occupational Therapy Association.

All, A. C., Loving, G. L., & Crane, L. L. (1999). Animals, horseback riding, and implications for rehabilitation therapy. *Journal of Rehabilitation, 65,* 49–57.

Bertoti, D. B. (1988). Effect of therapeutic horseback riding on posture in children with cerebral palsy. *Physical Therapy, 68,* 1505–1512.

Biery, M. J., & Kauffman, N. (1989). The effects of therapeutic horseback riding on balance. *Adapted Physical Activity Quarterly, 6,* 221–229.

Blinde, E. M., & McClung, L. R. (1997). Enhancing the physical and social self through recreational activity: Accounts of individuals with physical disabilities. *Adapted Physical Activity Quarterly, 14,* 327–344.

Bliss, B. (1997). Complementary therapies: Therapeutic horseback riding? *RN, 60,* 69–70.

Bracher, M. (2000). Therapeutic horse riding: What has this to do with occupational therapists? *British Journal of Occupational Therapy, 63,* 277–282.

Cawley, R., Cawley, D., & Retter, K. (1994). Therapeutic horseback riding and self-concept in adolescents with special educational needs. *Anthrozoös, 7,* 129–134.

DePauw, K. P. (1986). Horseback riding for individuals with disabilities: Programs, philosophy, and research. *Adapted Physical Activity Quarterly, 3,* 217–226.

Egger, M., & Smith, G. D. (1997). Meta-analysis: Potentials and promise. *British Medical Journal, 315,* 1371–1374.

Engel, B. T. (1997). *Rehabilitation with the aid of a horse: A collection of studies.* Durango, CO: Barbara Engel Therapy Services.

Foto, M. (1996). Nationally Speaking—Outcome studies: The what, why, how, and when. *American Journal of Occupational Therapy, 50,* 87–88.

Geyman, J. P., Deyo, R. A., & Ramsey, S. D. (Eds.). (2000). *Evidence-based clinical practice: Concepts and approaches.* Boston: Butterworth-Heinemann.

Haehl, V., Giuliani, C., & Lewis, C. (1999). Influence of hippotherapy on the kinematics and functional performance of two children with cerebral palsy. *Pediatric Physical Therapy, 11,* 89–101.

Heine, B. (1997). Hippotherapy. A multisystem approach to the treatment of neuromuscular disorders. *Australian Physiotherapy, 43,* 145–149.

Holm, H. A. (2000). Our mandate for the new millennium: Evidence-based practice. [2000 Eleanor Clarke Slagle Lecture]. *American Journal of Occupational Therapy, 54,* 575–585.

Land, G., Errington-Povalac, E., & Paul, S. (2001). The effects of therapeutic riding on sitting posture in individuals with disabilities. *Occupational Therapy in Health Care, 14,* 1–12.

Law, M. (Ed.). (2002). *Evidence-based rehabilitation: A guide to practice.* Thorofare, NJ: Slack.

MacKinnon, J. R., Noh, S., Laliberte, D., Lariviere, J., & Allan, D. E. (1995). Therapeutic horseback riding: A review of the literature. *Physical and Occupational Therapy in Pediatrics, 15,* 1–15.

MacPhail, H. E. A., Edwards, J., Golding, J., Miller, K., Mosier, C., & Zwiers, T. (1998). Trunk postural reactions in children with and without cerebral palsy during therapeutic horseback riding. *Pediatric Physical Therapy, 10,* 143–147.

McKibbon, A. (with Eady, A., & Marks, S.). (1999). *PDQ: Evidence-based principles and practice.* Hamilton, Ontario: B. C. Decker.

Ottenbacher, K. J. (2002, May). Evidence-based practice in rehabilitation. In Boston University (Ed.), *Faculty Summer Institute: Teaching evidence-based practice in rehabilitation professional curricula.* Boston: Boston University.

Ottenbacher, K. J., & Hinderer, S. R. (2001). Evidence-based practice: Methods to evaluate individual patient improvement. *American Journal of Physical Medicine and Rehabilitation, 80,* 786–796.

Platford, L. (1999). *The multiple effect of therapeutic horseback riding on adult patients with physical disabilities.* Unpublished master's thesis, Touro College, Dix Hills, New York.

Sackett, D. L., Straus, S. E., Richardson, W. S., Rosenberg, W., & Haynes, R. B. (2000). *Evidence-based medicine: How to practice and teach EBM* (2nd ed.). New York: Churchill Livingstone.

Sterba, J. A., Rogers, B. T., France, A. P., & Vokes, D. A. (2002). Horseback riding in children with cerebral palsy: Effect on gross motor function. *Developmental Medicine and Child Neurology, 44,* 301–308.

Sykes, M., Gouge, D., Newstead, A., Freeman, G., Tomberlin, J., & Mossberg, K. (1997). The effects of therapeutic horseback riding on balance in persons with brain injury. In B. T. Engel (Ed.), *Rehabilitation with the aid of a horse: A collection of studies* (pp. 127–144). Durango, CO: Barbara Engel Therapy Services.

Tickle-Degnen, L. (2002). Communicating evidence to clients, managers, and families. In M. Law (Ed.), *Evidence-based rehabilitation: A guide to practice* (pp. 221–254). Thorofare, NJ: Slack.

Whalley, K. R. (1980). Riding for the disabled: Improving the quality of life. *Occupational Therapy, 43,* 267–268.

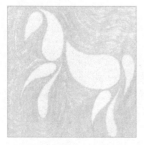

*Love means attention, which means
looking after the things we love.
We call this stable management.*
—George Morris

CHAPTER 9

Interrater Reliability of the GREAT Postural Rating Scale for Therapeutic Riding

*Linda A. Frease, MHS, OTR/L; Kay Walker, PhD, OTR/L, FAOTA;
and Orit Shechtman, PhD, OTR/L*

At the Fourth International Congress on Therapeutic Riding in 1982, the program committee recognized that it would be necessary to distinguish among distinct disciplines evolving under the umbrella term of therapeutic riding. The conference was divided into three topic areas: hippotherapy, remedial–educational riding and vaulting, and riding as sport (Klüwer, 1992).

Because therapeutic riding presents so many options for tailoring the intervention to the rider, it meets criteria for the three propositions central to the theory and practice of occupational therapy as summarized by Jarus (1994): "The client must be an active participant in the therapeutic process. Intervention should consist of purposeful activities in a structured environment. Adaptation of the environment and task presentation should produce desired responses in the client" (p. 810). Gliner (1985) suggested that the common ground between occupational therapy and motor control theory is the concept that the individual, the task, and the environment are inexorably linked. Shumway-Cook and Woollacott (2001) argued that "movement emerges from the interaction of three factors: the individual, the task, and the environment" (p. 2). The classically correct posture and alignment [task] of the rider [individual] is intended to facilitate the rider's adjustment of his or her own center of gravity [task] to the equilibrium changes of the horse [environment] while minimizing the energy expended by the rider (Seunig, 1956). Every movement of the horse elicits a reaction, or task solution, from the rider. Even at a standstill, a weight shift by the horse cues the rider to find a new strategy. The rider must perceive the weight shift and act to move his or her own weight to stay balanced over the horse.

Without doubt, the best sitting posture is obtained on horseback. The body is extremely well balanced above its seat base, and only small adjustments have to be made to its center of gravity to maintain this balance in posture. "On horseback there is a fixed amount of abduction increasing hip flexion and, therefore, an effective stabilization of the pelvic area" (Stewart & McQuilton, 1987, p. 137).

Sitting on the back of a moving horse is perhaps the only technique for improving posture and alignment that offers a rhythmically moving base of support in the context of a meaningful activity. Posture is a dynamic component of human function. It is not illogical to suggest that a dynamic technique, such as riding a horse, could be an effective modality for learning postural control.

Attempts to obtain evidence of functional improvement in posture as a result of participation in therapeutic riding programs have been marginally successful. Inconsistencies may be credited at least in part to insufficient research controls, small sample size, and inadequate measurement devices (Bertoti, 1988; Biery & Kauffman, 1989; Brock, 1985; Fox, Lawlor, & Luttges, 1984; MacKinnon et al., 1995). Several researchers have called for the development of instruments specific to the expected changes from riding horses (Brock, 1985; MacKinnon et al., 1995). Development of reliable measurement instruments could increase the statistical power of subsequent studies without requiring large groups of homogeneous participants (Leon, Marzuk, &

Portera, 1995). MacKinnon and colleagues (1995) cited the scarcity of "meaningful and responsive measures for therapeutic horseback riding" and recommended "development of measurement tools to assess and quantify meaningful improvements specifically related to therapeutic horseback riding" (p. 31). Brock (1985) had previously recommended the measure of posture in the riding position.

This chapter describes a study assessing the *Gainesville Riding* through *Equine-Assisted Therapy* (GREAT) scale, an instrument designed to assess the postural alignment of riders with disabilities sitting astride a horse and to determine the internal consistency and interrater reliability of the instrument.

Population

The postural alignment scale was designed for use with riders participating in therapeutic riding programs. It is applicable for use with riders of any age or disability who are able to sit independently, mounted astride and facing the horse's head. Raters were licensed practitioners of physical and occupational therapy who had completed the basic hippotherapy course offered by the American Hippotherapy Association (AHA).

Definitions

Correct postural alignment is defined as the alignment of body parts that results in minimum stress on the structures of the body. The operational definition for the study was the alignment of the body in which the head, shoulder, hip, and heel of a person mounted astride a horse and facing forward could be connected by an imaginary straight line with the line perpendicular to the support surface; this alignment earned a score of 0 in all categories on the GREAT scale (Figure 9.1).

Disability can be defined as any restriction resulting from an impairment of ability to perform an activity in the manner or within the range considered normal for humans (Hopkins & Smith, 1993, p. 784). The operational definition of disability for this study was the inability to maintain correct postural alignment, represented by scores other than 0 in all categories on the GREAT scale, while seated astride a horse (Figure 9.2).

Therapeutic riding is defined as the use of equine-oriented activities for the purpose of contributing positively to the cognitive, physical, emotional, and social well-being of people with disabilities. It is a generic term that encompasses all forms of equine-assisted therapy and incorporates hippotherapy. Hippotherapy is defined as the most passive form of therapeutic riding, in which

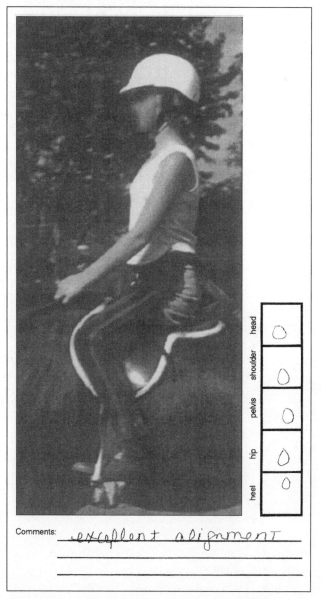

Figure 9.1. A rated sample image of rider without disabilities.

the movement of the horse is combined with positioning of the client/rider to facilitate appropriate reactions of the rider. Appropriate reactions vary depending on the rider but might include such items as postural alignment, relaxation of spastic muscles, weight shifts, or stability during gait transitions.

A *saddle* is defined as a piece of equipment secured to a horse's back for the purpose of increasing the comfort and security of a rider; it is attached by a girth that wraps around the horse. The saddle may be equipped with metal stirrups to support the rider's foot at the correct elevation. The stirrups are attached to the saddle

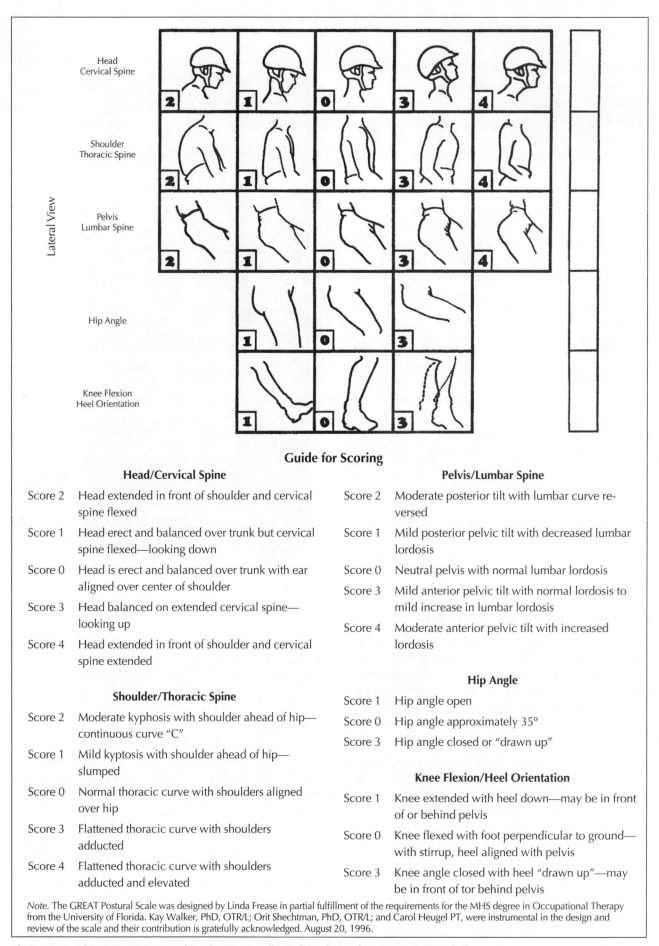

Guide for Scoring

Head/Cervical Spine

Score 2 Head extended in front of shoulder and cervical spine flexed

Score 1 Head erect and balanced over trunk but cervical spine flexed—looking down

Score 0 Head is erect and balanced over trunk with ear aligned over center of shoulder

Score 3 Head balanced on extended cervical spine—looking up

Score 4 Head extended in front of shoulder and cervical spine extended

Shoulder/Thoracic Spine

Score 2 Moderate kyphosis with shoulder ahead of hip—continuous curve "C"

Score 1 Mild kyptosis with shoulder ahead of hip—slumped

Score 0 Normal thoracic curve with shoulders aligned over hip

Score 3 Flattened thoracic curve with shoulders adducted

Score 4 Flattened thoracic curve with shoulders adducted and elevated

Pelvis/Lumbar Spine

Score 2 Moderate posterior tilt with lumbar curve reversed

Score 1 Mild posterior pelvic tilt with decreased lumbar lordosis

Score 0 Neutral pelvis with normal lumbar lordosis

Score 3 Mild anterior pelvic tilt with normal lordosis to mild increase in lumbar lordosis

Score 4 Moderate anterior pelvic tilt with increased lordosis

Hip Angle

Score 1 Hip angle open

Score 0 Hip angle approximately 35°

Score 3 Hip angle closed or "drawn up"

Knee Flexion/Heel Orientation

Score 1 Knee extended with heel down—may be in front of or behind pelvis

Score 0 Knee flexed with foot perpendicular to ground—with stirrup, heel aligned with pelvis

Score 3 Knee angle closed with heel "drawn up"—may be in front of tor behind pelvis

Note. The GREAT Postural Scale was designed by Linda Frease in partial fulfillment of the requirements for the MHS degree in Occupational Therapy from the University of Florida. Kay Walker, PhD, OTR/L; Orit Shechtman, PhD, OTR/L; and Carol Heugel PT, were instrumental in the design and review of the scale and their contribution is gratefully acknowledged. August 20, 1996.

Figure 9.2. The GREAT Postural Scale (*Gainsville Riding through Equine Assisted Therapy*).

with leather or fabric straps that may be adjusted in length. The operational definition is the all-purpose English-style synthetic (i.e., nonleather) saddle equipped with "Webber" stirrup leathers manufactured by Wintec and peacock-style safety stirrups. The alternative is a leather dressage saddle, model "Aherlich," manufactured by the Hopfner Company and equipped with stirrup leathers and stainless steel Fillis stirrups with angled treads or with offset Fillis stirrups with nonangled treads. Both types can be adjusted for length in increments of 1 inch.

Surcingle is operationally defined as a leather or elastic band fastened around the horse in front of the rider and used to secure a pad or series of pads placed on the horse's back to protect the horse and rider. The surcingle may be an elastic band approximately 3 inches wide that fits smoothly against the horse with no padding or protrusion, or it may consist of a padded leather loop that protrudes above the horse's back and serves as a handhold for the rider.

Literature Review

Heipertz, Heipertz-Hengst, Kroger, and Kuprian (1977) maintained that hippotherapy and riding therapy inhibited spasticity and resulted in more normalized muscle tone. Heipertz also stated that riding was able to stimulate static and dynamic equilibrium reflexes, improve coordination and proprioception, and complement techniques such as neurodevelopmental treatment (NDT). Heipertz was medical director of the Orthopedic University Clinic in Frankfurt and chaired the Scientific Committee of the Kuratorium for Therapeutic Riding. His observations were based on his experience but were not supported by systematic inquiry.

The department of aerospace engineering at the University of Colorado built a device to evaluate gains in balance, coordination, and strength of patients in a therapeutic riding program. For the pilot study, 19 participants, ages 7 to 14, participated in two 10-minute testing sessions. One session was before and the second after a 2-hour riding lesson. Results of the tests were combined to obtain preliminary estimates of the effects of the riding session. The authors reported increases in balance and coordination, arm strength, and leg strength and an improvement on measures of spinal curvature and symmetry (Fox et al., 1984). Specific details about some of the measures, participants, and test sequence were not included in the report; however, detailed drawings and permission to replicate the instrument were obtained by Brock (1985) to test the effects of a

program of riding therapy on adults with physical disabilities. The author reported significant improvement ($p < .01$) for arm and leg coordination using the instrument designed at the University of Colorado. Bertoti (1988) reported significant improvement in posture for children with cerebral palsy after a program of riding therapy. A postural scale was used to assess standing posture before and after riding. Insufficient control over threats to validity and lack of a control group were limitations noted in this study.

MacKinnon and colleagues (1995) improved on design for a study to determine the effects of therapeutic horseback riding on children with cerebral palsy but failed to reach significance on measures of fine and gross motor function and activities of daily living. Because of the variation in the ages of the study participants, the researchers faced a dilemma in the selection of assessment instruments and were not able to use the same instrument for all participants. The authors suspected that the failure to reach statistical significance was the result of a lack of assessment tools with the sensitivity to detect the subtle changes expected from this population. The difficulties with measuring subtle improvement in heterogeneous populations over time are common problems and not unique to therapeutic riding and hippotherapy.

Why are posture and postural control considered so important? *Posture* is defined as the position or bearing of the body, whether characteristic or assumed for a special purpose (*Webster's Medical Desk Dictionary*, 1986, p. 569). Shumway-Cook and Woollacott (2001) presented postural control as a motor task incorporating both the position and orientation of the body. The orientation considers the arrangement of the body segments and their relationship to the environment. A person may determine optimal orientation of the body for the task, but adjustments are usually made without conscious thought. Postural adjustments are "automatic, anticipatory, and ongoing" to "enable an individual to maintain balance against gravity, optimal alignment between body parts, and optimal orientation of the head, trunk, and limbs" (Trombly, 1995, p. 500). Postural adaptation is "the ability of the body to maintain balance automatically and remain upright during alterations in position and challenges to stability" (p. 678).

Normally, posture is a dynamic and constantly changing component of human functioning in response to the demands of the environment and the intentions or actions of the individual. Duncan, Studenski, Chandler, Bloomfeld, and LaPointe (1990) defined *dynamic postural control* as "the ability to maintain an upright position in motion by either moving the center of mass within the base of support or moving the base of support under the center of mass." Shumway-Cook and Woollacott (2001) preferred the term *adaptive postural control* (p. 166) because it hints at the complexity of system interactions involved in learned postural responses. They emphasized that, in addition to muscular and sensory components, automatic cognitive processes are involved in modifying sensory and motor systems in response to changing demands.

Haley (1986) discussed the importance of onset age and sequence of automatic postural reactions in assessment, intervention, and outcome measures. At the same time, he pointed out that little empirical data corroborated these widely accepted developmental sequences, which were originally based on clinical observations. After completing his study, he reported that his results were generally in agreement with previously described sequences. Horak and Nashner (1986) investigated automatic postural accommodations to determine whether people demonstrate consistent patterns. They hypothesized that people develop a repertoire of postural responses, as a result of experience, that simplify demands on the central nervous system and enable rapid response to changing task demands. These response patterns are referred to as *postural synergies,* defined as "functional coupling of a group of muscles . . . acting together as a unit" (Shumway-Cook & Woollacott, 2001, p. 597).

Although "many scientists believe that concepts important for stance postural control will be shown to be equally valid for understanding the control of seated posture" (Shumway-Cook & Woollacott, 1995, p. 138), few attempts have been made to verify similarities or assess differences. Preliminary support was offered when Harbourne, Giuliani, and MacNeela (1993) determined that infants used postural synergies in response to perturbation in the sitting position at 2 months of age. By the age of 5 months, the infants were adopting one of two postural synergies using the lumbar paraspinal and either the rectus femoris or the lateral hamstrings. They concluded that control of the muscles around the hip joint seemed to be a prerequisite for independent sitting. When Reid, Sochaniwskyj, and Milner (1991) investigated postural sway in children while seated on a bench with differing angles and without back support, they found that postural control increased as a function of age for normal children.

Sitting was defined by Waksvik and Levy (1979) as a posture requiring "dynamic maintenance of a mixed pattern of flexion and extension" (p. 147). Harms (1990) found that the "literature offers no single logical basis for the definition of correct sitting posture" (p. 266). Smith and Emans (1992) defined a "normal" sitting pattern as one in which weight is taken primarily on the ischial tuberosities and equally distributed between right and left sides. They defined *sitting stability* as the ability to sit independently with both arms in the air and to regain the original posture after being pushed off balance in any direction.

The majority of the studies examining sitting posture and balance have been done on people with abnormal postural controls who were seated in wheelchairs. Reid and colleagues (1991) noted no statistically significant differences in seated postural sway between children with and without head injury. Clinical observation did reveal an apparent rigidity, thought to be indicative of postural fixing, in children with head injuries. Similarly, Reid and associates found no statistically significant differences in sway between children with and without cerebral palsy, but when analyzed individually, half of the children with cerebral palsy were observed to display more upright posture when on a seat with an anterior inclination of 10°. The other half of the children with cerebral palsy exhibited increased sway on the anteriorly inclined seat but also had improved posture, leading the authors to conclude that an analysis of sitting in children with neurological impairments must include functional postural outcomes.

Nwaobi, Brubaker, Cusick, and Sussman (1983) measured the activity of extensor muscles of the lumbar spine in children with spastic cerebral palsy in a variety of seated positions. They cited a number of references to reduced hypertonicity as a result of the angle of hip flexion and expressed the desire to identify a combination of seat and back angles for wheelchair seating that might reduce hypertonicity and result in improved functional ability. They concluded that the angle of hip flexion may not be the sole determinant and acknowledged the "possibility that orientation of the head and neck and/or body in general relative to gravity, i.e., righting responses, plays an equal or perhaps more important role in controlling extensor activity." Nwaobi's (1986) study of the effects of body orientation in space supported the earlier observation of decreases in tonic activity of extensor and hip adductor muscles when in an upright as opposed to reclined position. Nwaobi speculated that the children's attempts to orient themselves to their environment may have resulted in some increase in muscle tone.

A functional sitting posture for children with cerebral palsy, defined by Myhr and von Wendt (1991) as one in which the weight was equally distributed on the ischial tuberosities with the upper body (head and trunk) positioned anterior to the fulcrum at the ischial tuberosities, was compared with a variety of positions in the wheelchair. They noted improvement in function for children positioned in the functional sitting posture when a tray table was provided to permit stabilization with upper extremities. In a 5-year follow-up, Myhr, von Wendt, Norrlin, and Radell (1995) found that 8 of the original 10 children studied were sitting in accordance with the sitting posture and demonstrated improved control of head, trunk, arm, and hand function.

Stewart and McQuilton (1987) maintained that conventional sitting posture, with the chair back upright and the seat at a 90° angle to the back, places the center of gravity of the upper body (located in front of the 12th thoracic vertebra) behind the base of support (ischial tuberosities). They observed that it is difficult for children without disabilities to maintain this posture while working and noted the tendency to flex at the trunk and lean on a support surface or to tilt the entire chair forward in an attempt to move the center of gravity over the base of support. They also observed that children with cerebral palsy seemed to respond well "when straddled across an adult's thigh with the upper trunk supported, inclined forwards of the pelvis with lower limbs slightly flexed and hips abducted. This position strongly resembled a person sitting astride a horse and leaning forward" (p. 137). Based on these observations, they designed a prototype straddle seat that provided a three-point fixation of the pelvis to minimize pelvic instability. They reported positive results on the 10 children who had used the chair but had not completed any objective studies to verify their observations.

Thus, no consensus exists as to "correct" sitting posture, particularly for people with conditions that restrict their ability to move independently. The only premise to which it is likely that all would agree is that each patient must be evaluated independently. As implied by Stewart and McQuilton (1987), sitting is a dynamic posture that typically entails frequent weight shifts and position changes.

Many of the assessment instruments used by therapists include components of postural control and balance. The Milani-Comparetti Motor Development (Milani-Comparetti & Gidoni, 1967) and the Movement Assessment of Infants (Chandler, Andrews, & Swanson, 1980) are two commonly used tools to track emerging postural reactions in infants and very young children. The Bruininks–Oseretsky Test of Motor Proficiency (Bruininks, 1978) includes measures of static and dynamic stance balance. The DeGangi–Berk Test of Sensory Integration (Berk & DeGangi, 1983) and the Sensory Integration and Praxis Tests (Ayres, 1989) include evaluation of balance and coordination. These tools are limited to use with certain ages and provide information on other relevant motor and sensory aspects of function.

Gilfoyle, Grady, and Moore (1990) maintained that assessment tools provide only part of the information needed for a complete assessment and "must be supplemented with other problem-solving processes, such as . . . observations of performance and environmental interactions." Qualitative observation requires a description of what is being seen. Quantitative observations are guided by a detailed and specific definition of the trait or behavior being observed. Salvia and Ysseldyke (1995) advocated five goals of observational assessment, which included observation of specific, precisely defined behaviors with procedures developed to gather objective information.

Postural rating scales have been used to assess both postural alignment and the ability to move in and out of postures. Bertoti (1988) designed a postural rating scale that graded the position of head and neck, shoulders and scapula, trunk, spine, and pelvis. Mulcahy, Pountney, Nelham, Green, and Billington (1988) described a scale with six levels of sitting ability, which evaluated the ability to assume a position, maintain the position, move within the position, and move into and out of position. Sandin and Smith (1990) referenced "the standard technique for evaluating static and dynamic sitting balance" (p. 82). Smith and Emans (1992) described a clinical measure to assess sitting balance for patients with spinal deformities, which included sitting stability (stable, poor, unstable), sitting patterns (normal, asymmetric, tripod, pubic), and sitting balance (static balance = mean % imbalance and dynamic balance = sum of differences from mean). They maintained that the standard technique described by Sandin and Smith (1990) did not provide an accurate assessment for the population with spinal deformities.

Myhr and von Wendt (1991) presented a sitting assessment scale for people seated in wheelchairs. The scale evaluated head control, trunk control, foot control, arm function, and hand function on a 4-point scale in which 1 designated *no control* and 4 designated *good control*.

Fife and colleagues (1991) presented a "clinical measure of postural control for assessment of adaptive seating in children with neuromotor disabilities" (p. 981). They decided to limit their measure to static postural alignment and functional movement after reviewing the postural components of several standardized assessment tools and discovering a lack of items specifically related to postural alignment. Their scale consisted of 22 items of postural alignment in the sitting position. The pilot study of the rater reliability of this scale revealed a need for refinement and further testing.

The GREAT postural scale for therapeutic riding was based on a combination of elements from Bertoti (1988) and Fife and associates (1991), as well as the author's experience as a consumer and provider of riding instruction. Consultation with other therapists was important in refining the categories. The GREAT postural scale considers the position of the head and neck, shoulders and thoracic spine, pelvis and lumbar spine, hip angle, and alignment of heel in a visual assessment by the therapist. The elements were selected for two reasons. First, they are commonly used as reference points for correction of riders' posture, regardless of disability. Second, they are the areas in which riders commonly demonstrate observable deviations. The rider is assessed in the lateral plane; the rater is parallel to the center of the rider to eliminate distortions that might result from an oblique viewing angle. In a discussion of the criteria that guided the development of their seated postural control measure, Fife and colleagues (1991) cited Kirshner and Guyatt's (1985) assertion that "a clinical evaluation scale should include all items assumed likely to be affected by the intervention" (p. 983). Both lateral and posterior views should be considered when assessing rider posture. In developing the GREAT scale, consideration was given to expanding it to include a scale to assess lateral balance (asymmetry) of the rider, but it was decided to focus on the alignment of the posture as viewed in the lateral plane.

Method

A convenience sample of people participating in a hippotherapy program in north central Florida was used to represent riders with disabilities. Participants with disabilities were selected on the basis of the ability to maintain upright sitting posture without assistance. Participants without disabilities were experienced riders. The sample included a total of 12 riders ranging in age from 2 years, 10 months, to age 30 years.

Three children were between age 2 years, 10 months, and age 6 years. One child was diagnosed with cerebral palsy (mild spastic quadriparesis), one was diagnosed with a developmental delay (pervasive), and one had no specified diagnosis and presented with mild hypotonia. No experienced riders in this age range were included.

Eight children were between ages 9 and 16. Two were diagnosed with cerebral palsy (one with mild hypotonia, the second with mild athetosis and cognitive involvement), and one rider was diagnosed with a genetic disorder resulting in coordination and flexibility deficits. Five riders had no known disability.

Finally, one adult rider had an incomplete spinal cord injury. No adult riders without disability were included.

The study involved five observer–raters. Two were physical therapists and three were occupational therapists. All raters had completed the basic hippotherapy course offered by the AHA. Completion of the basic hippotherapy course was thought to offer a measure by which the therapists' experience in assessment of the postural alignment of horseback riders could be quantified.

Four of the raters were from different areas of the United States and were not informed as to the identities of the other raters to decrease the likelihood of collaboration on the scoring of images. Rater 4 was the local physical therapist treating the riders and was representative of scale users in that she rated riders with whom she was familiar (i.e., typical users would not be blinded to identity and diagnoses). Her rating also would be used to provide some indication as to whether prior knowledge of the rider would affect the visual rating assigned. Each rater received an identical packet of images, the postural scale, and written instructions.

Data Collection

The decision was made to use photographs for the ratings because a photograph essentially captures and "freezes" the position of the rider. Use of videotapes or other moving images would increase the difficulty of ensuring that all the raters were assessing the same thing. Photographic images of riders with disabilities were selected from the progress photos maintained by a physical therapist with a private hippotherapy practice in north central Florida. Photographic images of riders without disabilities were taken of riders who were members of the local pony club. Informed consent was obtained in accordance with the requirements of the University of Florida Institutional Review Board prior to inclusion of any photographs in the assortment to be rated. All photographs were taken from a distance of approximately 33 feet and a height of approximately 64 inches. The camera was a Nikon Zoom

Touch 500 with an 80 mm lens setting. The horse was walking or at a halt. Only lateral views, taken from a position perpendicular to the center of the rider, were used to eliminate any optical distortion that might result from an oblique angle.

Riders in hippotherapy sessions were photographed on a regular basis and were accustomed to the presence of cameras. Because the riders were not informed as to the exact times that photographs were taken, most did not appear to make any attempt to change their posture for the picture. The animals, equipment, background, and helpers were the same for riders with and without disabilities. A representative assortment of images was selected to illustrate the full range of variation observed, but all riders were in a straddle position with one leg on each side and facing the horse's head.

The horses were equipped with saddles or with bareback pads, depending on the equipment normally used by each rider. Equipment and modifications used were considered to be representative of customary and normal variations found in the therapeutic riding environment. Variations such as side sitting, lying prone or supine on the horse, and positions assumed at gaits other than walk and halt were not used because the scale was not designed to assess those postures.

The original photographs were viewed and coded for identification by the primary researcher. Images were scanned into an Adobe Photoshop program on a Macintosh computer, then digitized and enlarged to facilitate clarity and focus on the position of the rider. No changes were made to the background features of the selected images, but the background itself was cropped out. In focusing on the rider, it was hoped that the presence or absence of sidewalkers in the background would be less obvious. Where possible, sidewalkers were cropped out of the final image. Sidewalkers are a normal aspect of the therapeutic riding environment, but their use was not consistent from rider to

rider. Riders who did not need sidewalkers did not have them, and some riders were pictured both with and without sidewalkers. To people familiar with therapeutic riding, the presence or absence of a sidewalker could prejudice an observer concerning the presence or absence of disability. The goal was to blind the raters as to which riders had disabilities. Facial features of the riders were blurred to protect identity and to prevent facial expression from distracting or influencing the rater. Figure 9.2 shows an image of one of the riders without disabilities, with rater comments.

All raters received identical packets of photos and instructions. Each rater received an excerpt from this paper explaining the design of the scale, a request for information concerning their experience, and the following instructions:

> Each of the thirty-two (32) photographs has a preprinted area to the left of the rider image. Please write the number which represents your rating in the appropriate boxes. There is an area provided for any comments you may wish to make about that particular image. The comment section is not part of the study. You may elect not to comment. A self-addressed stamped envelope is included for the return of the ratings. Please return all photographs and the rater information sheet. The primary researcher did not rate the photographs.

Results

The two hypotheses tested were (1) that raters of similar background would reliably score the postural alignment of riders using the GREAT postural scale and (2) that internal consistency of the GREAT postural scale as a homogeneous assessment of postural alignment would be demonstrated. To demonstrate similarity of background, raters were asked to provide information about their experience. Table 9.1 summarizes their experience

Table 9.1. Discipline and Experience of Raters

Rater	Discipline	Experience as Therapist	Experience in Hippotherapy/ Therapeutic Riding	Experience as Rider	Hippotherapy Training
1	OT	15 years	8/15 years	25 years	AHA
2	OT	19 years	11/20 years	33 years	Germany
3	OT	11 years	2/15 years	35 years	AHA
4	PT	18 years	6/14 years	20 years	AHA
5	PT	10 years	9/11 years	30 years	Germany

Note. OT = occupational therapy; PT = physical therapy; AHA = American Hippotherapy Association.

in four areas. The raters had an average of 14.6 years of experience as therapists. Their experience with hippotherapy ranged from 2 to 11 years. They had been involved with therapeutic riding for an average of 15 years. All were experienced riders (an average of 28.6 years). All raters had completed the basic course in hippotherapy offered by the American Hippotherapy Association, a section of the North American Riding for the Handicapped Association. Two raters also had received advanced hippotherapy training in Germany.

The intraclass correlation coefficient (ICC) was used in the analysis of ratings. Streiner (1995) stated that because the ICC is sensitive to both agreement and association among raters, it overcomes some of the deficits of other commonly used techniques. It would detect any systematic bias among raters. As suggested by Portnoy and Watkins (1993), an acceptable value of interrater reliability was established as .90 or more. Failure to achieve an ICC of .90 for all body parts resulted in additional analysis to determine what variation among raters might have affected the average of the raters. ICCs are presented in Table 9.2.

The five body areas were treated separately, and a Multivariate Analysis of Variance (MANOVA) was used to test for significant differences among raters ($\alpha = 0.01$). By treating this as five closely related instruments, we could look at each body area separately. ICCs were generated in this manner for each separate body part but not directly for the total. Rider scores were transformed to sequential numbers to establish values meaningful for the data analysis.

Because of patterns in the raw data, it was decided to calculate results several ways. The results of the MANOVA indicated significant variability among the five raters. No significant differences were found between the average occupational therapy ratings and the average physical therapy ratings. Significant rater differences persisted without Rater 1, but the coefficient values increased slightly. Without Rater 4, who had

extensive personal exposure to the participants and may have been biased, no statistically significant rater differences were found and the coefficient values were lowered. The comparison between Raters 2 and 5 was calculated because both raters had advanced hippotherapy training. The two raters were in agreement on several images, and the statistical analysis revealed no significant differences between them. With the exception of the head and heel, the correlation coefficients were higher for Raters 2 and 5 than for all raters.

Internal Consistency

Cronbach's coefficient, or coefficient alpha, was calculated to assess the internal consistency of the scale. According to Ary, Jacobs, and Razavieh (1990), Cronbach's alpha is a widely used measure of internal consistency that serves to "estimate the proportion of variance in a scale that is not attributable to internal inconsistency among multiple items of the scale" (Leon et al., 1995, p. 866) and is applicable to tests in which each test item has multiple possible scores. Kraemer (1991) compared the effect of instrument reliability on statistical power and reported that reliability of .80 should be satisfactory. Any increase over that level contributes little to statistical power. Each body area was scored separately and then combined for the entire instrument.

Significant rater variance contributed to the low Cronbach's alpha for all sections. Portnoy and Watkins (1993) defined *variance* as "a measure of the variability of differences among scores within a sample. The larger the variance, the greater the dispersion of scores, the smaller the variance, the more homogeneous the scores" (p. 57). When alpha is evaluated for Raters 2 and 5 (no significant rater differences), all values increase except for the head, in spite of the small sample size ($n = 2$). This comparison was included to highlight the impact of rater variability on instrument reliability. The values for Cronbach's alpha in all configurations are shown in Table 9.3.

Table 9.2. Intraclass Correlation Coefficients

Section	All Raters	Occupational Therapists vs. Physical Therapists	Without Rater 1	Without Rater 4	Raters 2 and 5 Only
Head	0.664	0.646	0.665	0.63	0.282
Shoulder	0.714	0.696	0.817	0.665	0.757
Pelvis	0.903	0.895	0.912	0.879	0.91
Hip	0.865	0.853	0.848	0.844	0.802
Heel	0.717	0.698	0.814	0.666	0.762

Table 9.3. Values for Cronbach's Alpha

Section	α for All Raters	α for Raters 2 and 5
Head	0.271	0.182
Shoulder	0.309	0.668
Pelvis	0.632	0.860
Hip	0.542	0.678
Heel	0.314	0.625
Entire instrument	0.475	0.564
Entire instrument without head	0.532	0.794

Portnoy and Watkins (1993) offered guidelines for interpretation of reliability coefficients. They suggested that "coefficients below .50 represent poor reliability, coefficients from .50 to .75 suggest moderate reliability, and values above .75 indicate good reliability" (p. 58). They also recommend reliability coefficients of at least .90 for clinical trials. No section of the GREAT instrument reached a .90 level. Without the head and neck component, the instrument met criteria for moderate reliability. The results do not support the hypotheses that similar raters would reliably score the postural alignment of riders using the GREAT postural scale and that the internal consistency of the scale would be demonstrated.

Discussion

The assumptions made while designing the scale and examining reliability included the following:
- A representative sample of rider postures could be obtained.
- Scale graphics would adequately describe the range of postural alignment variations normal within the population of riders.
- Raters of similar background would complete a visual assessment consistently.

Limitations of the scale design and reliability are as follows:
- The model for the scale graphics consisted of riders without disabilities.
- There was a small sample of riders with and without disabilities.
- Minimal training on the use of the scale was provided.

Design of the Scale

Comprehensive descriptions of all the variations that alter a rider's position may be found in texts on riding instruction and therapeutic riding. After extensive consideration of postural nuances, the scale was designed to assess the position of the rider at the walk and halt. The

riders must be seated in the center of the horse's back with one leg on each side and facing the horse's head. The rider may use a saddle or a bareback pad, with or without surcingle. Caution must be used in selection of the saddle and care must be taken to avoid special-use saddles that encourage other than balanced postures, such as side-saddles, jumping saddles, and racing saddles.

It is common for classical riding instructors to use verbal cues to correct the position of the rider by referencing the rider position in relation to the vertical (i.e., behind or in front of the vertical). Based on this practice, the vertical line framed a conceptual reference for graphic organization of the scale. The correct positions of the head, shoulder, pelvis, hip, and heel are located at the center vertical axis of the scale. Postures that would place the rider's body in front of the vertical line are located on one side of the axis, and those that place the rider's body behind the vertical are on the opposite side.

As a base of support for the upper body, the pelvis forms the framework upon which everything else is built. Conceptually, a horizontal line at the level of the pelvis was the point of reference used to determine the range of positions of the body above and below the horizontal line. Two increasingly angular pelvic deviations from the neutral pelvis, arbitrarily defined as mild and moderate, are described on each side of the vertical axis. It is at this horizontal line that the biomechanical limitations imposed by the horse on the human are considered. Because the area below the horizontal axis has fewer possible deviations than the area above it, one level of hip-and-knee deviation, arbitrarily defined as flexed or extended, is described on each side of the vertical axis.

An ordinal scale is used to score each segment of the body. The correct alignment earns a score of 0 at all five segments. Posterior pelvic deviations and the shoulder and head alignment deviations most often associated with them were assigned values of 1 and 2 and are located "behind the vertical." Similarly, values of 3 and 4 were assigned to anterior pelvic deviations and associated upper body alignment, located "in front of the vertical." The smaller numbers on both sides (1 and 3) are used to designate a mild deviation, and the higher numbers (2 and 4) designate a moderate deviation. Because less variability is expected at the hip and knee, the pattern of increased extension, which would fall in "behind the vertical," earns a score of 1, and the pattern of increased flexion, which would place the leg in front of the vertical, earns a score of 3.

Some riders may exhibit relatively static postural alignment throughout the riding session, but the nature of the intervention is to encourage dynamic postural accommodation. Movement in the rider's pelvis will occur, even when the alignment deviates from neutral. The observer must record the prevailing alignment at the time of assessment. The rider may make observable changes at one or two alignment points, the entire alignment may change, or multiple changes could occur in a single session. It also is possible for a rider to demonstrate trends during a single session. For example, a rider with spastic muscles may exhibit one alignment pattern early in the riding session. As the rider's muscles relax, a different postural alignment may be observed. To effectively record the variation of alignment patterns demonstrated by a rider in a single session, the assessment must be completed quickly. Because the scores for each alignment point are similar and cluster on one side of the vertical or another, it was hoped that raters familiar with the scale would be able to assess a rider's postural alignment in seconds. A field trial was completed in which the scale was used to assess rider postural alignment at 5-minute intervals during a 30-minute session. It was possible to observe and record the initial and interval postural alignment of the rider in less than 1 minute per observation.

Analysis of Results

High interrater reliability implies that raters are consistent in their scoring of the study participants. Causes of low reliability might include confusing photographs, inadequate rater training, rater bias, or problems with the instrument. Although the interrater reliability coefficients were generally acceptable, significant differences were found among the five raters. The differences were manifested in all body areas and reflected in the low Cronbach's alpha. The low correlation of the head scores for Raters 2 and 5 is the best demonstration of the effect of rater variation on instrument reliability (Cronbach's alpha). Although Raters 2 and 5 agreed most of the time, when they disagreed on head scores, their ratings were far apart. Their disagreement was not always in the same direction (i.e., Rater 2 was not consistently higher than Rater 5 and vice versa). Similar disagreement occurred among the five raters but was not isolated to one body position.

Portnoy and Watkins (1993) provided guidelines for interpretation of ICC values: Above .75 indicates good reliability, and below .75 indicates poor to moderate reliability. ICCs for the head, shoulder, and heel failed to reach the recommended level (>.75) but could be considered moderate because they were close to the recommended level. This result indicates that the instrument could be a useful tool, provided that interrater reliability is established for each setting in which the scale is used. The discussion that follows addresses the possible factors contributing to the reported correlation coefficients. Suggestions for revisions follow.

Ratings of the head position generated the lowest correlations (.664) for all raters. Because the facial features were blurred, raters were not able to use facial landmarks to judge position. Safety helmets, which are a required piece of safety equipment, also obscure landmarks (ear) in some instances. This observation appears to be chiefly applicable to the bicycle and soft helmets used by the smaller children. It is possible that raters were not able to rate head position consistently because of poor visibility of facial and head landmarks. The descriptions and illustrations of head positions may have been confusing. In particular, Positions 2 and 4 may be too similar to allow raters to make clear distinctions from the photographs. Also, it is possible that, by using a rider without disabilities as a model for the various positions, the primary researcher and scale designer failed to capture meaningful variations of the head position. Including the head and the neck as a single component also may have contributed to rater variance. Consideration should be given to evaluating the head and neck as separate components.

The shoulder and thoracic spine area generated the second-lowest (.714) correlation coefficient. Based on feedback from the raters, this area was difficult to assess because of the loose clothing worn by riders in many instances. Additionally, the verbal descriptions in the guide for scoring may have failed to provide sufficient direction for how to rate the variations represented.

The heel-area ratings yielded a correlation coefficient similar to that of the shoulder (.717). Because that area is clearly visible in the photographs, it is probable that the descriptions in the scoring criteria were inadequate and probably confusing.

The ratings for hip angle and pelvis yielded fairly high correlations (.865 and .903, respectively). It is possible that loose clothing or unclear photos may have contributed to some of the variation for those areas. Several raters commented that they had difficulty deciding which rating to assign, particularly in the pelvic area, because the position was "in between" two scores. Fife and colleagues (1991), while examining interrater reliability of a postural alignment scale for wheelchair seating, experienced similar difficulties with visual assessment. They argued that therapists support the reliability of visual assessment, and they planned to examine the clarity of item descriptions. Fife and associates also had anticipated that a module for training raters would be required.

Baker (1992) concluded that, even though changes in posture during riding are difficult to assess, it is critical to do so. Improvements in sitting position on horseback were presented as qualitatively assessed changes noted by MacKinnon and colleagues (1995). No measures were available to quantify these changes at the time of their study.

The GREAT Postural Scale begins to address those concerns. Acceptable interrater reliability results reported here indicate that the scale could be used in settings in which reliability is independently established by participating raters.

Recommendations for Scale Development

The graphic images and descriptions in the GREAT scale should be reevaluated on the basis of a larger sample of rider images. Representative postural variations should be redefined in the context of the larger sample. Provisions should be made for rating "in-between" postures.

A training manual for the scale needs to be designed. The manual should include samples with an analysis explaining why ratings were assigned to each image as they were. The training package should include actual examples (photos) of riders exhibiting the range of variation for each possible rating. In future studies to establish interrater reliability and internal consistency, riders should wear clothing that fits snugly.

Clinically, it is unlikely that most users would be able to consistently control the type of clothing worn, so consideration must be given as to how to instruct raters for these situations. Participants recruited for future studies in which photographs are used should be advised of and agree to the use of their full image, including the face.

Future studies could include comparisons between riders with and without disabilities to determine whether the scale differentiates between the two groups. Because it is not uncommon for riders without disabilities to exhibit incorrect alignment, depending on the level of experience, such variation must be considered. The scale also could be used to document postural changes during a single riding lesson and over a specified period of time.

References

Ary, D., Jacobs, L. C., & Razavieh, A. (1990). *Introduction to research in education.* Fort Worth, TX: Holt, Rinehart & Winston.

Ayres, A. J. (1989). *Sensory Integration and Praxis tests.* Los Angeles: Western Psychological Services.

Baker, E. A. (1992). A comparison of change in flexible kyphosis pre- and post-hippotherapy—A research approach. In B. T. Engel (Ed.), *Therapeutic riding programs: Instruction and rehabilitation.* Durango, CO: Barbara Engel Therapy Services.

Bertoti, D. B. (1988). Effect of therapeutic horseback riding on posture in children with cerebral palsy. *Journal of the American Physical Therapy Association, 68,* 1505–1512.

Berk, R. A., & DeGangi, G. A. (1983). *DeGangi–Berk Test of Sensory Integration.* Los Angeles: Western Psychological Services.

Biery, M. J., & Kauffman, N. (1989). The effects of therapeutic horseback riding on balance. *Adapted Physical Activity Quarterly, 6,* 221–229.

Brock, B. J. (1985). Effect of therapeutic horseback riding on physically disabled adults. *Therapeutic Recreation Journal, 22,* 34–43.

Bruininks, R. H. (1978). *Bruininks–Oseretsky Test of Motor Proficiency.* Circle Pines, MN: American Guidance Service.

Chandler, L., Andrews, M., & Swanson, M. (1980). *The Movement Assessment of Infants: A manual.* Rolling Bay, WA: Infant Movement Research.

Duncan, P. W., Studenski, S., Chandler, J., Bloomfeld, R., & LaPointe, L. K. (1990). Electromyographic analysis of postural adjustments in two methods of balance testing. *Physical Therapy, 70,* 88–96.

Fife, S. E., Roxborough, L. A., Armstrong, R. W., Harris, S. R., Gregson, J. L., & Field, D. (1991). Development of a clinical measure of postural control for assessment of adaptive seating in children with neuromotor disabilities. *Physical Therapy, 71,* 981–993.

Fox, V. M., Lawlor, V. A., & Luttges, M. W. (1984). Pilot study of novel test instrumentation to evaluate therapeutic horseback riding. *Adapted Physical Activity Quarterly, 1,* 30–36.

Gilfoyle, E. M., Grady, A. P., & Moore, J. C. (1990). *Children adapt: A theory of sensorimotor–sensory development* (2nd ed.). Thorofare, NJ: Slack.

Gliner, J. A. (1985). Purposeful activity in motor learning theory: An event approach to motor skill acquisition. *American Journal of Occupational Therapy, 39,* 28–34.

Haley, S. M. (1986). Sequential analysis of postural reactions in non-handicapped infants. *Physical Therapy, 66,* 531–536.

Harbourne, R., Giuliana, C., & MacNeela, J. (1993). A kinematic and electromyographic analysis of the development of sitting posture in infants. *Developmental Psychobiology, 26,* 51–64.

Harms, M. (1990). Effect of wheelchair design on posture and comfort of users. *Physiotherapy, 76,* 266–271.

Heipertz, W., Heipertz-Hengst, C., Kroger, A., & Kuprian, W. (1977). *Therapeutic riding: Medicine, education, sport.* Ottawa: Greenbelt Riding Association for the Disabled.

Horak, F. B., & Nashner, L. M. (1986). Central programming of postural movements: Adaptation to altered support-surface configurations. *Journal of Neurophysiology, 55*, 1369–1381.

Hopkins, H. L., & Smith, H. D. (Eds.). (1993). *Willard and Spackman's occupational therapy* (8th ed.). Philadelphia: Lippincott Williams and Wilkins.

Jarus, T. (1994). Motor learning and occupational therapy: The organization of practice. *American Journal of Occupational Therapy, 48*, 810–816.

Klüwer, C. (1992). The federation of riding for the disabled international. In B. T. Engel (Ed.), *Therapeutic riding programs: Instruction and rehabilitation.* Durango, CO: Barbara Engel Therapy Services.

Kraemer, H. C. (1991). To increase power in randomized clinical trials without increasing sample size. *Psychopharmacology Bulletin, 27*, 217–224.

Leon, A. C., Marzuk, P. M., & Portera, L. (1995). More reliable outcome measures can reduce sample size requirements. *Archives of General Psychiatry, 52*, 867–871.

MacKinnon, J. R., Noh, S., Lariviere, J., MacPhail, A., Allan, D. E., & Laliberte, D. (1995). A study of therapeutic effects of horseback riding for children with cerebral palsy. *Physical and Occupational Therapy in Pediatrics, 15*, 17–31.

Milani-Comparetti, A., & Gidoni, E. A. (1967). Routine developmental examination in normal and retarded children. *Developmental Medicine and Child Neurology, 9*, 631–638.

Mulcahy, C. M., Pountney, T. E., Nelham, R. L., Green, E. M., & Billington, G. D. (1988). Adaptive seating for motor handicap: Problems, a solution, assessment and prescription. *British Journal of Occupational Therapy, 51*, 347–352.

Myhr, U., & von Wendt, L. (1991). Improvement of functional sitting position for children with cerebral palsy. *Developmental Medicine and Child Neurology, 33*, 246–256.

Myhr, U., von Wendt, L., Norrlin, S., & Radell, U. (1995). Five-year follow-up of functional sitting position in children with cerebral palsy. *Developmental Medicine and Child Neurology, 37*, 587–596.

Nwaobi, O. M. (1986). Effect of body orientation in space on tonic muscle activity of patients with cerebral palsy. *Developmental Medicine and Child Neurology, 28*, 41–44.

Nwaobi, O. M., Brubaker, C. E., Cusick, B., & Sussman, M. D. (1983). Electromyographic investigation of extensor activity in cerebral palsied children in different seating positions. *Developmental Medicine and Child Neurology, 25*, 175–183.

Portnoy, L. G., & Watkins, M. P. (1993). *Foundations of clinical research: Applications to practice.* Norwalk, CT: Appleton & Lange.

Reid, D. T., Sochaniwskyj, A., & Milner, M. (1991). An investigation of postural sway in sitting of normal children and children with neurological disorders. *Physical and Occupational Therapy in Pediatrics, 11*, 19–35.

Salvia, J., & Ysseldyke, J. E. (1995). *Assessment* (6th ed.). Boston: Houghton Mifflin.

Sandin, K., & Smith, B. (1990). The measure of balance in sitting in stroke rehabilitation prognosis. *Stroke, 21*, 82–86.

Seunig, W. (1956). *Horsemanship: A comprehensive book on training the horse and its rider.* New York: Doubleday.

Shumway-Cook, A., & Woollacott, M. W. (1995). *Motor control: Theory and practical applications.* Baltimore: Williams & Wilkins.

Shumway-Cook, A., & Woollacott, M. H. (2001). *Motor control: Theory and practical applications* (2nd ed.). Baltimore: Lippincott Williams & Wilkins.

Smith, R., & Emans, J. (1992). Sitting balance in spinal deformity. *Spine, 17*, 1103–1109.

Stewart, P. C., & McQuilton, G. (1987). Straddle seating for the cerebral palsied child. *British Journal of Occupational Therapy, 50*, 136–138.

Streiner, D. L. (1995). Learning how to differ: Agreement and reliability statistics in psychiatry. *Canadian Journal of Psychiatry, 40*, 60–66.

Trombly, C. A. (Ed.). (1995). *Occupational therapy for physical dysfunction* (4th ed.). Baltimore: Lippincott Williams & Wilkins.

Waksvik, K., & Levy, R. (1979). An approach to seating for the cerebral palsied. *Canadian Journal of Occupational Therapy, 46*, 147–153.

Webster's Medical Desk Dictionary. (1986). Springfield, MA: Merriam-Webster.

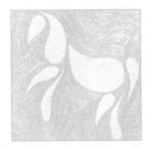

*The eternal and wonderful sight of
horses at liberty is magical to watch.*
—Bertrand Leclair

CHAPTER 10

Use of Sensory Integration in Equine-Assisted Therapy: An Occupational Therapy Perspective

Rebecca Gewurtz, MSc, OT Reg (Ont), and Ashleigh Eccles, OT Reg (Ont)

Equine-assisted therapy (EAT) is the use of horse-related activities for clients with physical, mental, cognitive, social, or behavioral problems. The goals and focus of an EAT program depend on each client's individual therapeutic needs.

Hippotherapy is a specialized area of EAT that relies on the three-dimensional movement of the horse to provide a movement challenge to the rider (Heine, 1997). Hippotherapy in North America is carried out directly by a rehabilitation or health care professional such as an occupational therapist, physical therapist, or speech pathologist, depending on the client's specific therapeutic needs and goals. In contrast, therapeutic riding and horsemanship activities (such as bridling and grooming) are areas of EAT that can be carried out directly by a therapist riding instructor with consultation provided by a licensed therapist, such as an occupational therapist. It is the unique combination of the horse; the horse's movement; and the stimulating, nonclinical environment that makes all forms of EAT so motivating for clients and effective in treating multiple body systems. This chapter discusses how occupational therapists can use EAT to assist clients with sensory processing dysfunctions using the principles of sensory integration (SI) theory.

Role of Occupational Therapists

An occupational therapist working in an EAT setting is part of a therapy team that includes the horse, the client

and his or her family, other therapists, the therapeutic riding instructor, sidewalkers, and horse leaders. It is important to distinguish the role of the occupational therapist from the other members of this team. Occupational therapists have a broad knowledge base in physical, cognitive, psychosocial, behavioral, and emotional rehabilitation and development that uniquely qualifies them to work in an EAT setting. This knowledge enables them to adapt the riding program to meet the multiple needs of a diverse clinical population. The skills involved in riding can be graded to enable successful experiences while providing the "just-right" challenge. The activity of horseback riding presents a unique opportunity for occupational therapists to target various physical, cognitive, psychoemotional, social, and behavioral skills simultaneously in a social and recreational environment.

Sensory Integration

The neurological process of SI, which consists of receiving and organizing sensations, contributes to the development of self-regulation, comfort, motor planning, gross and fine motor skills, attention, and readiness for learning (Yack, Sutton, & Aquilla, 1998). People with SI dysfunction may display a wide range of behaviors and symptoms, including a disregard for or exaggerated response to sensory stimulation, inconsistent ability to attend to tasks, distractibility, poor impulse control, motor planning and motor coordination problems, delays in speech and language development, poor self-concept, limited frustration tolerance, and fluctuating emotional reactions (Viviano, 1997; Yack et al., 1998).

Reprinted by permission of Canadian Association of Occupational
Therapists Publications, ACE.

Treatment programs that use strategies based on SI theory incorporate movements and activities that provide tactile, vestibular, and proprioceptive stimulation. The goal of SI intervention is to improve the way people who experience SI dysfunction receive, process, and organize sensations, thus improving their ability to interact with their environment.

Tactile Inputs

Clients with SI dysfunction may be hyper- or hyposensitive to touch or may have trouble with tactile discrimination. EAT can provide diverse opportunities for direct tactile input that can be graded by the occupational therapist to meet the individual needs of the rider. The most unique tactile experience provided during EAT comes from the horse's movement, which gives the rider constant tactile input. The horse's gait can be used to provide a gentle massage to the rider, depending on the rider's position on the horse. For example, if the rider is lying down on the horse (prone over the barrel, supine along the horse's back, or prone while lying backward), the tactile inputs are provided throughout the rider's trunk or back. The occupational therapist can specifically position a rider on the horse to provide tactile stimulation that meets the client's unique sensory needs.

Tactile stimulation can be provided through other activities involving the horse. For example, riders can be encouraged to pet the horse with their hands or participate in grooming the horse using different textured brushes and grooming tools. Participation in horse care activities can assist in developing body awareness, because the rider is encouraged to learn the different parts of the horse and how they compare with the rider's own body (e.g., "The horse has four legs and I have two legs"). Tactile "adventure bins" also can be set up in the ring: Riders can reach into the bins while on the horse and find a toy.

Vestibular Inputs

Satisfying a child's sensory needs through EAT activities can increase the child's ability to remain calm, alert, and attentive. At this point, the occupational therapists can create activities to target various cognitive and social communication skills. Some of the sensory processing benefits of EAT are as follows:
• Decreased sensory defensiveness

• Increased attention, concentration, and focus with decreased distractibility and impulsivity (i.e., "less fidgety")
• Increased coordination and motor planning
• Increased communication
• Increased responsiveness
• Increased self-concept and self-esteem
• Improved self-regulation.

Case Study

"Dara" is a 4-year-old girl with a global developmental delay. She started a one-on-one EAT session on a weekly basis with an occupational therapist. Her mother reported that Dara's biggest challenge was her short attention span. At her integrated nursery school, the teachers reported that Dara could attend to a task or activity for only a few seconds.

On the horse, the occupational therapist noticed that Dara appeared happy and attentive. She expressed joy at the different sensory inputs provided by the horse's movement. Dara could attend to a task for approximately 1 minute, respond to requests appropriately, and demonstrate appropriate social interaction. The occupational therapist realized that Dara was benefiting from the vestibular challenge provided by the height of the horse as well as from the tactile and proprioceptive inputs provided by the horse's movements. The sensory inputs were helping her organize incoming information from her environment, thereby enabling her to attend to the task at hand. The therapist began incorporating cognitive and fine motor activities that mirrored the skills she was working on at nursery school, such as matching and sorting. Gradually, the skills that Dara was learning during her EAT sessions carried over to the nursery school setting. This transfer resulted in a gradual increase in attention span, self-confidence, social interaction, orientation and awareness of her body in space, balance, and academic performance. Dara began initiating communication through words and hand signals that centered on her horse and her EAT experiences. It appeared that EAT had introduced joy and recreational pleasure into her life, enabled her to focus, and provided motivation for her to interact with the world.

Conclusion

Although organizing and processing sensory information is only one component of EAT, it can be an area that can have significant and long-lasting benefits for the rider. Moreover, those benefits can carry over into all aspects of the rider's life. It is important that an occupational therapist assess the sensory needs of each rider and incorporate those needs into an EAT program that is specifically designed to meet the client's therapeutic goals.

Acknowledgments

The authors are grateful for the assistance and support received from Karen McEwen and Ellen Yack through the process of writing and editing this chapter.

References

Heine, B. (1997). When is therapeutic riding hippotherapy? In B. T. Engel (Ed.), *Therapeutic riding II: Strategies for rehabilitation* (pp. 5–10). Durango, CO: Barbara Engel Therapy Services.

Viviano, A. (1997). Use of sensory integration treatment strategies in the hippotherapy setting. In B. T. Engel (Ed.), *Therapeutic riding II: Strategies for rehabilitation* (pp. 363–372). Durango, CO: Barbara Engel Therapy Services.

Yack, E., Sutton, S., & Aquilla, P. (1998). *Building bridges through sensory integration.* Toronto, ON: Print Three.

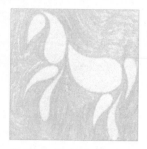

And I looked, and behold,
a white horse....
—Revelations, 6:2

CHAPTER 11

Postural Control Comparisons of Horseback Riders With and Without Brain Injury

Beatriz C. Abreu, PhD, OTR, FAOTA; Patricia Heyn, PhD;
Timothy A. Reistetter, PhD, OTR; Rita Patterson, PhD; William L. Bufford, Jr., PhD;
Brent Masel, MD; and Kenneth J. Ottenbacher, PhD, OTR, FAOTA

The high incidence and complex etiology of traumatic brain injury (TBI) and stroke demand a wide range of rehabilitation services. Conventional and alternative rehabilitation approaches are vital to the recovery of independence and improvement of function among people experiencing TBI and stroke.

Postural control impairment is a common problem associated with TBI and stroke, and current methods of postural control evaluation while seated are critical to help people maintain stability while seated and standing and while at rest and in motion in almost all daily activities. Hence, postural control assessment and training are key to rehabilitation interventions (DePauw, 1986; Ikai, Kamikubo, Takehara, Nishi, & Miyano, 2003). The acquisition of objective, systematic information about postural control through a portable pressure mapping system should benefit the process of rehabilitation for people with acquired brain injury.

Postural control is accomplished through a complex multilevel coordination of central and peripheral nervous system responses that are used to regain and maintain balance. The movement strategies are triggered by proprioceptive, vestibular, and visual cues concerning body imbalance. After brain injury, many people develop impairments in vision, proprioception, and the vestibular and musculoskeletal systems.

Therapeutic horseback riding is a term that encompasses a variety of activities for people with disabilities. The divisions of therapeutic riding, by goal, are education, recreation or leisure, sport, and therapy. Under the therapeutic goal are equine-assisted psychotherapy for clients with psychosocial disorders; Developmental Riding Therapy, a trademarked cognitive, motor, and affective sensory integration treatment; and hippotherapy, a technique that uses specific movements of the horse to mediate and improve riders' movement patterns.

Hippotherapy is a horse-mediated rehabilitation technique used to train postural control after brain injury (Biery & Kauffman, 1989; Heine, 1997). Many other physical and psychological benefits of therapeutic horseback riding have been reported (All, Loving, & Crane, 1999; MacKinnon, Noh, Laliberte, Lariviere, & Allan, 1995). Some of those benefits include improved strength and agility, muscle tone, weight-bearing ability (Bertoti, 1988), standing (MacKinnon et al., 1995), self-esteem, self-image, and interpersonal skills (Bliss, 1997). Limited studies, however, support the efficacy or efficiency of hippotherapy.

Hippotherapy uses the multidimensional movement of the horse to improve posture, balance, and function (Engel, 1997). During hippotherapy, the rider's body can smoothly and rhythmically move in a manner similar to the human gait, providing the rider with an ideal promoter of normal movement. Clinicians believe that the displacements of the rider's center of pressure while riding facilitate normal righting and equilibrium responses (MacPhail et al., 1998). This treatment approach can be implemented under the guidance of a variety of health care professionals, including occupational therapists, physical therapists, speech pathologists, and psychotherapists providing rehabilitation services (Bracher, 2000; DePauw, 1986; Heine, 1997; Whalley,

1980). These rehabilitation professionals may analyze and perceive the challenges of riding very differently from each other, because riding is a subtle skill, and it is not as easy as it looks.

A review of the literature reveals few experimental studies in hippotherapy. The published studies were limited methodologically, and none were randomized clinical trials; they lacked controls and were mostly pretest–posttest studies. The sample sizes are small, and the highest N was 29 (Cawley, Cawley, & Retter, 1994). The populations studied were primarily children with cerebral palsy and mixed physical and other disabilities. The length and frequency of the programs ranged from 5 to 24 weeks. Follow-up was minimal, and the outcome measures, mostly at the impairment level, were evaluated using videotape analysis and subjective movement assessments that included muscle tone, coordination, and postural control. The results describe subjective positive effects; however, given the level of evidence, the studies together do not provide sufficient support for the efficacy of hippotherapy. Although a few descriptive studies have reported improvement following hippotherapy in people with disability, few systematic, valid, reliable, and sensitive instruments are available to assess the outcomes of hippotherapy.

Bertoti (1988) evaluated 11 children with cerebral palsy before and after a 10-week therapeutic riding program that took place twice weekly for 1 hour. Bertoti designed an observational postural assessment tool for the study. She reported that muscle tone, posture, and balance improved, as evidenced by improved functional skills.

Biery and Kauffman (1989) studied 8 children and young adults with Down syndrome in a therapeutic riding program of 6 months' duration. They reported a subjective decrease in quadruped position test scores and no significant differences in standing test scores.

Cawley and colleagues (1994) studied 29 students between ages 11 and 17 who had educational needs. The duration of therapeutic riding was 8 weeks. They reported a small increase in self-concept as measured by the Piers Harris Children's Concept Scale.

MacPhail and colleagues (1998) performed a VHS camcorder kinematics analysis of horse and rider to investigate postural responses during horseback riding of 6 children with cerebral palsy and 7 children who did not have a disability. They found that the children with cerebral palsy displaced the trunk almost twice as much as the children without disability. In addition, the children with cerebral palsy responded with less frequent equilibrium reactions than the children without disabil-

ity. Another finding in the study was that the pelvic movement of the horse is a dual frequency sinusoidal curve rather than a simple sinusoidal curve. Kinematic reports in the literature attributed to Baumann describe similar vertical and lateral amounts of center of gravity displacement—about 0.5 cm—in both individual walking and horseback riding (cited in DePauw, 1986). However, Baumann reported that the degree of pelvic rotation from side to side was about 8°, which is less rotation than occurs in walking (DePauw, 1986). Additionally, the riders appeared to exercise the hip abductors with a minimal amount of stress to the spinal column.

Many of the case studies reported are descriptive in nature and measure the success of the program with minimal rigor (Osborne, 1998; Wingate, 1982). Haehl, Giuliani, and Lewis (1999) studied 2 children with cerebral palsy over 12 weeks using a two-dimensional video analysis of the cranial and caudal elements during the ride. They reported positive subjective effects in postural control and coordination; however, those effects did not generalize to functional performance in the Pediatric Evaluation of Disability Inventory (PEDI). Land, Errington-Povalac, and Paul (2001), in an 8-week study of 3 children with disabilities who were between 6 and 9 years old, measured the benefits of a therapeutic riding program using eight measures of sitting posture. They reported positive effects in four of the eight sitting postures, namely, head angle (front and side view), trunk angle (side view), and neck and body angle (front view). More recently, Sterba, Rogers, France, and Vokes (2002) studied the effects of 18 weeks of hippotherapy, once per week, in 17 children with cerebral palsy. Outcome measures used—the Gross Motor Function Measure (GMFM) and the WeeFIM—demonstrated improved overall gross motor function in the study sample. Blinde and McClung (1997), in a systematic qualitative study of 5 to 10 weeks investigating 23 adults ages 19 to 54 who had mixed physical disabilities, used open-ended interviews and reported that the hippotherapy participants experienced a positive, subjective benefit in sense of control in both their physical and their social lives.

Limited hippotherapy studies involve adults with TBI or stroke. A study identified in a secondary reference describes the changes in functional standing balance in four adults with TBI age 18 and older after a maximum of 20 weeks of hippotherapy intervention (Sykes et al., 1997). The outcome measure was a computerized balance platform and a functional balance assessment, as measured by a videotape analysis of gait. Results of the study demonstrated improvement trends in 2 of the 4 participants, and all clients demonstrated notable improvement in static balance as measured by the balance master center target test.

The purpose of this study was to quantitatively compare the effects of horseback riding in riders without disability and riders with brain injury. The authors hypothesized (1) that postural control, as measured by center of pressure distribution, will differ between the two groups of riders and (2) that a relationship exists among group classifications.

Method

The investigation proposed to study the center of pressure distribution as a measure of postural control. The study population included 12 experienced riders without disability, 14 novice riders without disability, and 7 clients with brain injury. Inclusion criteria for clients with brain injury were the diagnosis of severe TBI or cerebrovascular accident; age greater than 21 years but less than 80 years; receipt of acute care and discharge from hospital more than 30 days previously; ability to sit independently; and provision of informed consent by the client or guardian. Ages of clients with brain injury ranged from 19 to 51 (mean = 38.29, SD = 13.49). Mean height of clients with brain injury was 69.50 inches (range = 62.0–75.5, SD = 4.19); mean weight was 164.43 pounds (range = 127–186, SD = 21.27); and mean body mass index was 22.86 (range = 18–28, SD = 3.53). All clients with brain injury were right-handed and Caucasian. The initial Glasgow Coma Scale for clients with brain injury was < 8, indicating severe injury.

The clients required the ability to sit independently. Exclusion criteria included Transitional Learning Center (TLC) clients who had excessive lower extremity spasticity that precluded the amount of hip abduction, hip adduction, and hip internal rotation necessary to straddle the horse (Whalley, 1980). Clients who had a history of hip subluxation also were excluded. Sources of participant recruitment included staff at a community reentry center and a hippotherapy facility.

Inclusion criteria for control group participants included no history of central nervous system disease. The experienced riders had a minimum of 18 or more horseback riding experiences and ranged in age from 24 to 46 (mean = 32.42, SD = 6.52). The mean height of experienced riders was 66.21 inches (range = 63–73, SD = 2.79); mean weight was 147.17 pounds (range = 116–180, SD = 22.16); and mean body mass index was 23.91 (range = 21–30, SD = 2.47). Two experienced riders were Hispanic, and 10 were Caucasian.

The inexperienced riders had two or fewer experiences on a horse and ranged in age from 19 to 53

(mean = 31.79, SD = 10.49). Mean height of able-bodied inexperienced riders was 65.86 inches (range = 63–69, SD = 1.75); mean weight was 146.21 pounds (range = 115–210, SD = 22.76); mean body mass index was 23.79 (range = 19–35, SD = 4.08). One inexperienced rider was of Asian descent, and the remaining 13 were Caucasian.

Instrumentation

The horse used in the study was a 14-year-old Halflinger/Quarterhorse mare. She measured 14 hands, 1 inch. (This horse would technically be considered a large pony because she did not meet the standard threshold for a horse, i.e., 14.2 hands or larger.) The hand unit measures the height of the horse from the withers (the bony protrusion that marks the highest point of the horse's back) to the ground. A hand is a unit of 4 inches, supposedly equal to a hand's breadth. The horse weighed 1,200 pounds. This horse had been used for the past 12 years in the hippotherapy program at the center. A Western saddle supported the rider's seat, protected the horse's spine, and allowed the horse freedom of movement. A Circle Y barrel racer saddle measuring 15 inches was selected in order to accommodate to the highest number of people.

A Force Sensing Array (FSA) mat placed on the saddle was used to measure the rider's center of pressure distribution and frequency. FSA is a computer-based system that can map pressure distribution on any weight-bearing surface. A thin mat with sensors connected to a computer with FSA software was placed under the rider. The software received the data and created a visual representation of the rider's weight distribution. Data were displayed in topographical form with color gradations, three-dimensional schematics with peaks representing higher-pressure areas, or as numbers according to measured pressure. Reports on the validity of the transducers show that calibration characteristics are reliable, repeatable, durable, and accurate (Ferguson-Pell & Cardi, 1993). Main outcome indices of postural control were defined as (1) the number of sensors activated (NSA) and (2) body center of pressure dispersion area (BCOPD). The indices were measured using pressure-mapping technology from a mat placed over the horse's saddle. Manufacturer-reported accuracy with the interfaces was 90%. The BCOPD was computed from the x-axis (right–left) and y-axis (anterior–posterior) and standard deviations calculated over an elliptical area:

$$BCOPD = P_i \Sigma \left(2 \Sigma COPX\ SD \right) \Sigma \left(2 \Sigma COPY\ SD \right)$$

A repeated-measures research design was used to examine the influence of two independent variables on postural control—group classification (experienced riders without disability, inexperienced riders without disability, and riders with brain injury) and riding situation (right side, left side, clockwise, and counter-clockwise movement). The dependent variable was postural control as measured by NSA and BCOPD.

The investigation took place at a North American Riding for the Handicapped Association (NARHA)–certified therapeutic hippotherapy arena with NARHA-certified therapists. The therapists were also members of the American Hippotherapy Association, a subdivision of NARHA. These affiliations and accreditations ensured the experience and safety procedures used in the hippotherapy program. Consent forms were obtained from all riders. Confidentiality of the participants' identities was maintained by a coding system.

Procedures

We examined the pressure sensor readings and dispersion distribution during two laps at a NARHA-certified therapeutic hippotherapy arena. One lap was in a clockwise and the other in a counter-clockwise direction around the arena with clear views of identifiable location markers. Additionally, postural control indices were measured on the right and left sides of the body. Videos taken during the laps enabled the delineation of periods of interest (fragments) between the visible markers.

To maximize safety, each rider was fitted with an ASTM-SEI–approved (American Society for Testing and Materials–Safety Equipment Institute) riding helmet for head protection and was assisted in mounting and dismounting the assigned horse at a wheelchair-accessible mounting platform (Nelson, Rivara, & Condie, 1994). The riders mounted and dismounted from the horse's left shoulder while she was in a standing position. The rider mounted from the special platform to achieve a similar position on top of the pressure sensor map placed on top of the saddle. The riders were supervised by two sidewalkers positioned on each side of the horse for safety. An experienced horse handler long-lined the horse (i.e., professionally guided the horse using a standard lead rope while working a safe distance from the horse) along the edge of the arena in two sets of loops: clockwise and counter-clockwise. The arena was 130 feet × 66 feet with location markers.

The gait of the horse, which is the horse's natural foot movement, was standardized for the study. The horse used a walking gait, which is a rhythmic, even, four-beat sequence at about 8 km/hr or 3 mph. Each stride was of equal length. At least two feet were on the ground at the same time. The horse's walking speed was determined by timing the horse during each trial.

Data Collection

A 256-sensor (16 inches × 16 inches) pressure mat was placed between the saddle and the rider for each trial. The total outside dimensions of the mat sensing area were 17 inches × 17 inches, leaving 1.13 square inches for each sensor. A battery-powered FSA Interface Module was connected by cable to the FSA mat during each 30- to 40-second data collection trial. The pressure sensors were sampled 10 times each second. After completion of each data collection trial, the data were downloaded from the interface module to a notebook computer for subsequent analysis. Because of the small sample size, we calculated effect size, which is the magnitude of difference between means for 60 mmHg sensor pressure to minimize the likelihood of committing a Type II error. The *d* index indicated the *difference* between two group means expressed in terms of a pooled standard deviation (*SD*). The *d*-index equation is

$$d = X_1 - X_2 / \{(SD_1 + SD_2 / 2)\},$$

where X_1 and X_2 indicate group means and SD_1 and SD_2 is the average *SD*. A *d*-index value of 0.8 or greater reflects a large effect. Effect sizes of 0.5 and 0.2 indicate moderate and small effect sizes, respectively. Additionally, we computed U_3, which is the percentage of scores in the lower mean group that were exceeded by the higher mean group. Table 11.1 summarizes the effect sizes for all possible group comparisons.

Data Analysis

Body mass index (BMI) was calculated for each participant to examine homogeneity of groups with respect to height and weight influences on center of pressure and postural control. Independent-samples *t* tests were used to examine group composition. To test the effects of postural control on BCOPD for each group and direction of the ride (straight or curved), as well as all potential interactions, mixed repeated analyses of variance (ANOVA) were conducted using the postural control indices as the within-subject variable and the rider group as the between-subject variable. In conducting the analyses, all hypotheses were tested as two-tailed at the .05 α level. The global analysis was evaluated using a Greenhouse–Geisser calculation. Marginal mean analysis of main effect was performed using a Sidak adjustment. The center of pressure frequency and distribution were calculated and averaged for each rider. Finally, BMI was

Table 11.1. Effect Sizes for NSA and BCOPD

Comparison Groups	d Index	U₃ (%)
NSA effect sizes		
Experienced–inexperienced	0.74	77.0
Experienced–riders with brain injury	0.57	71.6
Inexperienced–riders with brain injury	1.18	88.1
BCOPD effect sizes		
Counter-clockwise left–counter-clockwise right	0.29	61.5
Counter-clockwise left–clockwise left	0.39	65.4
Counter-clockwise left–clockwise right	0.07	53.0
Counter-clockwise right–clockwise left	0.73	76.9
Counter-clockwise right–clockwise right	0.21	58.4
Clockwise left–clockwise right	0.47	68.3

Note. BCOPD = body center of pressure dispersion area; NSA = number of sensors activated.

calculated for each rider for independent-samples *t*-test analysis. The Statistical Package for the Social Sciences (SPSS 10.1, Chicago) was used for all statistical analyses.

Results

Examination of rider BMI showed no significant differences among groups. Data were obtained throughout the trajectory of the horse walking in two patterns along the edge of the arena: one pathway beginning in a straight line and culminating in a turn to the right; another pathway beginning in a straight line and culminating in a turn to the left. Significant differences between groups were identified ($F[2,29] = 4.26$, $p = .024$) in the NSA (Table 11.2 and Figure 11.1).

Marginal mean comparison using a Sidak adjustment revealed a significant difference between riders with brain injury and inexperienced riders (mean difference = 24.946, $p = .009$). Similarly, significant main effects were noted for the BCOPD within group variable ($F[2.3, 67.9] = 3.69$, $p = .024$; Table 11.2 and Figure 11.2). Sidak comparisons showed a significant difference between the counter-clockwise right and clockwise left riding situation (mean difference = .562, $p = .040$). Riders with brain injury had the highest NSA and the lowest BCOPD. Generally speaking, the results indicate that riders with brain injury showed a significantly higher activation of sensors in the mat at 60 mmHg than the inexperienced and experienced riders (Figure 11.3).

These findings are not surprising when taking into account the qualitative observations of the research team. The riders with brain injury showed less automatic or conscious postural adjustments, less variation in movements, and less awareness of the potential consequences of horseback riding. The data also indicate that, regardless of rider group, participants demonstrated the lowest BCOPD in the left-sided, counter-clockwise riding situation.

Observations of riders' positions showed that experienced riders sat deep in the saddle with their thighs and knees pressed down, close to the horse. Their arms hung relaxed. Their heads were up and looked forward, and they appeared symmetrical and their hips somewhat neutral. The inexperienced riders and, notably, the riders with brain injury showed more trunk and arm stiffness and more body asymmetry. The riders with brain injury collapsed in the seat with their thighs and knees forward on the horse. Their arms and elbows were tense on the side. Their heads were slightly down and looked down. They appeared asymmetrical, with

Table 11.2. ANOVA Summary Table for Sensor Pressure at 60 mmHg, by Rider Group

Source	df	SS	MS	F	p
Between Riders					
Rider group	2	12534.23	6267.11	4.257	.024
Error (between)	29	116.933	3.341		
Within Riders					
Stability ratio	3	21.91	21.91	.241	.627 NS
Stability ratio by group	6	66.44	33.22	.365	.697 NS
Error (within)	87	2637.78	90.96		

Note. df = degrees of freedom; SS = sums of squares; MS = mean of squares; NS = not significant.

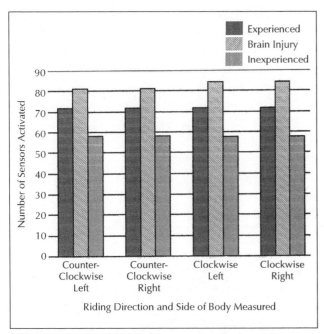

Figure 11.1. Amount of pressure into 60 mmHg sensors during riding by group.

their hips posteriorly tilted. The inexperienced riders, however, showed the largest BCOPD.

Because of limitations in sample size, the authors used the calculation of effect size, which is the magnitude of difference between means for 60-mmHg-sensor pressure to minimize the likelihood of committing a Type II error. The *d* index indicated the difference

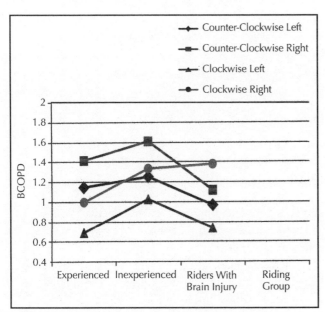

Figure 11.2. Body center of pressure dispersion area (BCOPD), by riding direction and group.

between two group means expressed in terms of a pooled standard deviation. The *d*-index equation is $d = X_1 − X_2 / \{SD_1 + SD_2\}/2\}$ (X_1 and X_2 indicate group means, and SD_1 and SD_2 is the average standard deviation). A *d* index of 0.8 or greater reflects a large effect. Effect sizes of 0.5 and 0.2 indicate moderate and small effect sizes, respectively. Additionally, we computed U_3, which is the percentage of scores in the lower mean group that were exceeded by the higher mean group. Table 11.1 reports the effect size values between all possible group comparisons.

Discussion

This pilot is one of the first to examine objectively postural control indices among riders with and without brain injury using pressure-mapping technology placed over the horse's saddle. The differences among riders can be partially explained by some qualitative observation noted among the riders. The inexperienced riders showed some apprehension and overadjustment in postural control movements. The riders with brain injury showed no apprehension about riding and underadjustment of postural control movement, and the experienced riders had a relaxed attitude and just-right adjustment of postural control movements. The observations and findings in postural control of the riders with brain injury are similar to those reported in the literature (Pauw, 2000); however, the differences among riders need further investigation.

Hippotherapy is a multisensory, complex rehabilitation approach that can be influenced by multiple variables emerging from the riding environment, including those related to rider and horse characteristics (Biery & Kauffman, 1989). For example, the horse's size, the horse's gait speed, the saddle type and size, and the rider's biomechanical and neuromuscular characteristics all can influence postural adjustments on the horse.

The generalization of the findings is limited by the small, heterogeneous sample size; the lack of randomization and the use of a single center; the predictable horse arena; and the riders' and horse's characteristics. Despite these limitations, the findings highlight and support the potential for the use of pressure mapping as an index of postural control during horseback riding. Pressure mapping analysis can contribute to the basis for better quantitative evaluation of postural control impairment. The creative transfer of technology by this research team can provide an additional tool that can maximize the analysis of postural control.

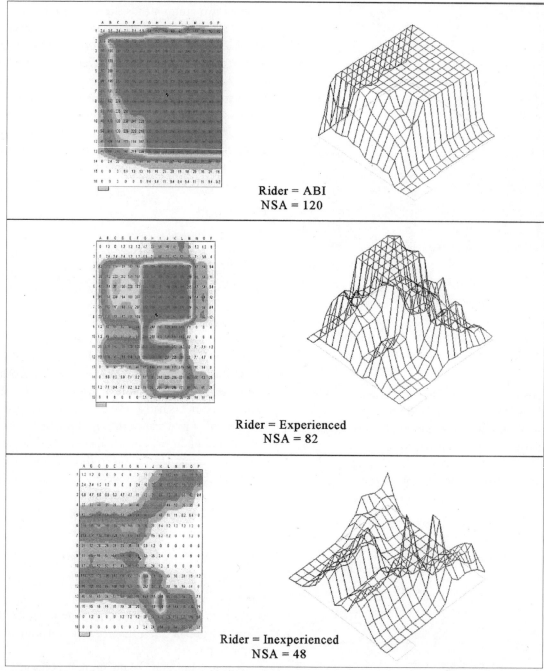

Rider = ABI
NSA = 120

Rider = Experienced
NSA = 82

Rider = Inexperienced
NSA = 48

Figure 11.3 Sample of number of sensors activated (NSA) in one point in time at 60 mmHg shown as two-dimensional and three-dimensional figures.

Conclusion

This pilot study allowed us to gain preliminary quantitative information about the differences in postural control among inexperienced riders, experienced riders, and riders with brain injury. Pressure mapping can illuminate the study of postural control as it relates to the effectiveness of hippotherapy as a rehabilitative technique. In conclu-

sion, pressure mapping can be used effectively as an index to compare postural control among riders with different capabilities.

Clients, families, and caretakers offered positive unsolicited information about their satisfaction with horseback riding as a rehabilitation technique. Comments such as these attest to the psychosocial aspects of animal–human bonding and the riders' perceptions of their increased mobility potential. These issues were not addressed in this study but need further study. Therapeutic horseback riding is a complex alternative rehabilitation technique that requires multifaceted investigation. Further qualitative and quantitative research methodologies at the impairment, functional activity, and participation level are needed to investigate the phenomena of hippotherapy for postural control after brain injury to expand the understanding of the benefits of therapeutic horseback riding.

Acknowledgments

This work was supported in part by the Moody Foundation Grant No. 2000-18; Research Supplement for Under-represented Minorities Grant No. 3R01AG17638-01A1S1 to Dr. Abreu from the National Institutes of Health; and postdoctoral fellowship to Dr. Heyn from the Interdisciplinary Rehabilitation Research Training Program Grant No. H133P99001, National Institute on Disability and Rehabilitation. We thank Karin J. Opacich for her guidance in the interpretation of results. We also thank Neil Huddleston; Kim Luppens, OTR; Becky Poehl, PT; Jean Minkel, PT; and Joanne Jones, OTR, for their collaboration during this study.

References

All, A. C., Loving, G. L., & Crane, L. L. (1999). Animals, horseback riding, and implications for rehabilitation therapy. *Journal of Rehabilitation, 65*, 49–57.

Bertoti, D. B. (1988). Effect of therapeutic horseback riding on posture in children with cerebral palsy. *Physical Therapy, 68*, 1505–1512.

Biery, M. L., & Kauffman, N. (1989). The effects of therapeutic horseback riding on balance. *Adapted Physical Activity Quarterly, 6*, 221–229.

Blinde, E. M., & McClung, L. R. (1997). Enhancing the physical and social self through recreational activity: Accounts of individuals with physical disabilities. *Adapted Physical Activity Quarterly, 14*, 327–344.

Bliss, B. (1997). Complementary therapies: Therapeutic horseback riding? *RN, 60*, 69–70.

Bracher, M. (2000). Therapeutic horse riding: What has this to do with occupational therapists? *British Journal of Occupational Therapy, 63*, 277–282.

Cawley, R., Cawley, D., & Retter, K. (1994). Therapeutic horseback riding and self-concept in adolescents with special educational needs. *Anthrozoos, 7*, 129–134.

DePauw, K. P. (1986). Horseback riding for individuals with disabilities: Programs, philosophy, and research. *Adapted Physical Activity Quarterly, 3*, 217–226.

Engel, B. T. (Ed.). (1997). *Rehabilitation with the aid of a horse: A collection of studies.* Durango, CO: Barbara Engel Therapy Services.

Ferguson-Pell, M., & Cardi, M. D. (1993). Prototype development and comparative evaluation of wheelchair pressure mapping system. *Applied Research, 5*, 78–91.

Haehl, V., Giuliani, C., & Lewis, C. (1999). Influence of hippotherapy on the kinematics and functional performance of two children with cerebral palsy. *Pediatric Physical Therapy, 11*, 89–101.

Heine, B. (1997). Hippotherapy. A multisystem approach to the treatment of neuromuscular disorders. *Australian Physiotherapy, 43*, 145–149.

Ikai, T., Kamikubo, T., Takehara, I., Nishi, M., & Miyano, S. (2003). Dynamic postural control in patients with hemiparesis. *American Journal of Physical Medicine and Rehabilitation, 82*, 463–469.

Land, G., Errington-Povalac, E., & Paul, S. (2001). The effects of therapeutic riding on sitting posture in individuals with disabilities. *Occupational Therapy in Health Care, 14*, 1–12.

MacKinnon, L. R., Noh, S., Laliberte, D., Lariviere, L., & Allan, D. E. (1995). Therapeutic horseback riding: A review of the literature. *Physical and Occupational Therapy in Pediatrics, 15*, 1–15.

MacPhail, H. E. A., Edwards, J., Golding, L., Miller, K., Mosier, C., & Zwiers, T. (1998). Trunk postural reactions in children with and without cerebral palsy during therapeutic horseback riding. *Pediatric Physical Therapy, 10*, 143–147.

Nelson, D. E., Rivara, F. P., & Condie, C. (1994). Helmets and horseback riders. *American Journal of Preventive Medicine, 10*, 15–19.

Osborne, M. B. A. (1998). Hippotherapy as an intervention modality for a patient with cerebellar dysfunction. *Physical Therapy Case Reports, 1*, 58–60.

Pauw, J. (2000). Therapeutic horseback riding studies: Problems experienced by researchers. *Physiotherapy, 86*, 523–527.

Sterba, J. A., Rogers, B. T., France, A. P., & Vokes, D. A. (2002). Horseback riding in children with cerebral palsy: Effect on gross motor function. *Developmental Medicine and Child Neurology, 44*, 301–308.

Sykes, M., Gouge, D., Newstead, A., Freeman, G., Tomberlin, J., & Mossberg, K. (1997). The effects of therapeutic horseback riding on balance in persons with brain injury. In B. T. Engel (Ed.), *Rehabilitation with the aid of a horse: A collection of studies* (pp. 127–144). Durango, CO: Barbara Engel Therapy Services.

Whalley, K. R. (1980). Riding for the disabled: Improving the quality of life. *Occupational Therapy, 43*, 267–268.

Wingate, L. (1982). Feasibility of horseback riding as a therapeutic and integrative program for handicapped children. *Physical Therapy, 62*, 184–186.

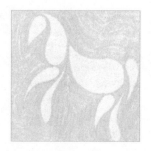

Riders who force their horses by the use of the whip
only increase their fear, for they then associate
the pain with the thing that frightens them.
— Xenophon

CHAPTER 12

Influence of Hippotherapy on Tonic Bite: A Case Study

Sandra L. Hubbard, PhD, OTR/L, ATP, and Dixie L. Carr-Heyn, MPT

Tonic bite is a frequent and painful occurrence for children with athetoid or dystonic cerebral palsy. This case study reports how hippotherapy was used as a treatment modality to decrease the incidence of tonic bite by (1) identifying the sequelae of events leading up to the event and (2) developing strategies to avoid the event.

Background: Developmental and Medical History

At the time of this study, Matt was a 6-year-old male with a clinical diagnosis of triplegia due to cerebral palsy. He presented with spastic and athetoid and dystonic muscle tone. Matt's gross and fine motor skills are disordered, at the 3- to 5-month age level; he is dependent in all activities of daily living. For mobility, he is carried or pushed in a manual wheelchair, which is equipped with tilt and recline. With support and assistance, Matt can stand and take a few steps; without assistance, he cannot sit or roll. He is fed a semisolid diet supported with tube feeding. Hearing and vision are within functional limits; cognitive level is unknown, but it appears to be in the normal range. Matt communicates with vocalizations and facial gestures, specifically with eye gaze and smile, although higher technology means were being pursued at the time of assessment.

Matt was carried full-term with no complications and delivered by Cesarean section (as was a previous sibling). During the pregnancy, his mother took phenytoin (Dilantin) to control seizures and resided in a community where a chemical spill leaked arsenic into the water supply, reaching peak levels in 1991, the year Matt was born. A few hours after birth, Matt experienced several episodes of apnea. A few days later, he was transferred to a specialty children's hospital. An electro-encephalogram and barium swallow showed normal results. He arrived home with an apnea monitor at 11 days old and continued to have episodes of apnea, always self-correcting. Matt's mother reported "a lot of movement" during his first 2 months, then at 3 months, a decrease in his progress and development of an extensor thrust pattern. Initially, physicians expected his development to "catch up."

By 5 months old, Matt was lacking trunk control and presenting with increased lower extremity adductor tone, making it difficult to change his diapers. Upon consult with a neurologist and a magnetic resonance image (MRI), Matt was found to have holoprosencephaly, a congenital defect resulting from an extra chromosome, either trisomy 13–15 or trisomy 18, which causes deficiency in the forebrain. Matt also developed diabetes insipidus, which was treated with hormone therapy. At assessment, he was receiving 0.6 cc of desmopressin acetate subcutaneously in the thigh every night to regulate body fluids. From the time he was 1 year old to age 2 years, 6 months, Matt was hospitalized four times for dehydration and once for pneumonia. During one dehydration episode, he experienced a seizure from receiving too much fluid too quickly, causing a significant reduction in sodium. He was placed on phenobarbital for 3 months. At age 2½, a gastrointestinal tube was surgically placed for feeding. Although Matt has taken various oral medications to reduce spasticity, he was not on medication to reduce spasticity at the time of this study.

At 5 months old, Matt began physical therapy and occupational therapy, twice weekly. At 6 months old, he began receiving early intervention program, including (at age 2) an inpatient stay at a rehabilitation hospital for family education. Matt began therapeutic riding before age of 3, and he began special education services at age 3. At the time of the study, Matt continued to receive physical, occupational, and speech-language therapies in school and in an outpatient clinic, and he received hippotherapy.

By age 2, Matt had received a manual wheelchair that provided head and trunk support. He was unable to progress to an electric power wheelchair because of poor head control and, thus, an inability to drive with a head switch. At age 4, Matt underwent surgical release of his adductors and hamstrings bilaterally. He began wearing ankle–foot orthoses bilaterally at age 5.

Tonic Bite

Normally developing infants demonstrate the phasic bite at about the age of 4 months (Ganz, 1987; Morris, Mueller, & Klein, 1987). The tonic bite reflex is abnormal: Stimulation placed in or around the mouth causes a tight closure of the jaw and an inability to open the mouth once the reflex has been initiated (Ganz, 1987; Morris et al., 1987). Biting has been found to be the most frequent abnormal oral reflex in people with cerebral palsy with spastic or athetoid tone (Ingram, 1962).

A literature search on Medline and the Cumulative Index of Nursing and Allied Health Literature (CINAHL) from 1966 to 2005 revealed a paucity of published, peer-reviewed literature on the tonic bite reflex. Although literature on the use of positioning to inhibit abnormal oral reflexes (Love, Hagerman, & Taimi, 1980; Morris et al., 1987; Ottenbacher, Bundy, & Short, 1983) exists, this literature does not address positioning in relation to the tonic bite.

Method and Intervention

Using a single-case study design, data were collected using direct observation and review of videotape over a period of 1 hippotherapy session per week for 3 months. Hippotherapy sessions were conducted by an occupational therapist, occupational therapy and physical therapy students, and trained volunteer horse handlers and sidewalkers. Limitations on ability to ride the horse included Matt's tight hip adductors, inability to sit independently, poor head control, and inability to reach and grasp (e.g., the reins). Factors that varied throughout the observation period included extraneous factors (e.g., weather), sidewalkers, home versus respite care, and medications (e.g., diphenhydramine, diazepam). Factors that remained consistent were the equipment used (surcingle, sheepskin, reins), horse, the presence of a backrider, and treatment-handling techniques.

Initially, and for the duration of this case study, Matt was backridden with sidewalkers during his therapy sessions.* Matt spent approximately 20 minutes on the horse each session. During the first 5 to 15 minutes of the hippotherapy session, the rhythmic movement of the horse and rotational activities initiated by the occupational therapist backrider facilitated a decrease in extensor tone of the trunk, resulting in upper and lower trunk dissociation, increased mobility of the pelvis, and release of tight lower-extremity adductors. The remainder of the session provided Matt with opportunity for functional and purposeful activities, his favorite being holding the reins. If and when Matt experienced extension, as his head extended back, his hands were drawn to his mouth as if it were one associated movement pattern. Thus, the question or problem was not why the jaws closed on the hands, but what caused the hands to be drawn to the mouth in the first place? Although answers to this question could not be found in the literature, techniques for inhibition (the intervention) were identified during hippotherapy sessions.

Once upper and lower truck dissociation and pelvic mobility were achieved, the occupational therapist backrider used her hip and trunk to maintain Matt in an assisted sitting position and used her hands to provide support to Matt's mandible, particularly at the gonial angle, using techniques described by Morris, Mueller, and Klein (1987). With the walking movement of the horse providing rhythms input to the pelvis and lower truck, the therapist could suspend Matt's upper trunk with slight pressure of two figures on either side of his lower jaw. Consequently, Matt's hands were free to reach for and maintain grasp on the reins, and he could rotate his head laterally, free from the effects of tonic neck reflexes. When this delicate balance was lost, Matt was overcome by extensor tone and his hands flew involuntarily back to his mouth. Once balance was re-achieved, Matt was able to use his hands to control the reins, perhaps the first time Matt had been observed to "reach."

This exercise then was taken one step further. While maintaining support to the mandible for the head and neck flexion, the therapist leaned forward

---

*During later hippotherapy sessions, a bolster attached to a surcingle and sidewalkers were used to maintain Matt's position on the horse in lieu of backriding; the horse ridden in those sessions was capable of a slow, consistent walk.

with her trunk, thereby shifting Matt's center of gravity forward while the horse continued at a rhythmical walk. Matt was able to support himself on one arm while using the other arm to grab the horse's mane and pat the horse.

Conclusion

A significant problem both on and off the horse was the tendency for Matt to bite his hands, a bite that was both involuntary and tonic and led to pain and risk of infection from puncture of his hands by his teeth. Matt had been provided with soft splints to protect his hands. It was observed that while riding on the horse, the incidence of tonic bite of his fingers decreased and functional hand use (i.e., holding the reins) increased.

References

Ganz, S. F. (1987). Decreasing tongue thrusting and tonic bite through neuromotor. *Physical and Occupational Therapy in Pediatrics, 7*, 57–75.

Ingram, T. S. (1962). Clinical significance of the infantile feeding reflexes. *Developmental Medicine and Child Neurology, 4*, 159–169.

Love, R. J., Hagerman, E. L., & Taimi, E. G. (1980). Speech performance, dysphagia, and oral reflexes in cerebral palsy. *Journal of Speech and Hearing Disorders, 45*, 59–75.

Morris, S. E., Mueller, & Klein, M. D. (1987). *Pre-feeding skills.* Tucson, AZ: Communication Skills Builder.

Ottenbacher, K. J., Bundy, A., & Short, M. (1983). The development and treatment of oral–motor dysfunction: A review of clinical research. *Physical and Occupational Therapy in Pediatrics, 3*, 1–3.

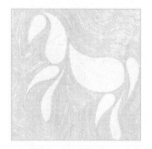

*Care and not fine stables
make a good horse.*
—Danish Proverb

CHAPTER 13

Efficacy of Hippotherapy as a Treatment Strategy for Children With Autism

Janine Stoner, MS, OTR

Autistic disorders are severe forms of pervasive developmental disorder (PDD); onset is in infancy or childhood, and the degree of impairment varies from child to child. The etiology of autism is unknown, and there is no known cure for the condition. The *Diagnostic and Statistical Manual of Mental Disorders, Fourth Edition* (*DSM–IV*; American Psychiatric Association, 1994) stated that children with PDD/autism are characterized by impairment in the development of reciprocal social interaction, in the development of verbal and nonverbal communication skills, and imaginative activity. They often have a restrictive repertoire of activities and interests, which are stereotyped and repetitive. Delays in development are common in intellectual skills; comprehension and speech production; posture and movements; patterns of eating, drinking, or sleeping; and responses to sensory input. Huebner (1992) pointed out that treatment of a child with autism must involve a team of professionals who can address potential social, cognitive, motor, attention, medical, and sensory deficits. Occupational therapists, as part of the treatment team, typically address sensory processing and modulation deficits.

Because a major symptom of autism is a disturbance of sensory processing, it is logical that sensory integration procedures would be used to ameliorate the autistic symptoms (Ayres & Tickle, 1980). *Sensory integration* is, according to Ayres (1979), "the organization of sensation for use" (p. 5). Watling, Deitz, Kanny, and McLaughlin (1999) reported that 99% of occupational therapists use a sensory integrative frame of reference in their treatment approach when working with children with autism.

This integrative frame of reference originated in the work of A. Jean Ayres, an occupational therapist and educational psychologist, in the 1960s and 1970s. Case-Smith (2005) stated,

> One of the most distinctive contributions that Ayres made to the understanding of child development was her focus on sensory processing, particularly with respect to the proximal senses: vestibular, tactile, and proprioceptive. In the sensory integrative viewpoint, these senses are emphasized because they are primitive and primary: they dominate the child's interactions with the world early in life. (p. 356)

Although therapy cannot cure a condition such as autism, it is aimed at the underlying capabilities and addresses sensory processing issues in children. Occupational therapists use specialized equipment such as suspension equipment, which consists of various swings, bolsters, and hammocks that are hung from overhead. This equipment provides rich opportunities for stimulating and challenging the vestibular system, along with a variety of somatosensory stimuli such as tactile, vibratory, and proprioceptive input (Case-Smith, Allen, & Pratt, 1996). The therapist arranges the clinic to be an environment rich in sensory opportunities. Case-Smith and colleagues stated,

> The child chooses the activity or equipment in which he or she wishes to engage. The therapist challenges the child by evoking increasingly complex adaptive responses. This is done by respecting the child's needs and interests while looking for opportunities to help the child successfully meet a challenge. (p. 308)

Families with children who have autism have attested to the benefits of treatment aimed at sensory processing to increase the child's ability to maintain focus, engage in tasks, and transition from one activity to another. The provision of sensory experiences throughout the course of the child's day often can help prepare the child to focus and tend to academic tasks. A sensory approach can affect a child's ability to tolerate transitions from one activity to another as well as social situations with classmates.

For there to be carry-over of benefits outside the therapeutic context, daily sensory processing activities are essential. Wilbarger (2002) indicated that therapy in isolation will not be enough—that a *sensory diet* is needed. The sensory diet consists of sensory-based activities that can be done throughout the day in a variety of settings. Recreational activities that provide a wealth of sensory input can help children with autism and their families improve their day-to-day function. Families are encouraged to schedule their lives around enjoyable activities related to their interests rather than around the therapy clinic. The inclusion of hippotherapy into an occupational therapy program can be part of a sensory diet.

The equine environment not only provides rich sensory opportunities but also has its own organizational structure, which is related to caring for and riding a horse. Providing a structural setting is beneficial to children with autism who have difficulty with organization (Hubbard, 1999). According to Shkedi (1991), in addition to providing proprioceptive and vestibular stimulation, the movement of the horse may provide other forms of sensory input, such as tactile, auditory, and visual stimuli, that may be beneficial to the rider.

Literature Review

In 1952, Madame Liz Hartel of Denmark, after being stricken with polio, had rehabilitated herself from wheelchair to horseback to win the silver medal for Grand Prix dressage at the Helsinki Olympics. Her achievement inspired the use of the horse for therapeutic purposes in Denmark, England, and Norway. In the 1960s, riding for people with disabilities spread to Canada and the United States. In 1970, the North American Riding for the Handicapped Association (NARHA) was established to set accreditation standards for riding programs and certification standards for instructors (Butt, 1970, cited in Engel, 1997).

The type of therapeutic riding varies in each country, often depending on the origin of its development. Therapeutic riding in the United States evolved from two directions—the British sports model and the more clinical models of Germany and Switzerland (Copeland, 1992). The British model uses riding as a recreational sport to improve mental and physical well-being, whereas the clinical model of Germany and Switzerland evolved from the medical world and focuses on postural alignment and physical rehabilitation of riding. The therapeutic aspect in its more scientific sense directed the early activities of therapeutic riding, including use of the Swiss term *hippotherapy*, which came into common use to describe therapeutic riding as a specialized medical treatment (Klüwer, 1982). In the United States, a third approach, which emphasizes educational goals, also has been developed. Although each model has a specific goals and approach, all three (sport/recreational, medical, and educational) overlap to integrate and support each other's objectives.

DePauw (1986) conducted a literature review of research conducted in the field of therapeutic riding and hippotherapy and found that prior to the 1980s, little scientific investigation had documented the benefits of therapeutic riding or hippotherapy. In addition, important studies conducted in Germany, Switzerland, and other countries were difficult to access because of translation difficulties.

Therapeutic riding grew out of the discipline of *dressage.* The term comes from the French word for *schooling* or *teaching.* This discipline aims to have the horse at its peak of balance and suppleness to perform specific movements. Many of the components involved in sensory processing also are involved in dressage (Engel, 1997). The client is engaged in purposeful activities that are movement-based to elicit a high-level adaptive response.

Tolson (1997) published a study of therapeutic horseback riding and behavior changes in children with autism. The study targeted three types of classroom behaviors of two children diagnosed with autism: echolalic speech, self-directed behavior (stereotypic or self-stimulatory behaviors), and other-directed behaviors (behavior directed at another student). Videotaped free play was used to observe behaviors. Tally marks were used with a time-sampling method. Results were plotted on a scattergram, and celeration lines were drawn for the intervention phase. Following 8 weeks of therapeutic riding 1 hour each week, it was reported that there was a decrease in echolalia. Kohn (1996) wrote,

> There is no one approach for working with autism. Because of the wide spectrum of characters are utilized. Many of these include behavior modification, speech-language therapy, vision therapy, sensory motor, and sensory

integration. All of these can and are addressed in therapeutic riding classes. (p. 6)

Kohn (1996) used the Treatment and Education of Autistic and Related Communication Handicapped Children (TEACCH) approach in her work. Students use visual schedule boards in their therapeutic riding endeavors. Riding Education of Autistic and Communication Handicapped Children (REACCH) grew out of the success seen in the practice of TEACCH. Children use their visual schedules to assist them with tasks such as putting on their helmets, mounting, and riding. In Kohn's research, children with tactile sensitivity had an opportunity to work through their defensiveness through the sensory processing work on horseback; teachers and parents noted that the children had improved in areas of sensory processing and seemed more aware of the world around them after riding.

Webb, Dean, Surgenor, and Jeffries (1997) found effects on social behavior and sensorimotor integration. In an experiment using therapeutic horseback riding with 11 men living in an institution in New Zealand, they measured length of arm reach, bilateral coordination, and balance on one leg with and without vision occluded. Results demonstrated significantly improved arm reach and bilateral coordination but no change in balance.

Sensory integration approaches to hippotherapy have emphasized the role of central processing to bring together kinesthetic, visual, and vestibular inputs to create the self-organization of new motor plans (Nettleton, 1997). The sensory input received during riding may have other beneficial effects, such as improved body awareness and visual perception. Shkedi (1991) noted that therapeutic riding provides proprioceptive and vestibular stimulation and has potential to provide other forms of sensory input, such as tactile, auditory, and visual stimulation. Adaptive motor responses are elicited through active participation of the rider. The participation in activities that are rich in vestibular, proprioceptive, and other sensory information is central to the theoretical frame of reference of sensory integration (Engel, 1997).

The preceding literature review indicates that research concerning the efficacy of hippotherapy as a treatment strategy for children with autism is needed. The current study, therefore, attempts to meet the needs of children with autism and their families by examining the use of hippotherapy as a treatment strategy and adding to the body of knowledge on hippotherapy as part of occupational therapy for children with autism.

Method

Twelve participants for the study were recruited from the waiting list at a therapeutic riding center and through local school systems. Participants were between ages 4 and 10 years and had a diagnosis of PDD or autism. To decrease threats to internal validity, the study used a true experimental research design (i.e., pretest, posttest, and control group). The 12 participants were randomly selected using a hat method from available candidates at the therapeutic riding center. They had no prior riding experience, were matched in pairs by age, and were randomly assigned (again, using the hat method) to either the experimental or control group. The mean age of the experimental group was 6.1; in the control group, it was 6.0. One rider in the experimental group was female, and 11 riders were male. All 12 riders were given a pretest and posttest at the beginning and end of the 10-week period.

The Riding Program

The 6 students in the experimental group participated in therapy that incorporated hippotherapy once a week for 10 weeks. Each session lasted 60 minutes and was divided into 30 minutes of premounted activities followed by 30 minutes of mounted activities. The posttest was the same as the pretest. Differences found, if any, among the experimental and control group can be attributed to the use of hippotherapy within occupational therapy.

All therapy sessions were conducted at the same therapeutic riding center. This facility follows guidelines established by NARHA for safety, and all instructors are NARHA certified. Each child had written permission from his or her pediatrician to participate in riding activities. Parents signed consent forms to include information regarding their child in the study. Sessions included hippotherapy activities that were validated for this research.

Procedures

The researcher administered a pretest and posttest, the Sensory Profile (Dunn, 1997b), to the 12 participants. The Sensory Profile is a standardized instrument that assesses the sensory processing skills of children on the basis of parent or caretaker observations of various tasks. The test consists of 125 items arranged in three sections: Sensory Processing, Modulation, and Behavioral and Emotional Responses (Dunn, 1997b). It uses a Likert scale to profile the effect of sensory processing on functional performance in the daily life of a child. Raw scores were translated into percentages for the purpose of this study. Studies of the Sensory Profile indicated that the items used as a measure were uncommon behaviors for children without disabilities and included atypical behaviors common with autistic children (Dunn, 1997a; Dunn & Ermer, 1998).

In addition to the Sensory Profile, a weekly questionnaire was given to parents and caretakers of the experimental group for 9 weeks. Following each therapy session that included hippotherapy, parents were given one question to answer: "Within the 12 hours following the session, did you notice a change in your child's behavior?" There were three possible choices: (1) Yes, a positive change, (2) Yes, a negative change, or (3) No change. Space was provided for additional comments. This format allowed for categorical data to be gathered to assess the effects of the program from a parent's point of view. This format also allowed for short-term effects of the program to be documented; the long-term effects would be documented through the use of the Sensory Profile.

Results

Sensory Profile scores were converted into percentages and entered into the computer program Statistical Program for the Social Sciences (SPSS, Chicago) for evaluative purposes. Tables 13.1, 13.2, and 13.3 show descriptive statistics, including the mean pretest and posttest scores, standard deviations, and changes in means, for the experimental and control groups.

The results indicate that test scores in the experimental group increased in the categories of multisensory processing, modulation related to body position and movement affecting activity level, modulation of sensory input affecting emotional response, modulation of visual input affecting emotional response and activity level, and behavioral outcomes of sensory processing. The control group did not have a positive change in mean of more than 3 percentage points, except in the area of vestibular processing. This information may support the claim that hippotherapy can improve modulation of sensory input and the ability to process auditory and multisensory input, but it does not support the claim that hippotherapy improves vestibular processing.

The program was arranged in such a way that the riders in the experimental group participated in an unmounted component that included sensory-based activities such as therapeutic listening, tactile activities, and vestibular and proprioceptive activities. The partici-

pants followed the unmounted time with an equal amount of mounted time. To determine whether the auditory processing scores in the experimental group differed as a result of the therapeutic listening program, data were entered into SPSS. Three participants from the control group and three participants from the experimental group were paired by age. Riders in both groups used a therapeutic listening program—the control group as part of their school therapy program and the experimental group during their therapy sessions at the therapeutic riding center. The scores increased in the experimental group by a mean of 14 percentage points (the mean pretest score was 71%, and the mean posttest score was 85%). In contrast, scores in the control group stayed the same at 65%. This may indicate that therapeutic listening, followed by an activity such as riding, will have a positive effect on auditory processing. A one-question weekly questionnaire was given to the parents of children in the experimental group to gather data. The results for each week and each of the subjects are in Table 13.3.

Given the data gathered in the weekly questionnaires, it appears that participants initially may have experienced what was interpreted by parents to be a "negative change" because the child seemed unorganized or had a change in energy level. This observed behavior, however, also could indicate that the central nervous system was taking in the experience and adjusting to it. After Week 3, identified changes were either "positive" or "no change." The percentage of "positive change" responses increased over the course of the 9 weeks: In Week 1, 2 of 6 responses (33%) were positive, but by Week 9, 5 of 6 responses (83%) were positive. This result may indicate that the short-term effects of therapy that incorporates hippotherapy include improved verbalization, improved verbal organization, increased attention and focus, and improved sleep patterns.

Discussion

This project revealed important information. The benefits of combining premounted sensory integration or sensory-based treatment followed by a mounted hippotherapy treatment appeared to have a positive impact on the participants, more so than either approach in isolation. Specifically, participation in a therapeutic listening program followed by riding activities resulted in an increase of auditory processing scores of 14%. Participants in a therapeutic listening program that was not followed with riding showed no change in auditory processing scores. The information used for evaluative purposes relied on parental observations. The Sensory

Table 13.1. Experimental Group Data (N = 6)

Category	Mean Pretest Score	SD	Mean Posttest Score	SD	Change in Mean (Percentage Points)
Auditory processing	71%	5.5	85%	13.3	14%
Visual processing	79%	13.6	75%	15.9	−4
Vestibular processing	75%	20.7	80%	6.8	5
Touch processing	76%	5.6	74%	6.9	−2
Multisensory processing	63%	9.5	71%	9.7	8
Oral sensory processing	78%	16.8	79%	19.2	1
Sensory processing related to endurance and tone	87%	12.1	87%	11.8	0
Modulation related to body, position, and movement	81%	11.8	78%	13.6	−3
Modulation of movement affecting activity level	65%	6.7	73%	11.3	4
Modulation of sensory input affecting emotional responses	69%	10.6	71%	11.0	6
Modulation of visual input affecting emotional responses and activity level	66%	10.8	72%	15.7	6
Emotional and social responses	73%	8.4	74%	8.6	1
Behavioral outcome of sensory processing	65%	11.9	68%	16.8	3

Note. Sensory Profile scores were converted into percentages. *SD* = standard deviation.

Table 13.2. Control Group Data (N = 6)

Category	Mean Pretest Score	SD	Mean Posttest Score	SD	Change in Mean Score (Percentage Points)
Auditory processing	67%	5.5	67%	13.3	0
Visual processing	79%	13.6	75%	15.9	−4
Vestibular processing	75%	20.7	80%	6.8	5
Touch processing	76%	5.6	74%	5.9	−2
Multisensory processing	72%	10.3	71%	6.9	−1
Oral sensory processing	75%	9.8	67%	14.4	−8
Sensory processing related to endurance and tone	82%	18.1	76%	15.1	−6
Modulation related to body, position, and movement	82%	10.9	72%	21.0	−10
Modulation of movement affecting activity level	57%	6.2	53%	10.3	−4
Modulation of sensory input affecting emotional responses	60%	6.3	61%	16.0	1
Modulation of visual input affecting emotional responses and activity level	71%	10.8	64%	5.8	−7
Emotional/social responses	73%	8.4	70%	15.9	0
Behavioral outcome of sensory processing	51%	18.7	51%	19.3	0
Items indicating threshold for responses	67%	13.1	69%	20.6	2

Note. Sensory Profile scores were converted into percentages. *SD* = standard deviation.

Table 13.3. Weekly Responses From Parents or Caregivers

	Positive Response	Negative Response	No Change
Week 1			
Participant 1	More jaunty, walking with a bounce. Talked for 20 minutes on car ride home in a sequential logical manner. Usually *very* bothered by flies in the car—didn't care about them on ride home.		
Participant 2		Seemed in need of a lot of sensory stimulation and unable to sit and work. By bedtime he was calmer and slept well.	
Participant 3			✓
Participant 4			✓
Participant 5			✓
Participant 6	We noticed a change. He was very content, very settled, and more agreeable.		
Week 2			
Participant 1	Was having a "bad" day prior to riding—he had been transitioning very poorly (in tears a lot). After his time at the riding center he was on a much more even keel for the rest of the day, more responsive, more interactive, more organized both physically and verbally.		
Participant 2	Positive, slept through the night, which is notable.	Negative change; very physically charged; required a lot of attention to keep focused.	
Participant 3			✓
Participant 4		Negative change; has had an abundance of energy, going to bed later and waking earlier.	
Participant 5		No questionnaire	
Participant 6	Positive change; he tried to verbalize his needs.		
Week 3			
Participant 1	Positive change; he sang to himself on the ride home.		
Participant 2	Positive change; more focused than usual.		
Participant 3		Negative change; had a tantrum, but it seems to be allergy related to the season.	
Participant 4	Positive change; he was very calm and relatively quiet most of the evening.		
Participant 5	More cooperative and engageable.		
Participant 6	Positive change; instead of humming along with songs, he tried to verbalize the words.		
Week 4			
Participant 1	Positive change; when he came home he told me and his father many imaginative stories. Usually he can only retell stories he has heard, not from his own imagination.		
Participant 2	Positive change; more focused and slept through the night.		
Participant 3			✓
Participant 4	Positive change; he was calm when we got home.		

(continued)

Table 13.3. Weekly Responses From Parents or Caregivers (*Continued*)

	Positive Response	Negative Response	No Change
Participant 5	Positive change; incredibly and wonderfully cooperative and social. Improved connection, language, and motor skills (drew an incredibly accurate picture).		
Participant 6	"Positive change; when he came home he tried to count objects verbally."		
Week 5			
Participant 1			✓
Participant 2	Positive change; slept through the night.		
Participant 3			✓
Participant 4	Positive change; he seemed calmer in the evening.		
Participant 5	Positive change; more cooperative, calmer affect.		
Participant 6	Positive change; had a good day. Spent more time interacting with his siblings, as opposed to "doing his own thing." Tried to verbalize words spontaneously.		
Week 6			
Participant 1	Positive change; more imaginative play and more verbally imaginative also.		
Participant 2	Positive change; calmer after his session and slept through the night.		
Participant 3	Positive change; more alert with more spontaneous language.		
Participant 4			✓
Participant 5	Positive change; very talkative about trotting and brushing the horse. Very cooperative at home after her session.		
Participant 6		No questionnaire	
Week 7			
Participant 1	"Positive change; Made up new and original verses to a song."		
Participant 2	"Positive change; he was more focused and slept through the night."		
Participant 3		No questionnaire	
Participant 4			✓
Participant 5	Positive change		
Participant 6			✓
Week 8			
Participant 1	Positive change		
Participant 2	Positive change		
Participant 3	Positive change		
Participant 4	Positive change		✓
Participant 5	Positive change, more easygoing, flexible, and enjoyable.		
Participant 6	Positive change		
Week 9			
Participant 1	No change noted, but the positive changes he has made appear to be lasting.		
Participant 2	Positive change		
Participant 3	Positive change		
Participant 4	Positive change		
Participant 5	Positive change		
Participant 6	Positive change		

Profile is a standardized tool, but it is dependent upon the observations of the parent or caretaker, as was the weekly questionnaire. Parents noted their satisfaction with the program and felt there were observable changes noted in their child's behavior. It is impossible to discern whether parental satisfaction with the program led them to answer the posttest questionnaire with an inflated positive response; however, it typically is inappropriate to evaluate children with autism using standardized assessments, which require completing various activities given verbal or one-time demonstrated instruction.

This study reinforced the notion that using functional or recreational activities to address therapeutic needs may be more motivating and satisfying for children with special needs and their families. Following this study, several participants continued in programs offered at the therapeutic riding center. One family made a formal request to their local school district to include hippotherapy as part of their child's occupational therapy program and be reflected in their individualized educational plan. The school district, as of this writing, was considering the request.

In conclusion, children with autism may benefit from hippotherapy to improve auditory processing, multisensory processing, and modulation of various sensory inputs.

References

American Psychiatric Association. (1994). *Diagnostic and statistical manual of mental disorders* (4th ed.). Washington, DC: Author.

Ayres, J. (1979). *Sensory integration and the child.* Los Angeles: Western Psychological Services.

Ayres, L., & Tickle, L. (1980). Hyperresponsivity to touch and vestibular stimuli as a predictor of positive response to sensory integration procedures by autistic children. *American Journal of Occupational Therapy, 34,* 375–381.

Case-Smith, J. (2005). *Occupational therapy for children* (5th ed). St. Louis, MO: Mosby Yearbook.

Case-Smith, J., Allen, A., & Pratt, P. (1996). *Occupational therapy for children* (3rd ed.). St. Louis, MO: Mosby Yearbook.

Copeland, J. (1992). Three therapeutic aspects of riding for the disabled. In B. Engel (Ed.), *Therapeutic riding programs* (pp. 19–20). Durango, CO: Barbara Engel Therapy Services.

DePauw, K. (1986). Horseback riding for individuals with disabilities: Programs, philosophy, and research. *Adapted Physical Activity Quarterly, 3,* 217–226.

Dunn, W. (1997a) The sensory profile: A discriminating measure of sensory processing in daily life. *Sensory Integration Special Interest Section Quarterly, 20*(1), 1–3.

Dunn, W. (1997b). *Sensory Profile user's manual.* Tucson, AZ: Therapy Skill Builders.

Dunn, W., & Ermer, L. (1998). The sensory profile: A discriminant analysis of children with and without disabilities. *American Journal of Occupational Therapy, 52,* 530–536.

Engel, B. (1997). Classic dressage as a treatment technique for persons with minimal brain and sensory integrative type dysfunction. In B. Engel (Ed.), *Therapeutic riding II: Strategies for rehabilitation* (pp. 421–432). Durango, CO: Barbara Engel Therapy Services.

Hubbard, S. (1999). Sensory integration as a frame of reference for the practice of hippotherapy with pediatric clientele. In B. Engel (Ed.), *Therapeutic riding I: Strategies for instruction* (pp. 273–284). Durango, CO: Barbara Engel Therapy Services.

Huebner, R. (1992). Autistic disorder: A neuropsychological enigma. *American Journal of Occupational Therapy, 46,* 487–501.

Klüwer, C. (1982). Zur psychologie des reitens-voitgierens. Therapeutisches reitens. In *Proceedings of the 4th International Congress of Therapeutic Riding* (pp. 371–378). Hamburg, Germany.

Kohn, D. (1996, Spring). *Strides Magazine,* P. Denver, CO: North American Riding for the Handicapped.

Nettleton, C. (1997). The effects of hippotherapy on attention and arousal. In B. Engel (Ed.), *Therapeutic riding I: Strategies for instruction* (pp. 390–396). Durango, CO: Barbara Engel Therapy Services.

Shkedi, A. (1991). Sensory input through riding. In *Proceedings from the 7th International Therapeutic Riding Congress* (pp. 129–132). Aarhus, Denmark.

Tolson, P. (1997). Therapeutic horseback riding and behavior change in children with autism: A single subject study. In B. Engel (Ed.), *Rehabilitation with the aid of a horse: A collection of studies* (pp. 15–23). Durango, CO: Barbara Engel Therapy Services.

Watling, R., Deitz, J., Kanny, E. M., & McLaughlin, J. F. (1999). Current practice of occupational therapy for children with autism. *American Journal of Occupational Therapy, 53,* 498–505.

Webb, W., Dean, E., Surgenor, L., & Jeffries, K. (1997). An integration of the effects of a one-year riding for the disabled program on some aspects of sensori motor behavior, and social behavior. In *Proceedings from the 9th International Therapeutic Riding Congress,* Denver, CO.

Wilbarger, S., & Wilbarger, P. (2002). Clinical application of the sensory diet. In A. C. Bundy, S. J. Lane, & E. A. Murray (Eds.), *Sensory integration: Theory and practice* (pp. 339–345). Philadelphia: F. A. Davis.

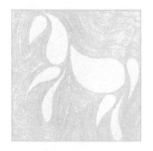

Of all creatures God made at the Creation,
there is none more excellent,
or so much to be respected as a horse.
—Bedouin Legend

CHAPTER 14

A Study of Therapeutic Effects of Horseback Riding for Children With Cerebral Palsy

Joyce R. MacKinnon, PhD, OT(C), OTR; Samuel Noh, PhD;
Judith Lariviere, MEd, OTR/L; Ann MacPhail, MSc, PT; Diane E. Allan, MA;
and Deborah Laliberte-Rudman, OT

The body of literature that pertains to the therapeutic benefits of horseback riding consists primarily of descriptive articles that contain the observations and subjective reports of therapists, riding instructors, relatives of riders, and riders (Biery & Kauffman, 1989; Dismuke, 1981). Although these descriptive articles have helped identify the variables that need to be empirically investigated, few investigators have objectively examined the therapeutic benefits of horseback riding (Biery, 1985). Moreover, the small number of studies designed to empirically examine the benefits of therapeutic riding* have methodological problems that make their findings inconclusive (Armstrong-Esther, Sandilands, Myco, & Miller, 1988; Brock, 1988).

The results of previous studies are described in detail in a prior paper, "Therapeutic Horseback Riding: A Review of the Literature" (MacKinnon et al., 1995). In the one study that focused exclusively on the psychosocial effects of therapeutic riding, the investigators concluded that the self-concept scores of control group children and experimental group children did not differ (Stewart, Moretti, O'Connor, Kates, & Doyle, 1988). For the most part, few investigators reported significant physical or psychosocial change. Aside from Dismuke (1984), all the studies in which improvements were reported failed to use a control group design. In addi-

tion, the majority of measurements were observational and thus failed to offer empirical support that horseback riding evokes physical and psychosocial changes. Therefore, what is lacking is the incorporation of standardized measures into studies involving therapeutic horseback riding.

The purpose of this study was to examine the physical and psychosocial therapeutic benefits that children with cerebral palsy derive from participation in a horseback riding program. The study attempted to answer the following research questions:
- Does a therapeutic riding program improve the physical abilities (e.g., posture, gross and fine motor control, activities of daily living [ADLs]) of children with mild to moderate cerebral palsy?
- Does a therapeutic riding program improve the psychosocial abilities (e.g., perceived self-adequacy, socialization, global behavior) of children with mild to moderate cerebral palsy?

Method

This study focused on children with mild to moderate cerebral palsy. Inclusion criteria included having a diagnosis of spastic-type cerebral palsy, being between ages 4 and 12, having IQ score greater than 70, having the ability to sit independently for 2 minutes in a chair, and being interested in riding. The exclusion criteria included riding instruction within the past 2 years, neurological or orthopedic surgery within the past 2 months, psychiatric problems, and other specific medical problems. The study included 19 children (10 girls and 9 boys); mean age was 6.5 years (standard deviation [SD] = 6.5) at the time of the pretest (Table 14.1).

Table 14.1. Description of Sample

Group	Sex	Age at Pretest	Group Mean of Age
Mild + Control	F	4	6.0 (SD = 1.87)
	F	9	
	M	6	
	M	5	
	M	6	
Mild + Experimental	M	7	6.8 (SD = 2.05)
	F	7	
	F	5	
	F	5	
	F	10	
Moderate + Control	M	5	5.7 (SD = 1.46)
	M	6	
	F	5	
	M	8	
Moderate + Experimental	F	6	7.2 (SD = 2.39)
	F	5	
	M	6	
	M	8	
	F	11	

Note. F = female; M = male; *SD* = standard deviation.

The sample was stratified into two groups: *mildly involved* and *moderately involved*. Mildly involved children were those who could walk independently, whereas moderately involved children were those who used wheelchairs or assistive devices for independent mobility. Within each group, children were randomly divided into control and experimental groups. The 10 children in the experimental group (7 girls, 3 boys) had a mean age of 6.8 years (*SD* = 2.05) for the mildly involved group and 7.2 years (*SD* = 2.39) for the moderately involved group. The 9 children in the control group (3 girls, 6 boys) had a mean age of 6.0 (*SD* = 1.87) for the mildly involved children and 5.7 (*SD* = 1.46) for the moderately involved children. The participation rate for the study was 94%. The attendance rate in the riding program was 93.1% (mild group, 93.8%; moderate group, 92.3%).

The children in the control group were not involved in the riding program but were placed on a priority list for riding following completion of the study. The children in the experimental group participated in a 6-month (26-week) horseback riding program. No attempt was made to stop routine therapies or activities in which the children were engaged.

The Riding Program

The riding sessions were conducted separately for the mildly and moderately involved children in the experimental group. The riding program focused on the development of functional riding skills, basic horse and stable knowledge, and skill at games on horseback (Exhibits 14.1 and 14.2).

Children in the mild group rode using saddles and were encouraged to use reins, holding one in each hand. The children in the moderate group did not use saddles but rode on saddle pads with surcingles, which provided handles for the children to hold onto for balance and support. The 6-month, 1-hour-weekly riding program was designed and implemented by a qualified therapeutic riding instructor and one physical therapist in consultation with members of the research team. External consultants, one with expertise in riding instruction for disabled children and the other, a physical therapist with qualifications in riding for disabled children, attended riding sessions on separate occasions to evaluate and to provide feedback approximately 3 months into the program. No significant changes were recommended for the program.

Procedures

Study participants were pretested and posttested by two testers who were unknown to the children and their parents and who were not aware of the group assignment of the children. The two testers were a pediatric physical therapy lecturer with expertise in assessment and an occupational therapy graduate student as the research assistant. The outcomes of the study were assessed by comparing the changes in pre- and posttest scores of the experimental group with the changes in the pre- and posttest scores of the control group and by examining qualitative data collected during the riding program. Analysis of variance procedure was used to analyze the quantitative data. For each outcome variable, the pretest scores were used as covariates. Two factors were the intervention and the severity (mild or moderate) of the children's physical condition.

Quantitative Measures

The physical outcome variables that were assessed included posture, gross motor function, fine motor function, and ADLs. Posture was assessed using a scale developed by Bertoti (1988). The scale involves ratings of body position and symmetry. Although the postural scale has not yet been subjected to rigorous testing of its

Exhibit 14.1.

Goals of the Horseback Riding Program With the Mildly Involved Group

Functional riding:
- Good degree of relaxation and mobility on horse
- Pelvis in neutral position
- Head up and relaxed

Maintain midline and balance without external support while steering the following patterns independently at the walk:
- Weaving through cones
- Three-loop serpentine
- Figure 8 through diagonals
- Slow and fast walk
- Speed changes within walk

Maintain and regain midline and balance without external support while on the lead at walk and performing the following exercises:
- Reach both hands towards ears
- Reach behind to touch horse's tail
- Touch hand to toe on same side and on opposite side
- Hands out to side, rotate

Working toward seat independent of hands:
- Do halt–walk transitions through use of voice, hands, and posture

- Trot sitting, half seat, rising with leader
- Know riding safety rules
- Be able to understand and describe school figures as well as ride them

Barn:
- Identify different items of tack, stable areas, equipment
- Know different types of horse feed
- Know names of grooming tools, understand their uses, and be able to use them effectively
- Know the parts of a saddle and bridle and how to put them on (assistance permitted with special pads and bridle)
- Know barn safety rules
- Know simple parts of the horse
- Know how to clean saddle and bridle

Games:
- Reinforce and apply riding skills
- Review stable management and horse knowledge questions incorporated into games

Improve social skills and interaction with peers and helpers as needed through choosing games, deciding riding order in teams, planning game approach with helpers, etc.

Exhibit 14.2.

Goals of the Horseback Riding Program With the Moderately Involved Group

Functional riding:
- Sense of responsibility for control over horse (adapted control if actual control not possible)
- Fair degree of relaxation and mobility on horse (relative to relaxation and mobility off horse)
- Pelvis able to attain neutral position
- Head up, eyes looking ahead

Able to maintain midline and balance with minimal external support while doing the following:
- Weaving through cones
- Riding large circle
- Figure 8 through diagonals
- Slow and fast walk

- Speed changes within walk
- One hand or both hands off handles
- Know riding safety rules

Barn:
- Identify different items of tack, stable areas, equipment
- Know barn safety rules
- Know parts of the bridle and saddle, if applicable
- Know simple parts of the horse

Games:
- Reinforce and apply riding skills
- Review stable management and horse knowledge
- Questions incorporated into games

Improve social skills and interaction with peers and helpers as needed through choosing games, deciding riding order in teams, planning game approach with helpers, etc.

psychometric properties, it was chosen because it was designed to assess the posture of children with cerebral palsy and had been used successfully in a previous therapeutic riding study.

The Gross Motor Function Measure (GMFM; Russell et al., 1990), which is appropriate for mildly, moderately, and severely impaired children with cerebral palsy, was used to measure the gross-motor skills of the participants. The authors indicated that major improvement is generally made in children under age 6.

Fine-motor function was measured by using one or two measures, depending upon the functional ability of each participant. The fine-motor component of the Peabody Developmental Motor Scale (PDMS; Folio & Fewell, 1983) was completed with all children. This scale was designed to be used with children from birth through 83 months. The four subscales of the fine-motor section cover grasping, hand use, eye–hand coordination, and manual dexterity. In addition, the response speed and the upper-limb speed and dexterity subtests of the fine-motor component of the Bruininks–Oseretsky Test of Motor Proficiency (Bruininks, 1978) were completed with children who obtained ceiling-level scores on the Peabody scale. The Bruininks–Oseretsky test is appropriate for use with children between ages 4.5 and 14.5 and therefore tests functional skills that are at a developmentally higher level than the skills measured by the PDMS.

The subscale of the Vineland Adaptive Behavior Scales (survey form; Sparrow, Balla, & Cicchetti, 1984) was used to measure ADLs. The daily living skills subscale of the Vineland scales assesses personal, domestic, and community living skills. This subscale is appropriate to use with people with disabilities at all ages.

The psychosocial outcome variables that were assessed included perceived self-adequacy, socialization, and global behavior. The teacher rating scale of the Harter Self-Perception Scale (Harter, 1985) was completed by the parents. This measure provided information about their child's perceived adequacy in the areas of scholastic competence, social acceptance, athletic competence, physical appearance, and behavioral conduct.

The Child Behavior Checklist (CBC; Achenbach & Edelbrock, 1983) was used to evaluate the global behavior of the children. This measure examines the social competencies, emotional adjustment, and behavior problems of children ages 4 to 16.

Qualitative Measures

In addition to the quantitative measures, four sources of qualitative assessment were collected:

- First, the riding instructor kept a journal of each child's weekly performance. Included in the records were comments about each child's physical, functional, social, and horsemanship status.
- Second, the physical therapist provided an end-of-program summary based on documented observations of each child's progress collected during the program; the summary commented on initial physical, functional, and social problems; equipment adaptations; gains; plateaus; and significant periods of improvement.
- Third, changes parents observed in their children were obtained using report sheets that were completed on three occasions during the program. The forms asked parents to report any physical, functional, and social changes that they believed might be related to the horseback riding program.
- Fourth, each child was videotaped from the mounting block (i.e., the platform where the children mounted their horses) at three different intervals during the study. The children were videotaped as they passed the mounting block. No prompting cues were given to the children. In fact, the children were following one another on their horses and apparently were not aware of when they were being videotaped.

Quantitative Results

Gross Motor Control

Although total GMFM scores showed improvements in each of the four participant groups, the results did not verify benefits from the riding program. Analyses on the subdimensions of the GMFM (standing, sitting, and walking) also revealed no statistical support for therapeutic benefit from riding (Table 14.2).

Posture

The Bertoti scale was completed with each child in a sitting position; no differences existed between the riding and nonriding groups. A difference, however, was noted between the mildly and moderately involved groups; the moderate groups showed gains, whereas the mild groups showed a slight decrease in scores.

Fine Motor Control

The only significant result from the PDMS fine-motor tests occurred in grasping. The differences found among the four participant groups were great enough to produce a significant interaction effect ($p = .006$). Subsequent analyses showed a significant result ($t = 2.44$,

Table 14.2. Test Score Changes Within Each Group

Measure	Moderate Experimental	Moderate Control	Mild Experimental	Mild Control	p
Physical Measures					
GMFM (Sit)	−0.40	2.00	−0.20	−2.05	
GMFM (Stand)	0.40	−0.50	1.40	2.55	
GMFM (Walk)	0.40	0.00	0.60	0.50	
GMFM (Total)	0.40	1.50	1.40	1.00	
Bertoti	1.20	1.00	−0.20	−1.30	
Bruininks	—	—	−0.75	−1.67	
Bruininks	—	—	0.60	5.33	.00[b]
Peabody A	1.80	−0.50	0.00	0.60	
Peabody B	3.40	1.25	0.40	0.10	
Peabody C	4.20	4.50	2.60	2.30	
Peabody D	1.00	2.25	0.20	2.05	
Peabody Total	9.80	8.50	3.20	5.05	
Psychosocial Measurement					
Vineland ADL	−18.73	−19.33	1.80	−0.45	
Harter	−3.00	2.80	2.20	3.35	
Vineland Socialization	−3.00	−5.75	−2.80	−5.40	.02[a]
CBC Activities	−0.70	0.42	1.00	−0.62	
CBC School	0.63	−0.25	0.00	−0.25	.04[b]
CBC Social	−0.90	0.13	0.30	−0.97	
CBC Total Problems	−1.40	−4.67	3.20	2.40	
CBC Total Competence	−1.73	−9.50	−7.00	−10.00	

Note. ADL = activities of daily living; CBC = Child Behavior Checklist; GMFM = Gross Motor Function Measure.

[a]Main effect of severity (moderate vs. mild).

[b]Effect of the interaction between group (riding vs. control) by severity (moderate vs. mild).

$p = .045$) between the moderate–experimental and moderate–control groups, suggesting that the riding program may have had some benefit.

ADL

The ADL subscale of the Vineland Adaptive Behavior Scale failed to confirm statistically significant changes.

Psychosocial Changes

In general, analyses of the Harter Self-Perception Profile for Children, the Vineland Adaptive Behavior Subscale on socialization, and the five CBC subtests failed to confirm statistically the proposed benefits of the therapeutic riding program. Results indicated a main direct effect of severity on the changes in children's self-perception (Table 14.2). Children with mild cerebral palsy showed the most gain in self-perception. Findings on the activity subscale of the CBC showed that participation in the riding program may have a diverse influence on children. Children with mild cerebral palsy improved, whereas children with moderate cerebral palsy deteriorated following the intervention.

Qualitative Results

Riding Instructor's Evaluations

The charts and notes compiled by the riding instructor revealed changes not found with the quantitative measures. With a few exceptions, the children in the riding program (both mildly and moderately involved) showed weekly progress in their sitting position on the horse. The mildly involved group also was evaluated on their ability to use, hold, and maintain reins at the proper length. All 5 children used their reins without relying on the saddle's pommel for support. They also held the reins appropriately between their ring and little fingers, but 3 were not able to maintain their forearms in a neutrally rotated position. Most of the children could maintain the reins at the appropriate length throughout the riding session, with knots in the reins as a tactile cue.

Therapist's Evaluations

Generally, each child's final report from the therapist indicated progress in physical or psychosocial areas or both. The most frequently cited improvements involved posture, trunk control, attention span, pelvic mobility, hand control, social interaction, and confidence. For example, one of the moderately involved riders demonstrated poor trunk control and balance, which resulted in the child continually falling to one side of the horse. This rider had so much spasticity in the left arm that he could not reach the left handle of the surcingle. A midline larger surcingle was fabricated to allow the rider to adopt a more upright posture using both hands. After 3.5 months, this rider was able to use conventional surcingle handles while maintaining a centered sitting position on the horse.

Another rider from the mildly involved group demonstrated major psychosocial gains. Initially, this rider was very quiet and rarely interacted with the other children. At the end of the 6-month study, this rider was running around playing and joking—not only with other riders but also with the volunteers. Of course, the changes were individual, including the time when the change first started to appear; some children demonstrated the most progress in the initial months, others in the latter months, and still others showed change throughout the entire 6 months of the program.

Parents' Evaluations

Improvements in the physical skills of the mildly involved children included gains in balance, flexibility, and strength and a decrease in tone. Parents observed positive changes in functional skills such as gait and ADL. In addition, improvements in social skills and general behavior were reported in motivation, willingness to try other new activities, self-confidence, self-esteem, cooperation, and enthusiasm. The only negative observation described was an increase in aggression that seemed to parallel the child's improvement in self-confidence. Examples of some parents' comments included the following:
- My child is "getting dressed standing instead of sitting all the time."
- "He is more self-assured and feels very positive about himself."
- "She is very happy about riding and it has given her a new open field—horse books, posters of horses, etc."

All parents of children in the moderate group observed improvements in their child's physical skills of flexibility, balance, relaxation, and posture. Negative physical concerns were related to short-term pain and muscle cramping for two of the children. In addition, evidence indicated that most of the children's skills had improved in the functional areas of dressing skills and gait. Last, all of the parents reported improvements in their children's psychosocial functioning, which included greater enthusiasm, pride, willingness to try new activities, cooperation, and confidence. Parents identified changes as follows, for example:
- "Flexibility has improved since horse riding lessons . . . she will sit cross-legged on the floor more easily than before."
- "Walks taller and with more speed."
- "It's easier to get shoes on and off."
- "Seems to be very cooperative since this project began."

Videotape Evaluations

Videotapes of each child at regular intervals demonstrated obvious improvements (i.e., readily apparent to other colleagues, who could differentiate early from later videos) in position of head, neck, shoulder, elbow, hand, hip, calf, and heel. Also, each rider's facial expression seemed to demonstrate an improvement in his or her levels of satisfaction and self-confidence.

Discussion

The current project uncovered some important findings. Most parents and children who were approached for recruitment were eager to take part in the project, and the attendance among the riding group was extremely high. Minimal obstacles occurred in running the 6-month program, but a significant time commitment was required from the research team, which held regular meetings and sent a representative to each riding session. People at three agencies—the Special Ability Riding facility, the Thames Valley Children's Centre, and the University of Western Ontario—had to be kept informed. The parents, instructor, and attending therapist repeatedly recalled highly positive experiences.

In the planning phase of this study, the research team was aware of the challenges related to measurement and thus decided to include both qualitative observations and standardized quantitative measures. Indeed, the results of the two sources revealed classic contrasts between the two opposing measurement approaches. On the one hand, the qualitative results from parents, the attending physiotherapist, and the riding instructor generated highly positive, endorsing comments and maybe even "self-fulfilling prophecies." On the other hand, statistical analyses of the quantified measures produced results that suggest the riding program was unsuccessful in demonstrating therapeutic benefits. This typical contrast cannot be resolved at this point.

A most difficult challenge was the apparent problems in the ability to measure change with existing standardized measurement tools. Researchers are acutely cognizant of the complexities involved in developing instruments that are valid and are responsive enough to capture a reasonable amount of improvement in outcomes (Russell et al., 1989, 1990). Naturally, according to Banus (1971), the challenge is greater when the population of interest involves children with chronic disabilities such as cerebral palsy, who typically are slow to show improvements over a short period of time and frequently plateau despite interventions.

No evidence has reported that improvements in therapeutic horseback riding can transfer to improvements in physical and psychosocial functioning, especially in such a short period of time. We have, however, been able to document improved riding skills for both mildly and moderately involved groups of children in the riding program. What we can say with some confidence is that the children in the riding groups achieved better skills and self-confidence relative to riding a horse.

An additional problem was the heavy reliance on standardized tests that required parental responses (all the psychosocial measures and the ADL measure) rather than the child's response or direct observations. We were not always able to obtain tests that covered the age range of our sample, a problem that forced us, on occasion, to use two different tests (e.g., tests of fine-motor skills). In poststudy discussions, we determined that more accurate measures could be taken if the target population consisted entirely of either adolescents or young children (i.e., under age 6). With an older sample, researchers could use a self-report format rather than questionnaires completed by parents. This approach would eliminate any parental biases and offer a more factual assessment of psychosocial variables. Conversely, most physical change probably occurs in children before age 6 (Bruininks, 1978; Sparrow et al., 1984); therefore, a study involving a young sample may yield the physical outcomes that we attempted to capture in this study.

In conclusion, the significant findings of this study suggest that for children with moderately involved cerebral palsy, grasp improved and perceived self-adequacy increased as a result of the riding program. Although

entirely speculative, grasp in the moderately involved riding group may improve because of the constant use of grasp to hold onto the surcingle ring, which the mildly involved group did not use. On reexamining the raw data, we noted that 4 of the 5 moderately involved children demonstrated an improvement on one item, grasping a marker, consistently. The children were not involved in grooming of the horse or stable chores and often did not have the skill to use reins, but they consistently grasped the surcingle for support. The change in perceived self-adequacy may reflect improvements in the children's behavior, such as increased energy, assertiveness, and confidence, all of which may have been perceived as disruptive and negative by the parents. Given the number of outcome measures and associated statistical tests, however, the quantitative data provide relatively little evidence for a positive impact of the riding program for children with cerebral palsy.

Testers expressed some concern that parents inflated their child's ability, behavior, and social demeanor during pretesting in an attempt to ensure that their child was selected for the therapeutic riding program. Posttest scores, then, might be a truer representation of the child's psychosocial status. In addition, the timing of posttesting was not ideal because it took place in December and the children were excited about Christmas, parties, and other activities unrelated to testing. This contextual factor may partly explain the aberrations in some of the standardized test scores.

Until more meaningful and responsive measures for therapeutic horseback riding are available, assessing the clinical effects of therapeutic horseback riding upon children with cerebral palsy will be difficult. Even the Bertoti test, which was developed for testing the balance of children with cerebral palsy while riding, does not test simulated riding positions, such as those that could be performed on a wooden horse. More rigorous research should focus on the development of measurement tools to assess and quantify meaningful improvements specifically related to therapeutic horseback riding, rather than global, indirect measures of behavior. The next step would be to demonstrate whether improvements in therapeutic horseback riding do generalize to physical and psychosocial improvements in children with cerebral palsy.

References

Achenbach, T. M., & Edelbrock, C. (1983). *Child Behavior checklist and revised Child Behavior Profile.* Burlington: University of Vermont, Department of Psychiatry.

Armstrong-Esther, C. A., Sandilands, M. L., Myco, P. M., & Miller, D. (1988, August). Validation of horse riding as a therapy for physically and mentally handicapped adults. In *Proceedings of the 6th International Therapeutic Riding Congress* (pp. 1–43). Toronto, Ontario.

Banus, B. S. (1971). *The developmental therapist.* Thorofare, NJ: Slack.

Bertoti, D. B. (1988, August). Therapeutic riding conferences— Positive progress. In *Proceedings of the 6th International Therapeutic Riding Congress* (pp. 400–405). Toronto, Ontario.

Biery, M. J. (1985). Riding and the handicapped. *Veterinary Clinics of North America: Small Animal Practice, 15,* 345–354.

Biery, M. J., & Kauffman, N. (1989). The effects of horseback riding on balance. *Adapted Physical Activity Quarterly, 6,* 221–229.

Brock, B. J. (1988, August). Therapy on horseback: psychomotor and psychological change in physically disabled adults. In *Proceedings of the 6th International Therapeutic Riding Congress* (pp. 118–142). Toronto, Ontario.

Bruininks, R. H. (1978). *Bruininks–Oseretsky Test of Motor Proficiency.* Circle Pines, MN: American Guidance Service.

Dismuke, R. (1981). Therapeutic horsemanship. *The Quarter Horse Journal, July,* 34–37.

Dismuke, R. (1984). Handicapped riding. *The Quarter Horse Journal, August,* 34–37.

Folio, M., & Fewell, R. (1983). *Peabody developmental motor scales and activity cards.* Austin, TX: PRO-ED.

Harter, S. (1985). *The Self-Perception Profile for Children: Revision of the Perceived Competence Scale for Children* [Manual.] University of Denver.

MacKinnon, J. R., Noh, S., Lariviere, J. MacPhail, A., Allan, D. E., & Laliberte, D. (1989). A study of therapeutic effects of horseback riding with children with cerebral palsy. *Physical and Occupational Therapy in Pediatrics, 15,* 17–34.

Russell, D. J., Rosenbaum, P. L., Cadman, D. T., Gowland, C., Hardy, S., & Jarvis, S. (1989). The Gross Motor Function Measure: A means to evaluate the effects of physical therapy. *Developmental Medicine and Child Neurology, 31,* 341–352.

Russell, D. J., Rosenbaum, P. l., Gowland, C., Hardy, S., Lane, M., Plews, N., McGavin, H., Cadman, D. & Jarvis, S. (1990). *Gross Motor Function Measure manual.* Hamilton, Ontario: McMaster University Press.

Sparrow, S., Balla, D., & Cicchetti, D. (1984). *Vineland Adaptive Behavior scales: Survey form manual.* Circle Pines, MN: American Guidance Service.

Stewart, P., Moretti, P., O'Connor, K., Kates, B., & Doyle, D. (1988). Therapeutic riding and self-concept of disabled children. In *Proceedings of the 6th International Therapeutic Riding Congress* (pp. 181–201). Toronto, Ontario.

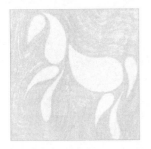

By reason of his elegance,
he resembles an image painted in a palace:
Though he is as majestic as the palace itself.
—Emir Abd-el-Kader

CHAPTER 15

Perceived Efficacy of Therapeutic Riding for Children With Autism

Nancy King, MS, OTR

In the past few decades, therapeutic horseback riding and hippotherapy have developed at a remarkable rate, especially among the pediatric population. Newspaper and magazine articles feature stories and photographs of children with various disabilities participating in a growing number of therapeutic riding programs (Hamish, 1998; Havas, 1999; Lawlor, 1999; Swanson, 2003). The programs aim to go beyond the more obvious recreational aspects by providing specific basic riding skills, such as balance and coordination, to benefit riders (Bassett, 2002).

Occupational therapists, along with physical therapists, speech pathologists, and psychologists, are increasing their practice in therapeutic riding and hippotherapy (Casady, 2003; Engel, 1992a). As the use of this treatment strategy increases in popularity, so does the need for occupational therapy to expand its body of knowledge by participating in research that examines hippotherapy's role within the realm of occupational therapy. Few studies on the effectiveness of hippotherapy have focused specifically on how this practice area relates to occupational therapy's domain of concern. This chapter examines the practice's potential benefits for a population frequently treated by occupational therapists: children with pervasive developmental disabilities, specifically autism.

Autism is difficult to categorize and presents significant treatment challenges for occupational therapists, who are constantly seeking effective intervention strategies for this population. The focus of occupational therapy intervention often is aimed at facilitating change in the social behaviors most typically associated with autism (Stancliff, 1996). Children with autism participate in an assortment of intervention services using various approaches (Case-Smith & Miller, 1999; Watling,

Deitz, Kanny, & McLaughlin, 1999). Treatment plans vary according to individual needs. Behavioral programs, communication, sensory integration, social skills training, and animal-assisted therapy are just part of the repertoire of approaches used for this population. Typically, two to three approaches are used simultaneously to address the complex nature of the disorder (Stancliff, 1996).

The purpose of this pilot study was to examine changes in the social and related behaviors of children with autism after participating in a therapeutic riding program. Occupational therapy concerns itself with these behaviors because they affect the child's ability to function in the social world, which includes the home, school, and play environments.

Literature Review

Autism is described as a pervasive developmental disorder with onset prior to age 30 months. It is characterized by abnormal development and functioning in the areas of communication, behavior, and social interaction (Kaplan & Sadock, 1998; Ruble & Sears, 2001). A clinical diagnosis of autism is categorized into the following five subclusters of disturbances, each of which have a continuum from mild to severe disruptions:

1. *Disturbances in relating to persons and things.* The child may be unreceptive to physical affection and may lack eye contact and social smiling. There is a lack of spontaneous seeking of shared enjoyment, interests, or emotional reciprocity with others. Children with autism may form unusual relationships and preoccupations with objects. Objects, parts of objects, and toys are not used in the manner for which they were intended and are manipulated in

highly unusual ways. Play style is often rigid, inflexible, uncooperative, and unimaginative.

2. *Disturbances in communication* may be characterized by immature patterns of speech, lack of speech or echolalia, and limited understanding of ideas. Words may be used without attachment to their usual meaning. The child may present as though he or she is deaf.

3. *Disturbances in motility* may be displayed by constant finger flicking, hand flapping, body rocking, and abnormal body motor patterns.

4. *Disturbances of developmental rate.* The child with autism may develop normally in one area and abnormally in another. Splinter skills and excellent ability in areas such as rote memory, music, and math may be present.

5. *Disturbances in sensory processing and perception.* These may manifest as abnormal responses to various sensation, such as tactile defensiveness. The child may be under- or overresponsive to stimuli such as sound and pain. He or she may become unusually focused on certain stimuli, such as the sound of the second hand on a watch (Case-Smith & Miller, 1999; Gerlach, 1993; Kaplan & Sadock, 1998).

A child with autism may display deficits in one subcluster but not necessarily in all. Other behavioral symptoms may include hyperactivity, sometimes alternating with hypoactivity; aggressiveness; and temper tantrums with no apparent reason. Self-injurious behaviors, highly stressful reactions to any change in routine, eating problems, and lack of fear response are other behaviors described in literature (Kaplan & Sadock, 1998).

Hippotherapy

The use of horseback riding for therapeutic purposes dates as far back as the 5th century B.C., when horses were used in the rehabilitation of wounded Greek soldiers (Mayberry, 1978). Of more recent significance, Liz Hartel of Denmark recruited her horse for the purpose of her own polio rehabilitation, and the pair won Olympic medals in 1952 and 1956. The world took notice of the extraordinary pairing of a horse and a rider with a disability (Griffith, 1992). Hartel was the inspiration for the first riding program for the disabled population, which began in 1954 in England and eventually was introduced throughout the world (Mayberry, 1978).

Children with pediatric conditions have become major candidates for hippotherapy and therapeutic riding (Engel, 1992b). Along with the proliferation of programs have been an increasing number of studies examining the benefits of hippotherapy and therapeutic riding for a variety of pediatric medical conditions. Wingate (1982), for example, studied 7 children with cerebral palsy. After a 5-week participation in a riding program, qualitative findings reported improved posture and gait, less falling when walking, improved head control, independence when taking a shower, and decreased hypertonicity.

Dismuke (1984) compared traditional speech therapy with speech therapy in a therapeutic riding setting. Thirty children (ages 6 to 10) with moderate to severe learning disabilities, language disorders, and mild physical impairments were divided into two groups of 15. The experimental group received speech and language therapy in a structured hippotherapy setting, and the control group received therapy in a clinical setting provided by the public schools. Significantly greater gains in speech and language were found in the children receiving the hippotherapy. Supplemental gains were evaluated by a physical therapist and an occupational therapist. Although a direct comparison of the two groups was avoided, each child was tested for physical and psychological gains. In addition, statistical analysis looked at whether the amount of gain might be attributed to chance, general maturation, or to environmental influences. When evaluating sensorimotor function using the California Tests of Sensory Integration, statistically significant improvement relative to muscle function of the lower back, legs, and trunk; visual perception; bilateral motor coordination; and left–right discrimination was found in the children in the riding program. Dismuke reported improvement of self-esteem as measured by the Piers–Harris Self-Concept Scale. Significant gains were not found in the control group.

Bertoti (1988) conducted a repeated-measures design study of 11 children with cerebral palsy. This study contained objective analysis of the effects of therapeutic riding on this population. Statistically significant improvements in posture were reported for 8 of the riders. Clinically subjective improvements in muscle tone, weight bearing, sitting balance, and self-confidence were reported by the author, parents, and physical therapists. They also reported decreased fear of movement and position change. Although the focus of the study was on the physical gains, observations of the psychosocial area were reported as dependent variables in the study.

Biery and Kauffman (1989) looked at the effects of therapeutic riding on balance. In a study of 8 people with mental retardation, significant improvement was seen in standing and quadruped balance. The authors attributed the improvements to the horse's movement being transmitted to the client in a smooth, rhythmical pattern that provided the necessary vestibular input and stimulation for the rider to make postural adjustments. This idea is consistent with the sensory integration frame of reference, which emphasizes the stimulation of the vestibular system as a powerful means for therapeutic remediation of sensory-integrative dysfunction (Engel, 1984; Lawton-Shirley, 2002).

In a study of 19 children with cerebral palsy, MacKinnon, Noh, Lariviere, et al. (1995; see Chapter 14 in this volume) conducted an ambitious study in response to the lack of empirical studies on the subject. The purpose was to examine physical and psychosocial benefits of therapeutic riding. The variables assessed included posture, gross motor function, fine motor function, and activities of daily living. The psychosocial variables assessed included perceived self-adequacy, socialization, and global behavior as reported by parents using the Harter Self-Perception Scale. Socialization was measured by a subscale of the Vineland Adaptive Behavior Scales, which addresses interpersonal relationships, use of leisure time, and coping skills. The Child Behavior Checklist measured global behavior, including social competencies, emotional adjustment, and behavior problems. Statistically significant improvements were not seen in the children of the therapeutic riding program, except for grasp skill in the moderately involved group. A number of qualitative results showed improvement. Riding instructors reported improved sitting position and ability to hold and maintain the reins for most of the children. The therapist reported progress in physical areas including posture, pelvic mobility, and hand control. In psychosocial areas, improvement was observed in attention span, social interaction, and confidence. Parents reported improvements in balance, flexibility, strength, and decreased tone. They reported improvements in activities of daily living, social skills, willingness to try other new activities, self-confidence, self-esteem, cooperation, and enthusiasm. Although MacKinnon, Noh, Lariviere, and colleagues reported that many of their findings were inconclusive, the study attempted to assess the intervention in an experimental manner. Rather than discount the qualitative results, the authors urged researchers to continue to find adequate measures.

The psychosocial aspects of therapeutic riding and hippotherapy are of particular interest to occupational therapists. The rationale for applying therapeutic riding to many psychosocial pediatric impairments is well documented (Griffith, 1992; MacKinnon, Noh, Laliberte, Lariviere, & Allan, 1995). For conditions involving sensory-integrative dysfunction, the unique characteristics of hippotherapy provides the sensory input into the nervous system necessary for functional sensory integration. As a result, children with sensory-integrative dysfunction have the opportunity to reorganize sensations from their own body and from the environment and make it possible to use the body effectively within the environment (Lane, Miller, & Hanft, 2000). The intent of using the sensory-integrative approach is to improve the efficiency of the nervous system and its ability to interpret and use sensory information for functional use and adaptive responses (Case-Smith, Allen, & Pratt, 1996).

Case-Smith and Bryan (1999) described the connection between autism and sensory-integrative dysfunction and how it relates to the functional social behaviors of children with autism. Problem areas include relating to others, difficulty communicating with adults and peers, not engaging in typical play behaviors, lack of perception of emotional gestures and expression, impaired attention, perseveration, stereotyped movement, self-stimulating behaviors, and relating to objects in unusual ways. These functional deficits are attributed to dysfunction in sensory processing and modulation.

Occupational therapists who treat children with autism often use a sensory-integrative approach, particularly for rededicating behaviors indicative of sensory defensiveness and intolerance. Proprioceptive input, vestibular input, and tactile media are frequently or always used as part of direct intervention. Activities using graded tactile, proprioceptive, and vestibular input are designed to decrease or increase arousal. The aim is for the child to modulate incoming sensory information, and achieve homeostasis so as to be able to focus on relevant stimuli, assimilate incoming sensory information, and respond in developmentally appropriate ways (Case-Smith & Miller, 1999; Watling et al., 1999).

In hippotherapy, the horse is the strategy for intervention and supplies the sensory input to the rider. The horse's natural movement transmits a precise, smooth, rhythmical pattern of movement to the rider (Bertoti, 1988). The three-dimensional movements of the horse's back during a walk consist of an up–down, side-to-side, and front-and-back motion. This movement pattern corresponds closely to the action of the human pelvis during a normal human gait (Lawton-Shirley, 2002; MacKinnon, Noh, Laliberte, et al., 1995). During the trot, proprioceptive stimulation of the trunk facilitates trunk extension, postural alignment, body awareness, and increased alertness (Lawton-Shirley, 1990). Vestibular input stimulating the balance mechanism and the continuous adjustments to the horse's movement lead to instigation of the righting and equilibrium reactions, resulting in improved postural control (Biery & Kauffman, 1989). The rider can experience normal weight shift and trunk mobility, sometimes for the first time. Adjusting to the horse's movement also involves the use of muscles and joints, leading to increased muscle strength, tone, bilateral motor control, balance, and range of motion (Biery, 1985; Lawton-Shirley, 1990, 2002).

Hippotherapy also provides a broad range of tactile experiences, including physical contact with the horse and input such as heavy touch pressure. Additional tactile experiences come from petting the horse and various grooming techniques (e.g., brushing facilitates proprioceptive input such as compression; Lawton-Shirley, 1990).

Hippotherapy also can provide the rider with the unique opportunity to move effortlessly through space and give him or her an opportunity to explore the environment. This experience of spatial awareness and sensory input is critical to the normal development of children's nervous systems (Lawton-Shirley, 1990). The unique smells, sounds, and visual environment stimulate the child's senses (Engel, 1984).

The warmth generated by the horse's muscles during movement is thought to promote muscle relaxation in the rider and help decrease abnormally high tone, especially when the child sits on the horse without a pad or saddle. This warmth may have a calming effect as well, particularly for children with hyperactivity (Lawton-Shirley, 1990). In the psychosocial area, the interaction among the therapist, child, and horse facilitates successful social interaction. Through various activities, such as learning to communicate commands to the horse and playing interactive games atop the horse, the child experiences a sense of mastery, confidence, and motivation (Lawton-Shirley, 2002; MacKinnon, Noh, Lariviere, et al., 1995).

These attributes of the horse and therapeutic riding combine to provide a sensory-rich environment for developing, selecting, and grading activities appropriate for occupational therapy treatment approaches (Lawton-Shirley, 2002).

Therapeutic Riding and Autism

Research examining the effects of therapeutic riding or hippotherapy for the autistic population is lacking. Biery

(1985) described an autistic child and the improvements seen in self-control and eye contact after developing a close relationship to a horse during therapeutic riding. He described the horse as unparalleled for teaching close relationships, communication, and sensitivity skills to this population. Brown (1996) provided a naturalistic description on the steady improvements in a child with autism who underwent a therapeutic riding program. Tolson (1997) presented a thorough single-subject design study on behavioral changes in two separate children with autism. She reported decreased echolalic speech and self-directed behavior and an increase in other-directed behavior after hippotherapy intervention.

Methodology

The parents of 5 children were contacted for a sample of convenience. Their children were pre-enrolled in a 10-week hippotherapy program. The children's special educator selected them for the program in accordance with each child's individual education plan and educational goals. Criteria for inclusion in the program included a diagnosis of autism and demonstration of social skill deficits.

The children attended the hippotherapy session once a week for 2 hours. The sessions used a team approach to address goals established by the child's teacher, parents, and occupational therapist. Each child was paired with one horse for the duration of the program. The horses were chosen on the basis of temperament and compatibility with the rider. Each child and horse had an on-foot leader and a spotter or sidewalker who walked on the opposite side from the leader. The team members consisted of program volunteers and three parateachers. A certified therapeutic riding instructor led the sessions.

The occupational therapist and teacher collaborated with the riding instructor to identify individual treatment needs. Intervention techniques emphasized sensory processing using sensory input and integration aimed at facilitating smooth transitions through a variety of tasks and activities, both on and off the horse. Improvements in social behaviors were emphasized as part of long-term goals and were integrated into purposeful activities, such as structured games and tasks based on interaction with the horse, the team, and the other children. In general, the sessions took place in an indoor riding ring and consisted of mounting the horse with assistance and walking around the ring several times. The children were instructed to do a variety of exercises, such as reaching one arm forward to touch the horse's ears and then reaching back to touch the tail. They were taught to say "walk" or "trot" to get the horse moving at a forward pace with varying gaits and "whoa" to make the horse stop. Games incorporated into the sessions included lining up in a row on the horses and throwing a softball to the rider next in line. The children also were asked to turn right and left around a barrel. At the conclusion of each session, the children were prompted to reach forward, hug the horse around the neck, and say "thank you" to the horse and to the leader by name. Each child brushed his or her horse after dismounting.

In addition to the routine exercises, the children participated in novel activities (e.g., creating collages using materials found at the stable such as hay, grass, and feed). After the riding sessions, they jumped on a trampoline and rolled on a barrel. They saw a movie about horses after one session. During a trail ride, the children took part in a scavenger hunt and were asked to identify various objects in the environment, such as "a flat rock" and "a bridge to make wishes that nobody knows."

Instrument

The riding program's effectiveness on social behavior deficits related to autism was evaluated by way of the parents' perceptions. The parents or guardians were chosen as respondents because they are the most intimately involved with the ramifications of the behaviors that result from the children's functional impairments. One parent or guardian of each child was asked to complete a pretest and posttest questionnaire, designed by the researcher, that compared their child's social behaviors before and after the riding sessions. The pretest–posttest research method was selected to compare ratings and observations of behaviors and how the hippotherapy might affect them. The questionnaire was accompanied by a cover letter explaining the purpose of the study and had a consent form attached. The questionnaires used a combination of Likert scales, multiple-choice, and open-ended questions that asked parents to provide information on the behaviors that had an impact on their child's social performance. The questionnaires were designed to yield both quantitative and qualitative data.

Data Collection and Analysis

Data collection occurred over a 10-week period. The school secretary distributed the questionnaire packets to each parent or guardian by hand during the first week of the program and again within 1 week of the final session. Each packet contained a self-addressed, stamped enve-

lope with instructions to return the questionnaire to the student researcher by a certain date (within 10 days of receipt of questionnaire). In addition, the researcher conducted telephone interviews with the parents of 5 children and the special education teacher.

Data analysis included a comparison of pretest and posttest responses to the questionnaires that were returned. Because of the small sample size, quantitative statistical analysis was not performed; however, the small sample was conducive to analyzing each participant individually to glean qualitative information that might relate to the functional status of his or her social behaviors and relate them to the therapeutic riding experience. This information, along with the teacher's report, is described in the results section.

Results

Although the quantitative results were inconclusive, the study did yield qualitative results, which were based on responses to the open-ended questions from the questionnaires, the telephone interviews with parents, and an interview with the classroom teacher. Qualitative data were collected on 5 participants. The following descriptions and quotations represent those responses.

The father of Child 1, a 9-year-old boy, reported that the boy "enjoyed and looked forward to it every week" and that "he talked with joy about his riding experience." During the telephone interview, the father stated,

> He doesn't usually interact well with other children or look forward to attending school. But to see that excitement in him due to the program was very gratifying to us . . . it's great to see eye contact. They have such a hard time with the eye contact and opening up. This really helped a lot—to see excitement and get a rise continually.

The father described how he usually gets one-word responses from his son at the dinner table when asked about other activities. He added that when asked about riding, his son excitedly talked about the day and verbally expressed details of riding "his horse, Joker," such as what games they played, who rode which horse, the horses' colors, and what the other children did during the riding activities. The father made a point of mentioning that his son had increased eye contact during the conversations relating to the riding experience. This was a source of great joy to him and his wife. He also mentioned improved self-confidence and the experience of caring for the animal as contributing to improved social behavior. He described his son's enthusiasm for attending school on the days he had a riding session.

The mother of Child 2, a 7-year-old boy, reported in the posttest questionnaire that her child responded "very positively" when asked about the riding sessions but did not provide details of the experience. She stated that she did not notice any significant changes in his behavior but that she did believe "he had a good time . . . and looked forward to going every week."

Child 3, a 7-year-old girl, was described by her mother as having "difficult" and "disruptive mood behavior." She remarked,

> The children benefit [sic] them in so many ways we cannot even begin to understand. The animals have a calming benefit, and their gentleness and companionship, like dogs, . . . is so therapeutic. . . . I always took . . . for short trips or long [sic] after school (if she had a hard day), and we would stop the car and pull some grass or bring carrots and feed the horses. . . . The animals all would always make us laugh and feel better!

The mother of Child 4, a 7-year-old boy, described her son as being "petrified of horses" and that she hoped the program would help him form other interests and increase his interaction with other people and animals. She said that at times he was "afraid of touch . . . he doesn't like or want it." She hoped that by learning to touch an animal he might "increase his ability to handle touch."

This same participant was reported by the special education teacher to have made "tremendous progress" as a result of the riding sessions. She recalled that initially, he refused to go into the barn and get on a horse. She invited him to watch the others as she fitted them with riding helmets. He then put the helmet on and proceeded, with assistance, to mount the horse and participate in the program. The mother reported to the teacher that on that day, he called a number of relatives and enthusiastically recounted his experience. She was amazed at his reaction and explained that he did not initiate that kind of social interaction. She said that he continued to speak about the horse, drew pictures of it, and talked about the other children by describing the horses they rode.

Child 5, a 9-year-old boy, was described by the teacher as initially resistant to the riding program; after spending some time in the barn area, he became more and more curious and became a regular and enthusiastic participant. This child also displayed olfactory sensitivity and repeatedly said he was going to "throw up" from the smells in the barn. He was easily distracted by such things

as birds chirping in the barn and the sound of trucks driving by. Although he was described as having ongoing sensory sensitivity, its level seemed to drop. According to the teacher, this improvement was demonstrated by a decrease in complaints, which she attributed, in part, to the focus he developed during the sessions.

Although this teacher stated that she was not fully supportive of the program at first, she described the children's improvements as undeniable. She cited less acting out, less impulsive behavior, being less physical with the other students, and being more open to trying new things as the most obvious functional gains.

The teacher attributed a number of additional benefits to the riding program. In particular, she observed a growing awareness and sensitivity to the horses' reactions and needs. For example, if the children scratched their horse's neck, the horse, in turn, might shake its head. When the horse had to urinate, the children learned that it was necessary to sit still. They learned to lean forward when riding uphill and to duck their heads when entering the barn on horseback. According to the teacher, this all contributed to increased body awareness in relationship to themselves and the environment. These experiences emphasized self-control and constraint, and the instructor observed carryover from the riding ring to other environments. For example, the children demonstrated increased awareness of their peers during play and school activities. The children's reactions to external events changed as well. She recalled a time when one of the horses sneezed and a child jumped in fear. Once it was explained that this was a natural event, just like in people, the child settled and did not have the same fear reaction during subsequent events.

The teacher described several other examples of how the riding experience translated into social gains in the school environment. Within the school, the children demonstrated a carryover of the functional language used in the program. For example, when the teacher used the term "walk on" in the hallway or "whoa" if the children were running, they recognized the phrases and reacted appropriately. Moreover, the children frequently use bikes and scooters in the hallways at school. The teacher recounted that she had no problems getting her students to put on their helmets, whereas she observed that children from other classes, who had not participated in the program, were more resistant to putting on the helmets and demonstrated greater intolerance for wearing them. She said that the children were more responsive within the school environment and demonstrated an increase in cooperative social behaviors.

Discussion

This study explored the impact of the riding session on the social behaviors of children with autism. Although statistical results were inconclusive, qualitative evidence, based on the accounts of the teacher and parents, suggests that riding provided benefits for the children in this sample group, who responded enthusiastically and eagerly in the presence of the horses. Of great importance is how those benefits may go beyond quality-of-life issues for individual children to affect their social environment by improving the nature of their interactions with family members, peers, teachers, and so on. These issues, which are related to role fulfillment and function, are at the core of occupational therapy (Mosey, 1996).

The study's results are consistent with the literature describing the rich sensory-integrative environment provided through horseback riding (Engel, 1997; Griffith, 1992; Lawton-Shirley, 1990, 2002; MacKinnon, Noh, Laliberte, et al., 1995). It has been shown that activities used in occupational therapy with a sensory-integrative approach often are used in treatment with this population (Case Smith & Bryan, 1999). Therefore, this study is consistent with the literature that describes the horse as a therapeutic strategy for providing a unique opportunity for intervention with children who have autism. The results of the study support the use of hippotherapy as a viable treatment option for occupational therapists when used in conjunction with other interventions for this population.

Although quantitative measures are necessary to target and measure specific performance components and how they affect function, this small group appeared to demonstrate qualitative evidence that therapeutic riding reinforces and strengthens function in the sensorimotor, cognitive, and psychosocial components that underlie a variety of functional skill areas for home, play, and school environments. Improvements were reported in the amount and quality of verbal interactions, level of focus and concentration to tasks, and willingness to participate in new activities. These behaviors were seen to contribute to improvements in role performance in school and at home. Additionally, riding appears to encourage children to develop the ability to care for other beings and to experience the sense of mastery and success that accompanies the various tasks performed atop a horse.

Although many previous studies focused on motor gains (e.g., in children with cerebral palsy; Bertoti, 1988; MacKinnon, Noh, Lariviere, et al., 1995), the improvements in psychosocial function noted in those studies are consistent with the current findings.

Limitations

This study had several limitations. The sample size was too small to conduct a meaningful statistical analysis of whether any improvements in social behaviors occurred as a result of hippotherapy. Future research might recruit a larger sample size by extending the survey to include classes from other schools or other riding programs. Other sampling limitations included lack of randomization and a control group of children not receiving therapeutic riding services. Including those features in the research design would have strengthened this study. Because the children were all in the same class, improvements in social behaviors may have been influenced by factors other than the riding, such as events in the classroom, home, or other extracurricular activities. Another limitation was that the parents' reports may have been biased to some extent. Parents may have permitted their children to participate in the hippotherapy sessions because they expected to see improvements; therefore, they may have displayed some form of self-fulfilling prophecy.

Implications for Future Research

Finding reliable and valid ways to measure gains in function poses an ongoing challenge for future researchers. In addition, more research is needed that applies occupational frames of reference to the studies. An examination of the generalization of learned skills to other situations also is warranted. The impact of financing, public support, educational goals, and health insurance on the use of hippotherapy also should be explored to determine whether its full potential is being realized or limited.

Conclusion

In conclusion, this pilot study explored the possibility of hippotherapy as an effective, innovative intervention strategy for children with autism. This pilot study offered support that riding has the potential for facilitating change in social behavior. Although further research will be needed before hippotherapy is placed into the mainstream of treatment options, its potential efficacy for children with autism is exciting. From an occupational therapy perspective, myriad therapeutic possibilities related to the hippotherapy approach have been raised. Although experimental methods are needed to provide quantitative support for hippotherapy's use, the qualitative approach used in this pilot study offers information to support hippotherapy's inherent qualities as a unique and promising intervention tool for occupational therapists and their clients with autism.

References

Bassett, J. (2002). Back in the saddle. *ADVANCE for Occupational Therapy Practitioners, 18*(14), 41–42.

Bertoti, D. S. (1988). Effect of therapeutic horseback riding on posture in children with cerebral palsy. *Physical Therapy, 68,* 1505–1512.

Biery, M. (1985). Riding and the handicapped. *Veterinary Clinics of North America: Small Animal Practice Journal, 15,* 345–354.

Biery, M. S., & Kauffman, N. (1989). The effects of therapeutic horseback riding on balance. *Adapted Physical Activity Quarterly, 6,* 221–229.

Brown, H. M. (1996). "Intrusion" and interaction therapy for riders with autism. *NARHA Strides, 2,* 17–21.

Casady, R. (2003). Building the evidence for hippotherapy. *Hippotherapy, 12*(3), 8–9.

Case-Smith, J., Allen, A. S., & Pratt, P. N. (Eds.). (1996). *Occupational therapy for children* (3rd ed.). St. Louis, MO: Mosby.

Case-Smith, J., & Bryan, T. (1999). The effects of occupational therapy with sensory integration emphasis on preschool-age children with autism. *American Journal of Occupational Therapy, 53,* 489–497.

Case-Smith, J., & Miller, H. (1999). Occupational therapy with children with pervasive developmental disorders. *American Journal of Occupational Therapy, 53,* 506–513.

Dismuke, R. P. (1984). Handicapped riding. *Quarter Horse Journal, 30*(12), 35–37.

Engel, B. T. (1984). The horse as a modality for occupational therapy. *Occupational Therapy in Health Care, 1,* 41–47.

Engel, B. T. (1992a). What are the disabilities riders might have? In B. T. Engel (Ed.), *Therapeutic riding programs: Instruction and rehabilitation* (pp. 213–230). Durango, CO: Barbara Engel Therapy Services.

Engel, B. T. (1992b). Therapeutic riding: Its benefits, professions, and divisions. In B. T. Engel (Ed.), *Therapeutic riding programs: Instruction and rehabilitation* (pp. 35–39). Durango, CO: Barbara Engel Therapy Services.

Engel, B. T. (1997). *Therapeutic riding II: Strategies for rehabilitation.* Durango, CO: Barbara Engel Therapy Services.

Gerlach, E. (1993). *Autism treatment guide.* Eugene, OR: Four Leaf.

Griffith, G. C. (1992). Chronicle of therapeutic horseback riding in the United States: Resources and references. *Clinical Kinesiology, 16*(9), 2–7.

Hamish, W. (1998, September 16). Kaatsbaan program helps handicapped: Horses serve as four-legged therapists. *Daily Freeman,* pp. A1, A4.

Havas, V. (1999, February). Remedial riding. *Hudson Valley, 27*(10), H8–H11.

Kaplan, H. I., & Sadock, B. J. (1998). *Synopsis of psychiatry* (8th ed.). Baltimore: Williams & Wilkins.

Lane, S. J., Miller, L. J., & Hanft, B. E. (2000). Toward a consensus in terminology in sensory integration theory and practice: Part 2: Sensory integration patterns of function and dysfunction. *Sensory Integration Special Interest Section Quarterly, 23*(2), 1–3.

Lawlor, V. (1999, June 6). Happy trails: Horseback riding programs are a therapeutic outlet for the handicapped. *Sunday Record,* pp. L1, L8.

Lawton-Shirley, N. (1990). The sensory integrative value of horseback riding therapy. *Sensory Integration Special Interest Section Newsletter, 13*(2), 3–4.

Lawton-Shirley, N. (2002). Hippotherapy. In A. C. Bundy, S. J. Lane, & E. A. Murray (Eds.), *Sensory integration: Theory and practice* (2nd ed., pp. 350–353). Philadelphia: F. A. Davis.

Mayberry, R. P. (1978). The mystique of the horse is strong medicine: Riding as therapeutic recreation. *Rehabilitation Literature, 39,* 6–7.

MacKinnon, L. R., Noh, S., Lariviere, L., MacPhail, A., Allan, D. E., & Laliberte, D. (1995). A study of therapeutic effects of horseback riding for children with cerebral palsy. *Physical and Occupational Therapy in Pediatric, 15,* 17–34.

MacKinnon, L. R., Noh, S., Laliberte, D., Lariviere, L., & Allan, D. E. (1995). Therapeutic horseback riding: A review of the literature. *Physical and Occupational Therapy in Pediatrics, 15,* 1–15.

Mosey, A. C. (1996). *The psychosocial components of occupational therapy.* New York: Lippincott-Raven.

Ruble, L. A., & Sears, L. L. (2001). Diagnostic assessment of autistic disorder. In R. A. Huebner (Ed.), *Autism: A sensorimotor approach to management* (pp. 41–48). Gaithersburg, MD: Aspen.

Stancliff, B. (1996, July). Autism: Defining the OT's role in treating this confusing disorder. *OT Practice,* 18–21, 23–29.

Swanson, B. (2003, November). Therapy Zone offers hippotherapy, much more. *Saddle Up!* pp. 16–17.

Tolson, P. (1997). Therapeutic horseback riding and behavior change in children with autism: A single subject study. In B. T. Engel (Ed.), *Rehabilitation with the aid of a horse: A collection of studies* (pp. 17–34). Durango, CO: Barbara Engel Therapy Services.

Wingate, L. (1982). Feasibility of horseback riding as a therapeutic and integrative program for handicapped children. *Physical Therapy, 62,* 184–186.

Watling, R., Deitz, J., Kanny, E. M., & McLaughlin, J. F. (1999). Current practice of occupational therapy for children with autism. *American Journal of Occupational Therapy, 53,* 498–505.

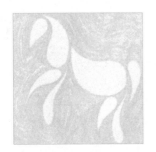

CHAPTER 16

*As often, be content of little,
reward always.*
—Nuno Oliveira

Using a Developmental Riding Therapy Approach to Provide Occupational Therapy to a Client With Traumatic Brain Injury: A Single-Case Study

Rebecca Cook, OTR, HPCS

According to Spencer (1988), lesions in the brain result in intellectual, personality, sensorimotor, communicative, physiological, and emotional changes. The rate of recovery and the final outcome of the adaptive level of function may vary from patient to patient. Recovery may plateau after 6 months or continue for several years. Outcome of rehabilitation also is related to the length of time the person was in a coma: The longer a patient is in a coma, the poorer the prognosis. Although a traumatic brain injury (TBI) is a nonprogressive brain lesion, the long-term impact may cause interference with learning ability, cognitive integration, social interaction and status, self-esteem, and motivation for personal goal setting and achievement.

Motor control and learning involves both biomechanics (the coordination of joints and muscles) and state of mind (such as alertness, motivation, and concentration; Brooks, 1986). A person needs to perform activities that are functional, challenging, and related to the real environment for lasting improvement in motor capabilities to occur (Barton & Black, 1989). Sietsema, Nelson, Mulder, Mervau-Scheidel, and White (1993) tested a principle of occupational therapy and motor learning theory. The results supported the use of an occupationally embedded intervention over traditional exercise for people with TBI. Lysaght and Bodenhamer (1990) proposed that impaired anxiety management and poor emotional control have a negative effect on the adaptive functioning of people with head injuries who are in the postacute stages of recovery. They found significant improvement in function when stress management and relaxation

were part of programs for persons with traumatic head injuries.

A head injury is a devastating disability that can require a long rehabilitation process, which can make patients frustrated and less motivated for therapy. To address those issues and revitalize the treatment process, a center in Florida began offering a dolphin-swim program to its clients (Fox, 1991). Another form of animal-assisted therapy that deals with this problem is equine-assisted therapy, a treatment approach using the horse and the equine setting by qualified health care professionals (Engel, 1992).

A fundamental concept in occupational therapy is that the activity (occupation) must be interesting and must promote the correct movement intrinsically (West, 1984). Mosey (1986) emphasized this need for structuring occupationally embedded exercise because the performance components are acquired through selective activity, not through mindless exercise or random tasks; they are acquired through active, goal-directed interaction with the environment. Developmental riding therapy (DRT) is a specialty system of equine-assisted therapy that can be used within the realm of occupational therapy. DRT is the integration of neurophysical and psychosocial treatment procedures with developmental positions and sequences in the form of purposeful activities, tasks, and games to gain specific medical goals in the treatment of clients with central nervous system disorders such as TBI (Spink, 1993). Spink noted that significant clinical changes or benefits to the neuromotor system (regarding postural control, alignment, and stability) seem to be most evident in children younger than age 6 or adults with recent brain injury. Therefore, young children with central nervous system deficits—especially those that are moderately to severely involved—or neurologically impaired adults with brain injuries within 3 months to 1 year (who may be more neurologically malleable) should be involved solely in treatment-focused approaches, if at all possible (Spink, 1993). This recommendation is supported by studies finding that most recovery is achieved by 6 or 12 months postinjury (Panikoff, 1983).

Case Study

The Client

Throughout her early life, "Dawn" enjoyed bike riding, basketball, softball, babysitting, and serving as class secretary. In December, 6 months after her high school graduation, Dawn was involved in a serious motor vehicle crash; she was 18 years old. The crash left her hospitalized for 7 months—in coma the first 6 weeks—and with the diagnosis of TBI. During the rescue, her vocal cords were injured, leading to a speech impairment. During hospitalization, a tracheotomy was required. Dawn was discharged to her parents' home with hand splints, ankle–foot orthoses, a wheelchair, air splints and Jobst stockings, and adult diapers for loss of both bowel and bladder control. Medications to control seizures and bladder infections also were prescribed. For 3 years post-accident, she attended physical, occupational, and speech therapies. She was discharged from all therapies because of her lack of further progress. Additionally, she identified feeling therapy "burnout."

Dawn's parents wanted to continue some type of therapeutic activity, and 3 months after discharge from traditional therapies, Dawn was enrolled in group therapeutic horseback riding lessons. After two 8-week group lessons, with several weeks between sessions, her parents obtained a physician's referral for private occupational therapy sessions using the horse. Dawn's insurance company agreed to reimburse treatment using the horse. Throughout the study period, the only formal therapy she received (with two exceptions) was her occupational therapy treatment, which used DRT techniques. The exceptions were two brief contacts outside of this setting, as follows:

1. An occupational therapist made a home visit for recommendations regarding home adaptations.
2. Her previous physical, occupational, and speech therapists reevaluated Dawn at the request of a new physician.

Table 16.1. Evaluation of Client-Identified Important Activities

	Favorite Activities	Client Rating of Helpfulness
1	Horseback therapy	2
2	Computer	"Not really that helpful."
3	Arts/crafts	"Not really that helpful."
4	Exercise bike	3
5	Swimming	1
6	School	"Not really that helpful."
7	Talking on Phone	"Not really that helpful."
8	Traditional Therapies	4

Note. 1 = great; 4 = worse.

During the study period, Dawn was actively involved in weekly swimming and began riding an exercise bike at home. She declined opportunities to participate in the group horseback riding lessons after beginning occupational therapy using the horse.

On the final evaluation date, Dawn was asked to list eight activities with a score according to how helpful she perceived them to be (Table 16.1). She stated, "I swim and ride my bike so I can ride my horse." She also attended developmental community college classes concurrently with the beginning of the therapy using the horse; she enrolled consecutively in political science, psychology, English composition, and keyboarding/computers.

Assessment

Initial evaluation occurred at Dawn's first one-on-one occupational therapy involving the horse (4 years' post-TBI), and the final evaluation occurred after 3 years of weekly one-on-one occupational therapy. Results are presented together for the sake of simplifying comparison of data. The three evaluations are presented in the following order: Scorable Self-Care Evaluation (SSCE), upper-extremity range of motion testing, and the Goodenough–Harris Draw-a-Person Test (Bakwin & Bakwin, 1960).

Initial Assessment

The initial assessment of Dawn was as follows:

1. Seizures controlled with medication (no seizures in more than a year)
2. No noted sensory deficits
3. No noted allergies
4. No skin breakdown
5. Hip adductor tightness with internal rotation
6. No history of dislocation

7. Infrequent bladder incontinence (for which a pad is worn)
8. Full control of bowels
9. No diabetes, heart condition, or recent surgery
10. Hemiparesis with abnormal (high) muscle tone on left side of body
11. Flexible postural asymmetry
12. Poor postural control with impaired balance responses
13. Impaired coordination
14. Decreased mobility (wheelchair dependent).

Scorable Self-Care Evaluation

Planning and design of the SSCE was directed at developing a measurable and quantifiable instrument using a numerical scoring method that could be standardized. The SSCE was structured to organize each task into 18 subtasks to provide a measure of self-care skills. These tasks are divided into four subscales: personal care, housekeeping chores, work and leisure, and financial management (Clark & Peters, 1984).

Each item of the SSCE is assigned a numerical value. A score is assigned for the inability to perform a specific action or task. Responses are specifically described in each subtask for each item to help eliminate subjectivity. The SSCE provides an objective measure of an individual's ability and disability (Clark & Peters, 1984). Table 16.2 summarizes Dawn's SSCE ratings at the initial and final evaluation.

SSCE Initial Evaluation

Personal Care: Dawn was clean and appropriately dressed. She requested that orientation form questions be read to her and answers be written for her. She was oriented to person, place, and time. At home, she has a tub and shower chair, a hand-held shower, and raised toilet seat. She requires assistance donning clothing, and with certain bathing, hair washing, and styling tasks. At therapy, she required assistance with toileting (opening door, pushing wheelchair up ramp, doffing pants, occasionally with wiping, donning pants, and exiting bath-

room). She was able, with the help of a grab bar, to stand and pivot-transfer to the toilet. She was unable to use a telephone book and was unable to state basic first aid procedures.

Housekeeping: Dawn could not recall meals eaten or the basic food groups. She recognized 50% safe versus unsafe pictures shown to her.

Work and Leisure: Dawn can state her interests and actively participates in leisure activities. She primarily relies on her family for transportation and has no future vocational plans.

Financial Management: Dawn's source of income is worker's compensation. She does not budget money and cannot read a bill or complete a checkbook register.

SSCE Follow-up 3 Years Later

All scores have shown improvement:

Personal Care: Dawn was clean and appropriately dressed at the time of the evaluation. She completed the orientation form independently; followed directions; and was oriented to person, place, and time. She continues to use adaptive equipment for bathing and toileting, as she did in Year 1 of the study. She is now independent with dressing, bathing, and toileting at home and at therapy, only occasionally requesting help with bra fastening or hair curling. She was able to look up six numbers in the telephone book. She continues to have difficulty, however, voicing basic first aid procedures, saying, "I have to take a first aid class."

Housekeeping: Dawn was able to plan 2 days of menus based on the four food groups, and she remembered what she had previously eaten. She was able to sequence cleaning and laundry tasks from the 10 picture cards given her, although arranging the cards took her about 10 minutes. She recognized 100% of safe versus unsafe pictures.

Work and Leisure: Dawn continues to actively pursue her interests. Her parents transport her to activities. She still cannot voice vocational plans.

Financial Management: Worker's compensation continues to be her source of income. She does not

Table 16.2. Dawn's Scorable Self-Care Evaluation (SSCE) Ratings

SSCE Subscale	Initial Evaluation Rating	Final Evaluation Rating
Personal care	Dysfunctional	Needs skill development
Housekeeping	Dysfunctional	Functional
Work and leisure	Needs skill development	Needs skill development
Financial management	Dysfunctional	Needs skill development
Total score summary	Dysfunctional	Needs skill development

budget her money but was able to complete a sample budget form successfully. She read a bill and was successful at filling out a checkbook register.

Upper-Extremity Range-of-Motion Testing

A goniometer was used to measure range of motion (ROM). Although normal ROM measurements are listed, it is important to note that "normal" varies in people of different ages, sex, and occupations. If one extremity is uninvolved, results of the involved extremity are compared with the results of the uninvolved extremity to determine what is "normal" for that person (Daniel, Strickland, & Strickland, 1992). Movement on Dawn's left (affected) side requires concentration, and during the initial evaluation, it was dominated by the tonic labyrinthine reflex and asymmetrical and symmetrical tonic neck reflexes. Also noted at that time were associated reactions with right hand use. No joint instability was noted. Spasticity on the left followed the typical pattern of internal rotation at the shoulder, flexion at the elbow with the forearm in pronation, ulnar deviation, flexion at the wrist, and adduction and flexion of the thumb. Amount of muscle tone was graded Moderate Impairment (visible stretch reflex elicited and resistance to passive motion beyond point of stretch

reflex; Daniel et al., 1992). Table 16.3 summarizes Dawn's ROM evaluations at the beginning and end of her DRT program.

Draw-a-Person Test

According to King (1982), the use of the person symbol as an assessment tool by occupational therapists must be considered part of a total framework of evaluation and treatment. The Goodenough–Harris Draw-a-Person Test was developed as an intelligence test for children ages 4 to 10. It is based on a point system; 1 point is given for each drawn detail. Each point represents three mental-age months, and a basic credit of 3 years is given as a starting point. The test corresponds closely to the Stanford–Binet test, with a few exceptions: Cerebral damage usually scores 2 or more years below the standard deviation, and people with schizophrenia usually test more advanced than the standard deviation (Bakwin & Bakwin, 1960). What makes the test feasible for use with an adult population is its spread of points, which can accommodate even a superior adult picture production, and that it is independent of artistic ability (King, 1982).

Another characteristic of the person symbol that is important in patient evaluation is that it is sensitive to

Table 16.3. Range-of-Motion Record: Upper Extremity Evaluation Form

	ROM in Degrees				
	Normal	Right	Left 1993	Left 1996	Change
Shoulder					
Extension/flexion	0–180	0–180	0–30	0–60	30
Hyperextension	0–50	0–50	0–10	0–40	30
Adduction/abduction	0–180	0–180	0–30	0–55	25
Internal rotation	0–90	0–90	70–90	0–90	70
External rotation	0–90	0–90	0	0	0
Elbow					
Extension/flexion	0–160	0–145	40–130	20–135	25
Forearm					
Supination	0–90	0–85	0	0–25	25
Pronation	0–90	0–90	20–90	0–90	20
Wrist					
Flexion	0–90	0–90	0–70	0–70	0
Dorsiflexion	0–70	0–70	0–10	0–60	50
Radial deviation	0–20	0–20	0–20	0–40	20
Ulnar deviation	0–30	0–50	0–5	0–20	15
Hand					
Thumb MP extension/flexion	0–50	10–80	0–30	0–60	30
Thumb IP extension/flexion	0–80	−5–85	20–80	0–90	30
Digit MP hyperextension/flexion	−30–90	−40–90	10–90	−30–90	40
Digit PIP extension/flexion	0–110	−5–110	20–110	0–110	20
Digit DIP extension/flexion	0–90	0–90	0–70	0–90	20

Note. ROM = range of motion. Passive ROM in shoulder extension/flexion: Initial to 60 (and after 3 years to 100). Adduction/abduction: Initial to 40 (and after 3 years to 115). Active ROM is measured unless otherwise noted. MP = metacarpophalangeal; PIP = proximal interphalangeal; DIP = distal interphalangeal.

dysfunction to the central nervous system, whether induced by trauma or by endogenous or exogenous chemical changes. The task of drawing a person is cognitive; that is, it depends on knowing and remembering. It involves the ability to be abstract and to use symbols, but it also involves visual–motor feedback loops, spatial organization, and sequencing. Thus, functions of both hemispheres, the cortex, the brain stem, and the cerebellum, along with other structures, all are involved in producing an integrated whole—the symbol of a person. Damage or dysfunction in any area or connecting pathway can be expected to interfere with the production of the picture. It follows that beneficial changes in central nervous system function will be reflected in improvements in the expression of the person (King, 1982).

When Dawn completed her picture during the final evaluation, she asked many questions: "Can I draw myself riding a horse?" "Can I write on it, too?" Each question was responded to by saying, "Draw a picture of yourself any way you would like." Dawn was not shown the picture that she completed during the initial evaluation until after she drew the final drawing, and she did not recall drawing it. The cognitive growth is quite evident between the two pictures (see Figures 16.1 and 16.2).

Goals and Course of Occupational Therapy

Spink's (1993) *Developmental Riding Therapy—A Team Approach to Assessment and Treatment* outlines the fundamental and distinctive elements of DRT. Therapists

using DRT must be trained in movement disorders, have mastery of a standardized set of horsemanship competencies, and possess credentials at the graduate level in psychomotricity, special education, social work, clinical psychology, or speech and language pathology, or possess a bachelor's degree with 2 or more years of clinical experience in physical or occupational therapy (Spink, 1993).

Each of the three DRT goal areas (sensorimotor, cognitive, and affective) covers a 3-year period (Spink, 1993). For each area, the therapist lists problems, a treatment consideration, goals, present level of performance, target objectives, and treatment strategies.

Sensorimotor

Dawn has impaired neuromuscular functioning, which needs improvement, along with sensorimotor integration to increase her independence in self-care, work, and leisure pursuits. Dawn will demonstrate improved neuromuscular functioning in ROM, muscle tone, endurance, posture, and coordination as evidenced by observation, increased mounted time, and a goniometer test.

First-Year Intervention Plan

Dawn uses a wheelchair for functional mobility. While sitting, she displays a posterior pelvic tilt and decreased muscle tone in the trunk. She has fair balance reactions when sitting and poor balance reactions while standing. She can place her feet with the assistance of two people and complete a pivot transfer. She has

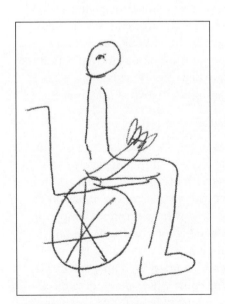

Figure 16.1. Dawn's Draw-a-Person test at initial evaluation; her score was 4 years, 9 months.

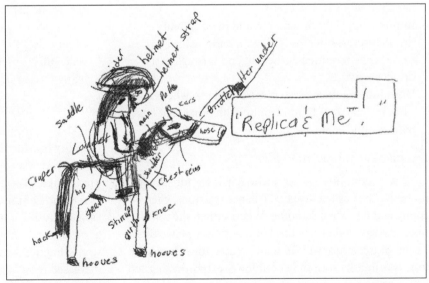

Figure 16.2. Dawn's Draw-a-Person test at final evaluation; her score was 11 years, 0 months.

increased tone throughout both lower extremities, most noted on the left. She has fair fine-motor coordination in her right upper extremity and increased tone with decreased ROM on the left. Sensation is intact, and Dawn has no history of skin breakdown. Equilibrium reactions appear slow and poorly developed, and pathological movement patterns are present. If Dawn attempts ambulation, her steps are uneven, and she displays unbalanced weight shifting.

Strategies to achieve the objective of *bilateral control* including the following:

1. Attend two therapy sessions weekly using surcingle and fleece pad, increasing mounted tolerance to 30 minutes.
2. Because of increased tone in lower extremities, bring client in wheelchair up mounting ramp, pivot transfer, and mount leg-over-crest. Allow a short amount of time before moving. Walk at a slow, low-amplitude pace, using a leader and two sidewalkers supporting arm over thigh on both sides of the horse.
3. Concentrate on correct alignment, postural symmetry, and tone reduction in lower extremities, walking the horse in long, straight lines.
4. Improve basic sitting and riding position and tolerance to graded movement shifts from horse at walk. Incorporate dynamic variance progression, gradually adding more challenging figures and more abrupt rhythm changes (e.g., lengthening and shortening stride, halt–walk–halt transitions while holding hands on thighs or crossed in front of body).
5. Increase proprioceptive and vestibular input through handling of horse and client.
6. Improve upper-body strength and hand stability through reverse sit-ups (going forward instead of back) while mounted at the halt and through cart-driving activities.
7. Dismount leg-over-crest, pivot transfer to wheelchair.
8. Choose a narrow- to moderate-width horse that has a flat and fluid walk.

Second-Year Intervention Plan

Dawn continues to use a wheelchair for functional mobility. She has fair-to-good balance reactions when sitting and fair when standing. When sitting, she sometimes displays either a neutral or a posterior pelvic tilt. Trunk musculature still shows decreased tone. Increased tone is primarily seen in her left lower extremity; her left upper extremity tightens when she applies effort. Volitional ROM is increasing in her left upper extremity. Pathological movement patterns are evident under stress when cognitive energy is directed elsewhere. She can walk slowly for 30 feet with two people assisting her.

Strategies to achieve the objective of *static and dynamic balance* include the following:

1. Attend one therapy session weekly, using English saddle with Devonshire boots, increasing mounted tolerance to 45 minutes. Use a triangle formation for walk and traditional leading position with two assistants using arm-over-thigh for trotting and balance exercises.
2. Have client walk up ramp with assist (i.e., using right hand railing) and mount right leg-over-croup. Dismount leg-over-crest and pivot transfer to wheelchair; be vigilant to signs of fatigue.
3. Improve muscle tone to maintain neutral pelvic alignment. Use low-amplitude, steady-rhythm walk in long, straight lines, grading progression to improve flexion and extension control reactions. Once those basic reactions are automatic, gradually add more (weight-shift) lateral flexion and rotational movements by using circles, serpentines, and simple leg yields to work on righting and equilibrium reactions. Begin two-point exercises at halt and then at walk. Progress to low-level sitting trot work, including transitions.
4. Decrease tendency toward plantar flexion via foot weight bearing using safety stirrups with extended base (Devonshire boot).
5. Choose a narrow- to moderate-width horse that has a fluid walk and a flat, low-amplitude trot.
6. Use a passive level of client–horse interactions when automatic balance reactions are being emphasized. One such activity is the Blind Walk, in which the client closes the eyes during various movements at the walk (this is used to determine whether balance is being integrated using alternative sensory input).

Third-Year Intervention Plan

Dawn continues to use a wheelchair for functional mobility outside the therapy setting. At therapy sessions, she is standing with one person assist for 10 minutes, walking 60 feet with a walker and one-person assist, and climbing stairs with railing and one-person assist. Equilibrium and balance reactions are fair to good during ambulation, and trunk muscles are strengthening. Dawn's left lower extremity still displays increased tone during effort. She is developing the ability to inhibit excessive tone in her left upper extremity and shows voluntary movement with increased range of motion.

Strategies to achieve the objects of *motor planning, crossing the midline,* and *environmental competency* include the following:

1. Attend three therapy sessions per month using rainbow reins and client's own tack (i.e., English saddle, Western saddle, or surcingle and pad), increasing mounted tolerance to 1 hour.
2. Have client walk 30 feet across arena floor to the mounting block with assistance, climb steps, and mount leg-over-croup. A leader holds and controls the horse, a spotter on the off-side offers assistance as needed, and mounting assistance is given as needed for balance on the mounting block. Dismount leg-over-croup and walk with walker or two-person assist 30 feet to wheelchair at exit of arena.
3. Increase riding challenge by adding two-handed rein use, using components of guiding the horse; halt–walk–halt transitions; and steering in and out of obstacles such as a maze, trail course, or simple dressage test.
4. Assist with grooming the horse (e.g., the neck and body of one side of the horse) using curry comb and body brush, gradually increasing working time to 15 minutes.
5. Have client ride a variety of horse sizes and widths. Horse should be quiet and responsive to reins and should display fluid walk and trot transitions.
6. Begin using a modified leading position at walk activities. Use a therapy triangle for trotting and balance activities.
7. Have client clean her equipment, focusing on slowly squeezing water out of tack sponge as a visual and kinesthetic aid to work on grading hand movements.
8. Perform horse knowledge games that require client to reach, gather, or match items (e.g., matching the word *pinto* to a colored picture of a horse and attaching it to the wall; gathering grooming items spread on a barrel to make a complete grooming kit located in another location of the arena; touching a part of her body and naming and locating the corresponding part on the horse, touching it if possible).

Cognition

Dawn has impaired cognitive functioning. She needs improved function to increase her performance in activities of daily living and respond to an unstructured environment. Dawn will demonstrate improved cognitive performance in attention span, sequencing, ability to follow commands, memory, reading concepts, judgment, problem-solving, and organization as evidenced by completion of a modified dressage test, improved

results in the SSCE, and increased cognitive age score in the Draw-a-Person Test.

First-Year Intervention Plan

Dawn is oriented to person, place, and time. Her attention span is dependent on others' direction or redirection because she turns inward to her thoughts or attends to nonessential stimuli, such as talking with the assistant or looking at cats. She is able to follow two-step verbal directions. Reading ability was untestable because she asked for questions to be read to her. She has impaired judgment in unfamiliar situations (e.g., placing her hand in a horse's stall to pet his nose). She has decreased volume of speech and a mild articulation problem. She has good receptive and expressive language skills, however. From the SSCE, it can be determined that she has difficulty with sequencing, is visually overwhelmed by certain stimuli, and has impaired memory.

Strategies to achieve the objectives of *memory, concentration and select attention, safety awareness,* and *procedures* include the following:

1. Emphasize learning the names of horse and helpers. Review safety and barn rules, ask client to name a "rule of the day," and pay special attention to that procedure.
2. Improve body awareness as it relates to self-protection and safety awareness around the horse by completing limited grooming from the ground, learning petting procedures, and learning how to feed treats to the horse.
3. Improve ability to focus attention for a 1-hour therapy session with progressively fewer prompts.
4. Take advantage of cognitive strength of language processing by verbally defining a task as it is demonstrated, starting with two steps and slowly adding more as task is learned. Repeat verbal input and ask client to repeat.

Second-Year Intervention Plan

Dawn still requires environmental structure to maintain attention for more than 10 minutes. She is able to follow three-step directions with the assistance of verbal or written prompts. She is able to articulate safe versus unsafe behaviors and practices safe behaviors with only an occasional reminder. Speech is still softer than normal, but language skills remain good. Visual perception skills appear to be increasing because she is not overwhelmed by parts of horse pictures, for example. She also has become involved in taking a community college developmental English composition class.

Strategies for achieving the objectives of *vocabulary and concept development, setting goals,* and *developing strategies* include the following:

1. Encourage verbal expression/explanation during select times of completing a task while mounted or unmounted.
2. Increase language within the context of the riding environment by having her identify or match parts of horse/tack and look through horse-related magazines as homework.
3. Allow her to choose between two or more activities as a start to the goal-setting process and slowly add more choices. Guide focus of goals toward showing a horse.

Third-Year Intervention Plan

Dawn's attention span now lasts for the entire therapy session. She is beginning to sequence and follow multistep tasks if given the opportunity to repeat directions and have them repeated. She eagerly demonstrates her horse knowledge of tack or parts of the horse. She is regularly reading horse books, magazines, and sales catalogues.

Strategies to achieve the objectives of *sequencing, animal husbandry,* and *problem-solving* include the following:

1. Increase responsibility for horse by giving client accountability for grooming tasks pre- and postride. Use sequencing tools and direction of use.
2. Encourage problem-solving skills by setting up a dressage ring or obstacle course and giving client a written card to follow. Allow practice time, and then ask her to perform the skills.
3. Increase awareness of complete stable management by discussing and reading about horse diet, diseases, vaccinations, hoof care, and more.

Affective

Dawn's impaired psychosocial skills need to be improved to increase her ability to become reintegrated into society and participate in productive living. Dawn will demonstrate improved psychosocial skills in self-concept, coping skills, self-control, and social interaction as evidenced by use of relaxation techniques, increased assertion, and a more complete figure drawing in the Draw-a-Person Test.

First-Year Intervention Plan

Dawn is socially outgoing, friendly, and spontaneously expressive with greetings. However, regarding her own feelings or thoughts, her personality style tends to be passive. She displays a willingness to try new things and shows trust in the therapist–instructor. About adjustment to her disability, she states, "I have learned to accept the things I can no longer do, and I have had to learn how to live in a wheelchair. . . . Even though I have had to learn to live through some very tough experiences, I am happy that I am well enough to make new choices."

Strategies to achieve the objectives of *self-regulation, relaxation,* and *self-image* include the following:

1. Increase client's ability to monitor her feelings about herself in regard to difficult tasks. Assist in analyzing a task and discuss it before performance. Acknowledge what client is feeling and give opportunities for discussion. Provide words for feelings as needed.
2. Begin sessions with an individual warm-up routine (that she helps create) to help stretch, relax, and open the body and mind to learning. Supplement the routine with visual imagery and relaxed discourse about the therapy session to come. Warm-up activity could include, for example, taking a large comb (12–18 inches) and, using both hands, combing the horse's mane while mounted, reaching up as far as she can go. This exercise could include combing an imaginary tail, reaching slowly up and down in front of her.
3. Incorporate music into activities to promote relaxation.

Second-Year Intervention Plan

Dawn continues to be engaging, a trait she sometimes uses as a means of controlling her environment (e.g., when she is completing a tiring or difficult activity, initiating a conversation enables her to rest and avoid having to say she is tired). She also seeks the therapist's approval and at times has been sarcastic or dominating to peers, parents, and other team members.

Strategies to achieve the objectives of *sharing success and failure, social risk taking,* and *friendly competition with others* include the following:

1. Decrease avoidance tendencies and empower client's self-esteem.
2. Improve client's ability to take appropriate controlled risks. Rely on her strong language skills to facilitate this goal by openly expressing concerns and strengths and discussing future events.
3. Adapt position, movement skills, and transition work for the purposes of public demonstration and friendly performance (first for relatives, then for a barn competition, and finally at the county fair in special adapted classes for disabled riders).

Third-Year Intervention Plan

Dawn states she is working on being assertive. She communicates with the entire team through the use of humor. She continues to be enthusiastic about therapy and riding. She engages others with eye contact, by recalling their names, and by sharing her acquired knowledge about saddles and parts of the horse.

Strategies to achieve the objectives of *accepting feedback, cooperation,* and *self-image* include the following:

1. Increase focus on learning the horse's basic needs as an assist with reining work. Teach to reward through petting; talking calmly to horses; and making slow, steady movements.
2. Pose questions about feelings, thoughts, wants, and needs and allow ample opportunity to express them with appropriate reactions and verbal exchange.

Results

The results of formal assessments after 3 years of occupational therapy using DRT indicated significant positive gains in all areas tested. The SSCE showed a 30% increase in function in self-care tasks, an increase that, depending on the area, gave Dawn from 0% dysfunctional to 30% needs skill development ratings. In the area of personal care, she showed a marked change from dependence to independence in dressing, bathing, and toileting. The change was probably to the result of increased motor and cognitive skills. Scoring continued to be low in the personal care category, however, because it is heavily influenced by first aid skills—an area in which she needed much development. The greatest SSCE change was in the area of housekeeping; this improvement is attributable to cognitive growth because these tasks require sequencing, memory, and judgment and safety skills. No change was demonstrated in the area of work and leisure because of Dawn's continued dependence on parents for transportation (note, however, that using public transportation while living in the country is not feasible) and her inability to voice future vocational plans. She would have scored considerably higher in the area of financial management if she had responsibility for budgeting or bill paying. Those skills are not out of her reach, but there is no immediate need for them.

ROM demonstrated an average of 26% increase. Dawn was persistently motivated to ride the horse well. She completed exercises at therapy and at home throughout the week. This dedication of stretching, strengthening, and "using," combined with the therapeutic movement of the horse, led to decreased spasticity, decreased abnormal reflex involvement, increased ROM and, finally, functional movement.

The Goodenough–Harris Draw-a-Person Test indicated a 6-year, 3-month gain in cognitive functioning. According to Piaget (cited in Papalia & Olds, 1981), the second learning stage is *preoperational intelligence* (ages 2 to 7), in which the use of imagery, memory, and rote learning contributes to skill development and in which the milestones in motor control progress from bilateral to unilateral to contralateral and activities become more language based (Papalia & Olds, 1981). Dawn's first figure drawing scored 4 years, 9 months, placing her in the preoperational stage. Her second figure drawing scored 11 years, 0 months, rising to Piaget's third, *concrete operational,* stage (ages 7 to 11). At this stage, most learning is completed through the cognitive and affective domains and the following skills are developed: classification, sequencing, patterning, conservation, and reversibility. The last stage Piaget identified (ages 11 to adult) is *formal operational intelligence;* it is in this stage that problem-solving, abstraction, and logic develop (Papalia & Olds, 1981). These emerging skills can provide a focus for future goals.

The Goodenough–Harris Draw-a-Person Test also can portray improvements in body image and body concept. Figure drawings show a strong tendency for people to mirror, often unconsciously, their own body characteristics. For example, a 25-year-old depressed man drew a figure that was unremarkable except that part of the lines indicating the right thigh were missing. They had not been erased; there was simply a gap in the lines. A search of the chart disclosed nothing in the physical exam or history that would explain this. When questioned about his right leg, the client revealed that he had recently been released from a hospital after long treatment of a complicated fracture of the right femur. He was unaware that he had left a gap in the lines of his drawing (King, 1982).

Dawn's first figure drawing (Figure 16.1) has clear gaps in the front of the neck, lower back, and heel. Review of the client's case revealed a history of tracheotomy, surgery for a ruptured spleen, lower body weakness with bowel and bladder incontinence, and casting of the foot and leg because of spasticity. Missing parts also can provide a clue to physical status. For example, if the ears are missing, one could suspect hearing problems, auditory discrimination difficulties, or auditory defensiveness (King, 1982). Missing parts in the first figure drawing include ears, nose, mouth, hair, and clothing. A final observation in the first figure drawing is the choice of arm placement and the lack of a shoulder, suggesting shoulder-girdle instability (King, 1982); indeed, this was accurate.

The second figure drawing (Figure 16.2) shows a more intact person, without gaps and complete with features. Body concept is the ability to conceptualize the body accurately. According to King (1982), conceptualizing a "map" of the body and understanding its movement capacities are the basis for *praxis*, or motor planning, and thus are a foundation or prerequisite for all the higher functions implied in object relationships, occupational role behavior, and even interpersonal relationships. From Ayres's research, as cited in King (1982), we can deduce development of body concept and, hence, that remediation of motor-planning deficits occurs through appropriate sensory and motor experiences. The positive changes between the two drawings suggest that occupational therapy using the strategy of DRT provided appropriate sensory and motor experiences.

Summary

The therapeutic process with people with TBI can continue for several years, with discharge generally occurring after a lengthy plateau in functioning. What, then, is the "barometer" of skill level achieved in occupational therapy combined with DRT that determines when a client is ready to transition out of a therapeutic setting? According to Spink (1993), there comes a strategic time when a client is psychomotorically ready to be shifted from the "control of the self" to control of something beyond and outside of the self (in this case, the horse). Reining a horse specifically requires the ability to extend boundaries connected to (a) cognitive functioning, (b) responsibility, (c) safety, (d) judgment cause and effect reasoning, (e) visual–spatial skills, (f) self-control, (g) coordination of both sides of body, (h) physical competency secondary to secure balance, (i) muscle tone abnormalities, (j) kinesthetic and position awareness, and (k) ability to grade hand movements. Once the client makes this distinct, though gradual shift, and is able to work steadily and progressively on control of the horse, he or she is ready to graduate to group or remedial work or horsemanship lessons. At the end of her DRT program, Dawn was working on the challenge of controlled rein use (a combination of balance and stabilization of the trunk combined with gross- and fine-motor coordination skills), and her choice was to continue in the therapy setting.

Sensorimotor Function

Dawn's goal in this area stated "Client will demonstrate improved neuromuscular functioning in range of motion/muscle tone/endurance/posture/coordination, as evidenced by observation, increased mounted time, and goniometer testing." According to the criteria outlined, this goal was being met at the end of the 3-year program. Neutral to anterior pelvic tilt was observed while mounted, mounted time increased from under 30 minutes to 1 hour, and goniometer testing showed increased ROM in the left (affected) upper extremity. Because progress continued to be shown (i.e., Dawn had not plateaued), this goal was still valid, and further treatment areas were identified through new objectives and strategies.

Cognition

The goal in this area states "Client will demonstrate improved cognitive performance in attention span, sequencing, ability to follow commands, memory, reading concepts, judgment, problem-solving, and organization, as evidenced by completion of a modified dressage test, improved results in the SSCE, and increased cognitive age score in the 'Draw-a-Person Test.' " According to the criteria outlined, this goal was being met at the end of the 3-year program. In Year 3 of therapy, Dawn completed the modified dressage test successfully as outlined in the Year 3's Strategy 2 (see chapter appendix), results on the SSCE showed improvement, and Dawn had an increased cognitive age score in the figure drawing test. Because progress continued to be shown, this goal was still valid, and further treatment areas were identified through new objectives and strategies.

Affect

The goal in this area states "Client will demonstrate improved psychosocial skills in self-concept, coping skills, self-control, and social interaction, as evidenced by use of relaxation techniques, assertion, and a more complete figure drawing in the 'Draw-a-Person Test.' " According to the criteria outlined, this goal was being met at the end of the 3-year program. This client begins each session with relaxation, assertion is emerging through the use of humor, and the second figure drawing shows a more complete person. Because progress continues to be shown, this goal was still valid, and further treatment areas were identified through new objectives and strategies.

Conclusion

Most people with TBI are young and active with long life expectancy (Panikoff, 1983). Questions arise regarding recovery, prognosis, and discontinuation of treatment. It is generally thought that most recovery is achieved in the first year of disability. This single-case study presents a person first seen 4 years' post-TBI, and assessment results demonstrate increased function in activities of daily living, ROM, and cognitive functioning after 3 years of occupational therapy using the DRT approach. This approach shifts attention from self to horse; it enhances strengths and defines target areas in a way that does not seem problem-focused to the client. This system cleverly disguises the therapeutic process through pleasurable tasks and challenging skills, thereby progressing clients through a series of meaningful, purposeful achievements that enable them to see themselves as competent. This system also parallels the maxim that people are most motivated to learn and to persevere when they are relaxed and happy within their learning environment (Spink, 1993).

Whether the recovery presented here is sensitive to the many variables that have an impact on goal attainment or can be accurately applied to another person's recovery will require further testing. Replication of these results and further investigation comparing the recovery over specific time periods of two groups receiving differing therapy interventions (one being animal-assisted therapy) also are recommended.

References

Bakwin, H., & Bakwin. R. M. M. (1960). Goodenough "Draw a Person Test." In *Clinical management of behavior disorders in children* (2nd ed.). Philadelphia: W. B. Saunders.

Barton, L., & Black, K. (1989). Setting functional outcomes for inpatient rehabilitation. In *Proceedings of the Forum on Neurological Physical Therapy Assessment* (Neurological Section). Alexandria, VA: American Physical Therapy Association.

Brooks, V. B. (1986). *The neural basis of motor control.* New York: Oxford University Press.

Clark, E. N., & Peters, M. (1984). *Scorable Self-Care Evaluation.* Thorofare, NJ: Slack.

Daniel, M. S., Strickland, R. L., & Strickland, L. R. (1992). *Occupational therapy protocol: Management in adult physical dysfunction.* Gaithersburg, MD: Aspen.

Engel, B. T. (1992). *Therapeutic riding programs: Instruction and rehabilitation.* Durango, CO: Barbara Engel Therapy Services.

Fox, S. (1991, January 21). Flippered specialists make therapy exciting. *Advance for Occupational Therapists.*

King, L. J. (1982). The person symbol as an assessment tool. In B. J. Hemphill (Ed.), *The evaluation process in psychiatric occupational therapy* (pp. 169–194). Thorofare, NJ: Slack.

Lysaght, R., & Bodenhamer, E. (1990). The use of relaxation training to enhance functional outcomes in adults with traumatic head injuries. *American Journal of Occupational Therapy, 44,* 797–801.

Mosey, A. C. (1986). *Psychosocial components of occupational therapy.* New York: Raven.

Panikoff, L. B. (1983). Recovery trends of functional skills in the head-injured adult. *American Journal of Occupational Therapy, 37,* 735–743.

Papalia, D. E., & Olds, S. W. (1981). *Human development.* New York: McGraw-Hill.

Sietsema, J. M., Nelson, D. L., Mulder, R. M., Mervau-Scheidel, D., & White, B. E. (1993). The use of a game to promote arm reach in persons with traumatic brain injury. *American Journal of Occupational Therapy, 47,* 19–24.

Spencer, E. A. (1988). Head injury. In H. L. Hopkins & H. D. Smith (Eds.), *Williard and Spackman's occupational therapy* (8th ed., pp. 474–480). Philadelphia: J. B. Lippincott.

Spink, J. (1993). *Developmental riding therapy: A team approach to assessment and treatment.* Tucson, AZ: Therapy Skill Builders.

West, W. L. (1984). A reaffirmed philosophy and practice of occupational therapy for the 1980s. *American Journal of Occupational Therapy, 38,* 15–23.

Appendix 16.A. Three-Year Treatment Plan

Table 16.A.1. Three-Year Treatment Plan to Improve Dawn's Sensorimotor Functioning

Category: Sensorimotor

Problem: Impaired neuromuscular functioning

Treatment Considerations: Improve neuromuscular function and sensorimotor integration to increase client's independence in self-care, work, and leisure pursuits.

Goal: Dawn will demonstrate improved neuromuscular functioning in ROM, muscle tone, endurance, posture, and coordination as evidenced by observation, increased mounted time, and goniometer testing.

Year	Objective	Present Level of Performance	Strategies
1	Bilateral control	Dawn uses a wheelchair for functional mobility. While sitting, she displays a posterior pelvic tilt and decreased muscle tone in the trunk. She has fair balance reactions when sitting and poor balance reactions while standing. She can place her feet with the assistance of two people and complete a pivot transfer. She has increased tone throughout both lower extremities, most noted on the left. She has fair fine-motor coordination in her right upper extremity and increased tone with decreased ROM on the left. Sensation is intact, and Dawn has no history of skin breakdown. Equilibrium reactions appear slow and poorly developed, and pathological movement patterns are present. If Dawn attempts ambulation, her steps are uneven, and she displays unbalanced weight-shifting.	1. Attend two therapy sessions weekly using surcingle and fleece pad, increasing mounted tolerance to 30 minutes. 2. Because of increased tone in lower extremities, bring client in wheelchair up mounting ramp, pivot transfer, and mount leg-over-crest. Allow a short amount of time before moving. Walk at a slow, low-amplitude pace, using a leader and two side-walkers supporting arm-over-thigh on both sides of the horse. 3. Concentrate on correct alignment, postural symmetry, and tone reduction in lower extremities, walking the horse in long, straight lines. 4. Improve basic sitting and riding position and tolerance to graded movement shifts from horse at walk. Incorporate dynamic variance progression, gradually adding more challenging figures and more abrupt rhythm changes (e.g., lengthening and shortening stride, halt–walk–halt transitions while holding hands on thighs or crossed in front of body). 5. Increase proprioceptive and vestibular input through handling of horse and client. 6. Improve upper-body strength and hand stability through reverse sit-ups (going forward instead of back) while mounted at the halt and through cart-driving activities. 7. Dismount leg-over-crest, pivot transfer to wheelchair. 8. Choose a narrow- to moderate-width horse that has a flat and fluid walk.
2	Static and dynamic balance	Dawn continues to use a wheelchair for functional mobility. She has fair to good balance reactions when sitting and fair when standing. When sitting, she sometimes displays either a neutral or a posterior pelvic tilt. Trunk musculature still shows decreased tone. Increased tone is primarily seen in her left lower extremity; her left upper extremity tightens when she applies effort. Volitional range of motion is increasing in her left upper extremity. Pathological movement patterns are evident when cognitive energy is directed elsewhere. She can walk slowly for 30 feet with two people assisting her.	1. Attend one therapy session weekly, using English saddle with Devonshire boots, increasing mounted tolerance to 45 minutes. Use a triangle formation for walk and traditional leading position with two assistants using arm-over-thigh for trotting and balance exercises. 2. Have client walk up ramp with assist (i.e., using right hand railing) and mount right leg-over-croup. Dismount leg-over-crest and pivot transfer to wheelchair; be vigilant for signs of fatigue. 3. Improve muscle tone to maintain neutral pelvic alignment. Use low-amplitude, steady-rhythm walk in long, straight lines grading progression to improve flexion and extension control reactions. Once those basic reactions are automatic,

138

gradually add more (weight-shift) lateral flexion and rotational movements by using circles, serpentines, and simple leg yields to work on righting and equilibrium reactions. Begin two-point exercises at halt and then at walk. Progress to low-level sitting trot work, including transitions.

4. Decrease tendency towards plantar flexion via foot weight bearing using safety stirrups with extended base (Devonshire boot).

5. Choose a narrow- to moderate-width horse that has a fluid walk and a flat, low-amplitude trot.

6. Use a passive level of client–horse interactions when automatic balance reactions are being emphasized. One such activity is the Blind Walk, in which the client closes the eyes during various movements at the walk (this is used to determine whether balance is being integrated using alternative sensory input).

---

3 | **Motor planning, crossing the midline, environmental competency**

Dawn continues to use a wheelchair for functional mobility outside the therapy setting. At therapy sessions, she is standing with one person assist for 10 minutes, walking 60 feet with a walker and one-person assist, and climbing stairs with railing and one-person assist. Equilibrium and balance reactions are fair to good during ambulation, and trunk muscles are strengthening. Dawn's left lower extremity still displays increased tone during effort. She is developing the ability to inhibit excessive tone in her left upper extremity and shows voluntary movement with increased ROM.

1. Attend three therapy sessions per month using rainbow reins and client's own tack (e.g., English saddle, Western saddle, or surcingle and pad), increasing mounted tolerance to 1 hour.

2. Have client walk 30 feet across arena floor to the mounting block with assistance, climb steps, and mount leg-over-croup. A leader holds and controls the horse, a spotter on the off-side offers assistance as needed, and mounting assistance is given as needed for balance on the mounting block. Dismount leg-over-croup and walk with walker or two-person assist 30 feet to wheelchair at exit of arena.

3. Increase riding challenge by adding two-handed rein use, using components of guiding the horse; halt–walk–halt transitions; and steering in and out of obstacles such as a maze, trail course, or simple dressage test.

4. Assist with grooming the horse (e.g., the neck and body of one side of the horse) using curry comb and body brush, gradually increasing working time to 15 minutes.

5. Have Dawn ride a variety of horse sizes and widths. Horse should be quiet and responsive to reins and should display fluid walk and trot transitions.

6. Begin using a modified leading position at walk activities. Use a therapy triangle for trotting and balance activities.

7. Have client clean her equipment, focusing on slowly squeezing water out of tack sponge as a visual and kinesthetic aid to work on grading hand movements.

8. Perform horse knowledge games that require Dawn to reach, gather, or match items (e.g., matching the word *pinto* to a colored picture of a horse and attaching it to the wall; gathering grooming items spread on a barrel to make a complete grooming kit located in another location of the arena; touching a part of her body and naming and locating the corresponding part on the horse, touching it if possible, etc.)

Table 16.A.2. Three-Year Treatment Plan to Improve Dawn's Cognition

Category: Cognition

Problem: Impaired cognition

Treatment Considerations: Improve cognitive function to increase client's performance in activities of daily living and respond to an unstructured environment.

Goal: Client will demonstrate improved cognitive performance in attention span, sequencing, ability to follow commands, memory, reading concepts, judgment, problem solving, and organization as evidenced by completion of a modified dressage test, improved results in the Scorable Self-Care Evaluation (SSCE), and increased cognitive age score in the Draw-a-Person Test.

Year	Objective	Present Level of Performance	Strategies
1	Memory, concentration and select attention, safety awareness, and procedures	Dawn is oriented to person, place, and time. Her attention span depends on others' direction or redirection because she turns inward to her thoughts or attends to nonessential stimuli, such as talking with the assistant or looking at cats. She is able to follow two-step verbal directions. Reading ability was untestable because she was asked for questions to be read to her. She has impaired judgment in unfamiliar situations (e.g., placing her hand in a horse's stall to pet his nose). She has decreased volume of speech and a mild articulation problem. She has good receptive and expressive language skills, however. From the SSCE, it can be determined that she has difficulty with sequencing, is visually overwhelmed by certain stimuli, and has impaired memory.	1. Emphasize learning the names of horse and helpers. Review safety and barn rules, ask Dawn to name a "rule of the day," and pay special attention to that procedure. 2. Improve body awareness as it relates to self-protection and safety awareness around the horse by completing limited grooming from the ground, learning petting procedures, and learning how to feed treats to the horse. 3. Improve ability to focus attention for a 1-hour therapy session with progressively fewer prompts. 4. Take advantage of cognitive strength of language processing by verbally defining a task as it is demonstrated, starting with two steps and slowly adding more as task is learned. Repeat verbal input and ask client to repeat.
2	Vocabulary and concept development, setting goals, and developing strategies	Dawn still requires environmental structure to maintain attention for more than 10 minutes. She is able to follow 3-step directions with the assistance of verbal or written prompts. She is able to articulate safe vs. unsafe behaviors and practices safe behaviors only with an occasional reminder. Speech still is softer than normal, but language skills remain good. Visual perception skills appear to be increasing because she is not overwhelmed by parts of horse pictures, for example. She also has become involved in taking a developmental community college English composition class.	1. Encourage verbal expression/explanation during select times of completing a task while mounted or unmounted. 2. Increase language within the context of the riding environment by having her identify or match parts of horse/tack and look through horse-related magazines as homework. 3. Allow her to choose between two or more activities as a start to the goal-setting process and slowly add more choices. Guide focus of goals toward showing a horse.
3	Sequencing, animal husbandry, problem solving	Dawn's attention span now lasts for the entire therapy session. She is beginning to sequence and follow multi-step tasks if given the opportunity to repeat directions and have them repeated. She eagerly demonstrates her horse knowledge of tack or parts of the horse. She regularly reads horse books, magazines, and sales catalogues.	1. Increase responsibility for horse by giving Dawn accountability for grooming tasks pre- and postride. Use sequencing tools with direction of use. 2. Encourage problem-solving skills by setting up a dressage ring or obstacle course and giving Dawn a written card to follow. Allow practice time and then ask her to perform the skills. 3. Increase awareness of complete stable management by discussing and reading about horse diet, diseases, vaccinations, hoof care, etc.

Table 16.A.3. Three-Year Treatment Plan to Improve Dawn's Affective Functioning

Category: Affective

Problem: Impaired psychosocial skills

Treatment Considerations: Improve psychosocial skills to increase client's ability to become reintegrated into society and participate in productive living.

Goal: Client will demonstrate improved psychosocial skills in self-concept, coping skills, self-control, and social interaction as evidenced by use of relaxation techniques, increased assertion, and a more complete figure drawing in the Draw-a-Person Test.

Year	Objective	Present Level of Performance	Strategies
1	Self-regulation, relaxation, self-image.	Dawn is socially outgoing, friendly, and spontaneously expressive with greetings. Regarding her own feelings or thoughts, however, her personality style tends to be passive. She displays a willingness to try new things and shows trust in the therapist-instructor. About adjustment to her disability, she states, "I have learned to accept the things I can no longer do and I have had to learn how to live in a wheelchair. . . . Even though I have had to learn to live through some very tough experiences, I am happy that I am well enough to make new choices."	1. Increase Dawn's ability to monitor her feelings about herself in regard to difficult tasks. Assist in analyzing a task and discuss it before performance. Acknowledge what Dawn is feeling and give opportunities for discussion. Provide words for feelings as needed. 2. Begin sessions with an individual warm-up routine (that she helps create) to help stretch, relax, and open the body and mind to learning. Supplement the routine with visual imagery and relaxed discourse about the therapy session to come. Warm-up activity could include taking a large comb (12 to 18 inches) and, using both hands, combing the horse's mane while mounted, reaching up as far as she can go. This exercise could include combing an imaginary tail, reaching slowly up and down in front of her. 3. Incorporate music into activities to promote relaxation.
2	Sharing success and failure, social risk taking, friendly competition with others	Dawn continues to be engaging, a trait she sometimes uses as a means of controlling her environment (e.g., when she is completing a tiring or difficult activity, initiating a conversation enables her to rest and avoid having to say she is tired). She also seeks the therapist's approval and at times has been sarcastic or dominating to peers, parents, and other team members.	1. Decrease avoidance tendencies and empower Dawn's self-esteem. 2. Improve Dawn's ability to take appropriate controlled risks. Rely on her strong language skills to facilitate this goal by openly expressing concerns and strengths and discussing future events. 3. Adapt position, movement skills, and transition work for the purposes of public demonstration and friendly performance (first for relatives, then for a barn competition, and finally at the county fair in special adapted classes for disabled riders).
3	Accepting feedback, cooperation, self-image	Dawn states she is working on being assertive. She communicates with the entire team through the use of humor. She continues to be enthusiastic about therapy and riding. She engages others with eye contact, by recalling their name, and by sharing her acquired knowledge about saddles and parts of the horse.	1. Increase focus on learning the horse's basic needs to assist with reining work. Teach to reward through petting; talking calmly to horses; and making slow, steady movements. 2. Pose questions about feelings, thoughts, wants, and needs and allow ample opportunity to express them with appropriate reactions and verbal exchange.

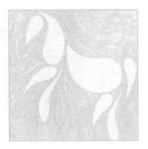

*The horse through all its trials
has preserved the sweetness
of paradise in its blood.*
—*Johannes Jensen*

CHAPTER 17

Therapeutic Horseback Riding and Reaction Time in Children With Disabilities: An Exploratory Pilot Study

Christopher Hipsher, MS, COTA/S

"Any riding program using horse-related activities for clients with physical, mental, cognitive, social, or behavioral problems is a therapeutic riding program" (Heine, 1997, p. 10). Therapeutic riding programs are occupational in nature. Although therapeutic riding has gained an increase in popularity, relatively little research has investigated its benefits in a controlled manner. This study measured reaction time in children who participated in a therapeutic riding program as well as in a group of children not participating in a therapeutic riding program. *Reaction time* is the length of time between the arrival of a stimulus and the moment a response to the stimulus is initiated (Schmidt & Lee, 1999). By measuring reaction time, it was my intent to determine whether therapeutic riding has positive effects on the child's central nervous system.

During a typical therapeutic riding session, the child engages in horseback riding while performing various occupations that address specific areas for the child's rehabilitation (Bracher, 2000). Depending on the facility, each session may last from 30 to 60 minutes. Generally, a trained leader and one or two trained sidewalkers are assigned to each rider. The leader's occupation during the session is to keep the horse moving at the proper speed and to lead the horse in the way in which the instructor asks. The instructor keeps the session moving by asking the riders to play certain games or do certain occupations while on the horse and by asking the leaders to lead the horses in certain directions and patterns, such as serpentines or circles. The sidewalkers are trained to watch the rider throughout the session to make sure that the child stays centered and balanced upon the horse, to assist the child with different games, and to be the child's friend and companion. Facilities often make an effort to match the same sidewalkers with the same riders in each session so that they can bond.

Therapeutic riding can help with a wide range of disabilities; it provides physical as well as psychosocial benefits. Psychological benefits include increased self-esteem, self-image, and interpersonal skills, and physical benefits include improved respiration, circulation, balance, and strength; reduced spasticity; and increased coordination and range of motion (Bliss, 1997). To maintain balance on the moving horse, the rider must constantly make adjustments, using many of the same muscles and joint movements used in walking (Lane, n.d.).

Nelson's Conceptual Framework of Therapeutic Occupation

According to Nelson (1994), "Occupation involves the doing of something. The 'doing' is the occupational performance, and the 'something' to be done is the occupational form" (p. 11). The occupational form includes not only the objects that are present in the physical environment during the occupation but also the sociocultural dimension. Nelson's ideas can be applied to therapeutic riding. One aspect of the occupational form is the horse.

The riding instructor must consider many areas when choosing the right horse to include in a therapeutic riding program. Different horses may suit a rider's special needs better than others. A horse with a rhythmic, balanced gait; good balance; a good base of support; and a strong, broad, short back should be chosen. Such a horse will help the child feel relaxed, secure, and symmetrical on the horse (Engel, 1992a; Kellon, 1992). As another example, a child "with spasticity will relax more easily on a horse with good [momentum], long stride, rhythmic gait [*sic*], and smooth transitions"

(Engel, 1992b, p. 92). The horse must be properly trained. A child with a disability may kick the horse, have poor balance, perform jerky or uneven movements, rock, and have poor reactions. The horse must be tolerant and gentle toward the child, and it also must be trustworthy. It must respond immediately and smoothly to requests in a predictable manner (Engel, 1992a; Sayler, 1992).

Other areas of a rider's physical occupational form include such things as the riding instructor, the other riders and their horses, and the actual setting in which the riding takes place (i.e., an indoor arena or outdoors). Depending on the needs of the rider, a saddle may be used, or the rider may ride bareback.

Another part of the physical dimension, according to Nelson (1994), is the temporal aspect. Many changes take place during the riding session, including the location of the horse and the game that is being played at the particular moment. For example, 22 minutes into the session, perhaps the horse is circling a barrel while the rider is in the process of balancing an egg on a spoon. At 23 minutes, maybe the rider has dropped the egg as the horse is walking over a cavaletti. In addition, a person's condition can change from day to day, especially with such disabilities as cerebral palsy.

A person may do well during riding one day and have a slight change the next time. These variations are part of the developmental structure and should be taken into account. Some of the sociocultural aspects of the occupational form include the role of the person while riding the horse: the role of being a rider. The rider is expected to follow certain rules, such as wearing a helmet while in the arena or sitting up straight and tall on the horse. The environment during the session is supportive and encouraging for the rider who receives praise and "high fives" from the sidewalkers when accomplishing a goal (e.g., catching a ball). The rider is encouraged to do things without assistance, but the sidewalkers are there to help when needed. All of these aspects of occupational form are important to the occupation.

A person's developmental structure includes "sensorimotor, cognitive, and psychosocial abilities and characteristics" (Nelson, 1994, p. 20). A rider's developmental structure needs to be carefully taken into account when planning the goals that are to be accomplished during riding and when choosing a horse and sidewalkers for the rider. The rider's strengths and weaknesses need to be considered so that those strengths can be used to work on the weaknesses. How is the rider's balance? Can he or she follow commands? How are the

rider's coordination and range of motion? These aspects of the person's developmental structure must be considered when determining what needs to be worked on during the program.

Before engaging in the occupational performance, the rider must first interpret the meaning of the occupational form and then find purpose in it (Nelson, 1994). This purpose may be intrinsic or extrinsic (e.g., in the latter, a child who is told to sit may do so to please the person who made the request).

Anecdotally, the riding experience has been documented to have an intrinsic purpose for the riders. One rider was quoted as saying, "I like to look like the riders do on the television. I feel big on a horse, [*sic*] I wouldn't miss my riding for anything" (Lane, n.d.). Another rider said, "When I ride I feel like a normal person" (Lane, n.d.). Therapeutic riding is enjoyable and allows the rider a chance to succeed at something (All, Loving, & Crane, 1999).

Occupational performances taking place during a typical session can vary greatly; one of the most important distinctions is whether the rider actually stays on the horse during the session as it moves about the arena. Another example is that of a child who makes a correction in posture when asked to by the instructor or sidewalker. Another performance may be a rider throwing a basketball into a hoop or playing catch with the sidewalker or a rider shouting "whoa" during a game of "Red Light, Green Light" after hearing the instructor shout "Red light!" A final example of occupational performance is the rider placing his or her foot in the stirrup while mounting the horse at the beginning of class.

"Adaptation is the effect of a person's purpose and/or occupational performance on the person's developmental structure" (Nelson, 1994, p. 28). The following studies demonstrate how the occupation of horseback riding can affect the rider's developmental structure.

General Studies

A limited number of controlled studies have investigated the effectiveness of therapeutic riding for the adaptation process (Bertoti, 1988; Encheff, 2002; Fox, Lawlor, & Luttges, 1984; Haehl, Giuliani, & Lewis, 1999; Land, Errington-Povalac, & Paul, 2001; MacKinnon et al., 1995; McGibbon, Andrade, Widener, & Cintas, 1998; Yack et al., 1997). McGibbon and colleagues (1998) studied gait, energy expenditure, and gross motor function in 2 girls and 3 boys with cerebral palsy who ranged in age from 9 to 11 years old. The riding program lasted 8 weeks. Each twice-weekly session lasted for 30 minutes, giving a total of 16 half-hour riding sessions. A repeated-measures, within-subjects design was used. The children were measured a total of three times: Two baseline measurements were taken 8 weeks apart prior to the program, and a final posttest was given after the program was complete. Each child was timed, and the number of steps taken while walking 10 meters was counted. Two trials were taken for free speed, and another two trials were taken for fast speed. The equation *stride length = velocity/*(0.5 *cadence*) then was used to assess each child's gait. Each child's energy expenditure was measured by measuring both resting and walking heart rate, then measuring the average heart rate and time while the child walked 10 meters. Each child's Energy Expenditure Index (EEI) then was calculated using the equation (walking heart rate–resting heart rate)/walking velocity. Finally, a third assessment, Dimension E of the Gross Motor Function Measure (GMFM), which assesses walking, running, and jumping, was conducted. Statistically significant decreases in the EEI and statistically significant increases in the GMFM scores occurred for each child following the riding program. Although improvements in the gaits of the children occurred, they were not statistically significant.

MacKinnon and colleagues (1995) used a pretest–posttest design to study 10 girls and 9 boys ages 4 to 12 who had spastic cerebral palsy. The participants were divided into two groups: *mildly involved* and *moderately involved*. The two groups were then randomly divided into control and experimental groups, for a total of four groups: mild–experimental, mild–control, moderate–experimental, and moderate–control. The experimental groups participated in separate 26-week riding programs consisting of one 1-hour session each week. The sessions focused on functional riding skills, basic horse and stable knowledge, and skill games. The children in the mild group used saddles and reins, whereas the children in the moderate group used saddle pads with *surcingles*, which are belts used to hold the saddle pads tightly onto the horse. Several variables were quantitatively measured. Gross motor control was measured using the GMFM. Improvements were seen in each area of the assessment, but the results were not significant. The Bertoti Scale (described below) was used to measure the children's posture. No differences were seen between the experimental and control groups, but the moderate groups showed improvements, and the mild groups showed decreases in scores.

Fine-motor control was tested using the Peabody fine-motor tests. Significant improvements were seen in

the area of grasping for the moderate–experimental group compared with the moderate–control group. The Vineland Adaptive Behavior Scale, which was used to assess activities of daily living, showed no significant changes. Last, psychosocial changes were measured using three assessments: the Self-Perception Profile for Children, the Vineland Adaptive Behavior Subscale on Socialization, and the Child Behavior Checklist. All three of the assessments failed to show significant results. Although the only quantitative measure showing significant results was for grasping, qualitative results showed many improvements in sitting position, posture, trunk control, attention span, balance, gait, and various psychosocial aspects. The qualitative results came from riding instructors, therapists, parents, and videotape evaluations.

Bertoti (1988) used a repeated-measures design and found significant improvements in posture with her study of 4 girls and 7 boys with spastic cerebral palsy, who ranged in age from 2 years, 4 months, to 9 years, 6 months. The riding program in this study lasted 10 weeks and consisted of two 1-hour sessions per week. A pretest was given 10 weeks prior to the beginning of the program and again at the beginning of the 10-week program. A posttest was given following the program. Bertoti used a posture assessment scale, which she designed, that allows the therapist to assess the child's standing posture in five areas: head and neck, shoulder and scapula, trunk, spine, and pelvis. Each area is rated on a scale of 0 to 3. The scores from the five areas are then added together. Bertoti also subjectively found other improvements in the children, including improved weight-bearing and balance, increased head control, and improved posture and self-confidence.

Fox and colleagues (1984) studied 19 children ages 7 to 14 who had various disabilities, including cerebral palsy, spina bifida, learning disabilities, and mental retardation. A novel testing instrument created by the Department of Aerospace Engineering Sciences at the University of Colorado–Boulder was used for the study. The instrument contained auditory and visual feedback components as well as objects used in horseback riding (reins, stirrups, and horse grooming brushes), which were attached to a balance beam. Balance and coordination were tested using the reins, stirrups, and brushes. The children were instructed to keep the beam balanced while using the various objects one at a time. Auditory and visual feedback was given. The stirrups were used to test leg strength, and the brushes were used to test arm strength. Testing was done before and after a 2-hour riding session, and the program lasted 6 weeks.

Improvements were found in all three areas tested for most of the children. It was found that accurate positioning of the balance beam increased by an average of 18.6%, arm strength increased 8.1%, legs showed a 13.8% increase, and increase in balance and coordination required to demonstrate stability increased 7.2% immediately following the riding session.

Haehl and colleagues (1999) studied 2 typically developing children and 2 children with cerebral palsy in a two-phase study. The Peak Performance System and a fourth-order 6 Hz Butterworth low-pass digital filter for motion analysis were used to assess the data collected with a 60 Hz camcorder in both phases. As a control group, Phase I studied postural control and coordination in 2 typically developing children, a 7-year-old boy who had never ridden a horse and a 9-year-old girl who had competed in riding before. Phase II studied a 9.5-year-old girl who had mixed spastic and athetoid quadriplegic cerebral palsy and a 4-year-old boy who had spastic diplegic cerebral palsy. In addition to the video recordings and analysis using the same equipment as in Phase I, the Pediatric Evaluation of Disability Inventory (PEDI) was given 1 week before and 1 week after the 12-week program. Both children in Phase II showed improvements in postural stability and postural coordination during the final week of the program. Both children improved on the PEDI as well, but only the boy showed significant improvement. According to Haehl and associates, riding "encourages the client to problem solve and discover new ways to coordinate a postural response" (p. 99).

Land and colleagues (2001) studied sitting posture using a pretest–posttest design. Three females (a 10-year-old with spastic cerebral palsy and a 19-year-old and a 40-year-old with developmental delays) were studied. Each participant's posture was measured using a super VHS video camera and motion analysis equipment. Measurements of both the frontal posture and side posture were taken twice before the 8-week session began and then twice again after the 8-week session was over. Significant sitting posture was shown in four of the eight measures using repeated-measures analysis of variance, a finding suggesting that riding had positive effects on the riders' sitting posture.

Yack and colleagues (1997) investigated standing and walking balance in a 9-year-old boy diagnosed with attention deficit disorder and mild cerebral palsy and a 10-year-old boy diagnosed with attention deficit hyperactivity disorder. Both boys had balance difficulties. During the 4-week program, they rode three times per week for 1 hour each session. Their balance was tested twice per week before the start of the program and thereafter during the program. The Pediatric Clinical Test of Sensory Interaction for Balance (P–CTSIB), the Bruininks–Oseretsky Test of Motor Proficiency (BOTMP), and an assessment of walking smoothness to test walking balance with accelerations were used. The results of the P–CTSIB showed the greatest improvement in balance with eyes open. An upward trend in data, demonstrating improvements, was observed for both participants. The study authors noted that the findings may show that therapeutic riding initially has the greatest influence on the integration of visual information for balance control. Additionally, an upward trend in data for the P–CTSIB was shown for Participant 1 with his eyes closed. For Participant 1, upward trends were shown in the smoothness of his walking; this finding suggests that the adjustments that he had to make to the motion of the horse carried over and had a positive influence on the smoothness of his walking. Both boys scored greater than 2 standard deviations (SDs) below the norm on the BOTMP before the riding program began. After the program, both boys scored within 1 SD, suggesting that the program had a positive influence on their balance.

Encheff (2002) compared the muscle activity of the gluteus maximus, gluteus medius, vastus lateralis, rectus femoris, gracilis, rectus abdominus, external oblique, and erector spinae (L3 level) during walking and during horseback riding in normal adults ages 25 to 40. Seven men and 1 woman participated in the study. Encheff found that all eight muscles are active during horseback riding, although at a lower level than during walking. Using a Noraxon Telemyo Telemetry Electromyography (EMG) system, the mean EMG activity for each muscle was calculated during the ambulation trial (AT) and horseback riding trial (HT). The AT and HT also were videotaped using a Panasonic Palmcorder Camcorder. The video and EMG data were combined. The AT and HT values were shown as "a percentage of the average level of EMG activity of the group for each muscle during the walking gait cycle" (p. 23). The AT and HT values are as follows: the rectus femoris during AT: 102.792 and HT: 20.470, vastus lateralis during AT: 113.332 and HT: 20.923, gracilis during AT: 101.191 and HT: 23.082, gluteus maximus during AT: 101.721 and HT: 26.305, gluteus medius during AT: 76.676 and HT: 24.158, external oblique during AT: 110.146 and HT: 9.281, rectus abdominus during AT: 94.278 and HT: 50.111, and erector spinae during AT: 92.983 and HT: 35.921. Three of the muscles—the rectus abdominus, gluteus maximus, and erector spinae—showed similar phasic patterns to those shown during walking. The author noted that this finding shows that therapeutic riding can help riders "who could benefit from postural control, trunk co-contraction and stabilization, and enhanced balance in order to improve their ambulation and functional mobility" (p. 44).

Potential Benefits for the Central Nervous System

Reaction time is a reflection of the length of time it takes for a movement to be planned (Wu, Wong, Lin, & Chen, 2001). According to Tortora (1999), the cerebellum plays a role in learning and performing movements. The cerebellum compares the information it receives about what movements are planned with sensory information it receives (Tortora, 1999). The cerebellum also contributes largely in the timing of learned movements (Salman, 2002). Thus, testing the reaction time of riders can provide an indication of whether therapeutic riding is helpful to the functioning of the central nervous system in general, including the cerebellum. Coordinated movements cannot take place if the cerebellum is not receiving the correct sensory information or motor feedback. If a child is not receiving proper proprioceptive information, for example, balance will not be maintained. A child will not correct his positioning on the horse if he does not feel him- or herself tilting or slipping to one side. The horse provides both movements and sensory stimulation.

The brain is highly interconnected. The pyramidal and extrapyramidal systems together are involved in the programming and execution of motor actions (Newman, 1995). The extrapyramidal system consists of prefrontal areas as well as the basal ganglia and reticular formation nuclei. One function of the extrapyramidal system is to maintain muscle tone. The extrapyramidal system receives input from such areas as the thalamus, the cerebellum, and the vestibular system (Drobny & Kurca, 2000). The nervous system receives proprioceptive sensory feedback from muscles (muscle spindles), joints (joint receptors), tendons (Golgi tendon organs), and the skin (cutaneous receptors). This proprioceptive feedback provides information about the position and motion of the limbs (Rosenbaum, 1991).

The pyramidal system drives voluntary movements. The basal ganglia are involved in initiation of movement, the motor cortex is involved with controlling the direction and force behind movements, and the premotor cortex is involved in motor preparation and selection of the movement path. The supplementary motor cortex plans sequences for extensive movements (Rosenbaum, 1991).

A boy waving to his mother and tracking her with his eyes as he rides past her on his horse is using his superior colliculi, which receives stimuli from the retina and coordinates eye movements (Newman, 1995). If the boy turns his head while keeping his eyes fixed on his mother, he is using the vestibulo-ocular reflex. This reflex uses the vestibular system, including the semicircular canals of the ear, as well as the nerves and centers of the brain that deal with vision (Rosenbaum, 1991).

For the brain to regain whatever is lost following a brain injury, the stimulation must be increased, and the child must be presented with that stimulation over and over again. For example, a common source of difficulty for a child with brain injury is poor tactility (Pennock, 1999). According to Pennock, without tactile awareness, it is difficult to control one's movements. With proper tactile stimulation, new tactile pathways can be created in the brain. Pennock advocates for increasing the intensity, frequency, and duration of various stimuli in order to bring about new pathways and connections in the nervous system.

In addition, the Rood approach (Stockmeyer, 1967) to treatment of brain injury makes several interesting contributions. Sensory and motor functions are highly related. "Treatment or therapy is not in the form of a motor act alone, but rather is the application of stimuli to activate a response, followed by sensory input from a correct response with additional stimuli given to facilitate or inhibit elements in the pattern" (Stockmeyer, 1967, p. 903).

Both Pennock's and Rood's approaches can be compared to therapeutic riding and the effects that the horse has on the rider. "The progression of development is a neurobiological process that begins with sensory registration" (Morin & Carrasco, 1994, p. 57). To develop motor planning, one must first develop body scheme and bilateral integration. This is achieved through sensory experiences, which can be experienced through therapeutic horseback riding (Morin & Carrasco, 1994).

According to Schultz (1999), in a typically developing child, proprioceptive and vestibular senses begin to develop within the womb. After birth, the senses continue to mature and "develop in close reciprocity to the motor activity and, later, to the locomotion of the child" (p. 47).

A horse allows exploration for the child just as a mother carrying her child without holding it fast allows her child to move and explore (Schultz, 1994). The horse's movement gives the rider many oscillating impulses every minute. Those impulses facilitate the child to erect himself and keep his balance. The movement of the horse encourages the child to look around and discover space and sensory awareness (Schultz, 1994, 1999).

These studies show that therapeutic riding provides the rider with a variety of benefits, including improved balance, coordination, proprioception, increased awareness, improved posture, increased strength, increased attention span, and improved gait. Motor control requires successful integration of several portions of the central nervous system. The stimulation from the horse, for example, can facilitate proprioceptive input, which in turn can cause improved coordination and motor control.

In this line of research, the next logical step was to investigate reaction time in therapeutic riding. Because studies have shown that therapeutic riding leads to improvements in other motor areas, and because reaction time is an indicator of central nervous system processing abilities, our first hypothesis was that in a pretest–posttest simple experimental design, a significant change in the reaction time of the children in the riding group would occur between the beginning and end of the riding program. Our second hypothesis was that the reaction times of the children in the riding group would be significantly different from the reaction times of the children in the nonriding group.

Method

This study was approved by the Medical College of Ohio's Institutional Review Board, and all participants gave informed consent before participating. In addition, all participants' legal guardians gave informed consent before the start of the research.

Participants

Boys and girls with various developmental disabilities ranging from age 7 to 17 were recruited from a riding center in the Midwest to participate in this study. The study originally had 9 participants enrolled. Before data collection began, however, 3 participants withdrew from the study. Of the remaining 6 children, 1 girl and 2 boys were in the riding group and participated in the therapeutic horseback riding program during the course of the study. The other 3 children, all girls, were in the

nonriding group, meaning they did not participate in the therapeutic riding program during the course of the study (Figure 17.1). All parents and guardians signed an informed-consent form, and all of the children signed an informed-assent form.

The pretest data collection took place in January 2004, and the posttest data collection took place during the last week of the riding session in March 2004. The inclusion criteria stated that the participants had to be capable of following the directions given to them, had to be able to clearly see a computer screen and be able to tell when a stimulus was given on that screen, and had to have the ability to use the Big Red Switch activation device after seeing the stimulus.

Apparatus

A Big Red Switch (AbleNet, Minneapolis, MN) was connected to an analog-to-digital board (model OKPCM–CIA–16AI, Keithley Instruments, Cleveland, OH) that was housed within a 366 MHz Pentium computer. Data were collected at 100 Hz. Custom data acquisition software collected the data and provided the stimulus for each of the participants (Figure 17.2). In addition, the custom software calculated the time from when the stimulus appeared to when the participant released the switch. Last, the custom software randomly selected an interval of time from 3 seconds to 6 seconds before providing the stimulus.

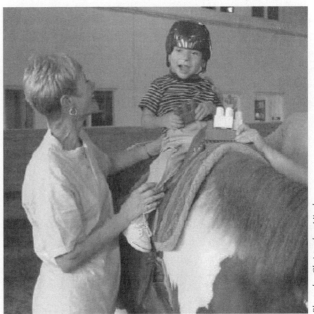

Photo by Christopher Hipsher

Figure 17.1. Boy stacking blocks while riding Rusty the horse, accompanied by his sidewalkers.

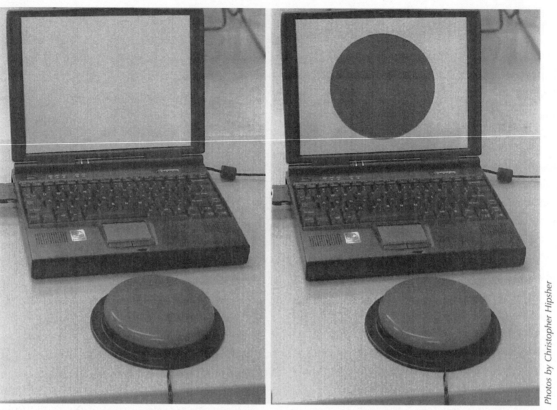

Figure 17.2. The laptop computer displays no stimulus (left) and displays the stimulus (right).

Photos by Christopher Hipsher

Procedure

The riding group participated in an 8-week therapeutic riding program. Two participants were not enrolled in the riding program during the study, but the other 2 participants were. During the 8-week period, the 2 children in the nonriding group did not participate in the therapeutic riding program. Each child's reaction time was tested using a laptop computer and a Big Red Switch before the riding session in Weeks 1 and 8. The laptop was set up with a program that caused a stimulus to appear and kept track of how long it took for the child to remove his or her hand from the switch. At the riding facility, either 3 or 4 riders were in each hour-long session, and the children rode once per week.

The testing took place in a private room free from distractions. Each child was tested individually while seated at a table with the laptop in front of him or her and with the Big Red Switch positioned so that the participant's hand of preference rested comfortably on it. The spatial orientation of the participant to the computer and to the Big Red Switch was recorded.

Once the participant had been physically oriented to the research setup, he or she was given 20 trials, a number chosen because it was assumed that this quantity would provide a stable baseline from which to make the comparison (Ottenbacher, 1986). A trial consisted of having the participant place his or her hand of preference on the Big Red Switch. Once the stimulus appeared, the participant removed his or her hand from the Big Red Switch, which marked the time from the appearance of the stimulus to the time the participant's hand was removed from the Big Red Switch. Once the participant's hand was removed from the Big Red Switch, the stimulus disappeared and the participant placed his or her hand back on the Big Red Switch to wait for the stimulus to appear again. For each trial, the investigator pressed a button on the computer to initiate the trial. Once the trial had been initiated, the amount of time until the stimulus appeared was either 3, 4, 5, or 6 seconds and was randomly selected through a computer algorithm across each of the 20 trials. Upon completion of the study, each participant received a packet of stickers and a ribbon as a token of appreciation for his or her participation.

Results

One participant in the riding group was unable to hold down the switch and wait for the stimulus to appear and was withdrawn from the study. After the completion of

Table 17.1. Mean Reaction Time of Participants Across 20 Trials of Pretest and Posttest

	Nonriding Participant 1		Nonriding Participant 2		Riding Participant 1		Riding Participant 2	
	Pretest	Posttest	Pretest	Posttest	Pretest	Posttest	Pretest	Posttest
RT (Sec)	0.639481	0.644431	0.601334	0.665679	1.062354	0.649547	0.581935	0.538415

Note: RT = reaction time.

the study, data from a participant in the nonriding group were discarded after it was determined that the participant had not understood the directions.

The remaining children, 2 in the riding group and 2 in the nonriding group, ranged in age from 8 years, 6 months, to 8 years, 11 months, at the beginning of the study. The 4 participants consisted of 3 girls and 1 boy, all of whom had cerebral palsy.

One participant had been in the therapeutic riding program for 2 years at the start of the study and had been on a break for 3 months. Another participant had been riding in the program for almost 4 years at the start of the study and had last attended a session in August 2003. A third participant began riding in a program in July 2002 and had last attended a session in October 2003. The fourth participant did not have any therapeutic riding experience.

Two of the 4 participants had had surgeries in their lifetimes, including a patent ductus arteriosus ligation, colostomy, reverse colostomy and repair of hernia, bilateral hip surgery, heel cord lengthening, and a thyroplaty. In addition, 2 of the 4 participants had had botox injections, the most recent being in October 2003.

Two of the 4 participants used assistive devices, including a wheelchair, walker, gait trainer, power wheelchair, and a SWASH (*S*tanding, *W*alking, *A*nd *S*itting *H*ip Orthosis) brace. Three of the 4 participants used ankle–foot orthoses at the time of the study.

Three of the 4 participants received outside therapy at the time of the study. One participant received speech therapy through school for 30 minutes per week. One participant received occupational and physical therapy only through school, each therapy session being once a week for 30 minutes each. The other 2 participants received both occupational and physical therapy in school and outside of school at intervals ranging from 30 minutes per week to 30 minutes daily. One participant missed one riding session and five therapy sessions during the study because of illness. The other participants did not miss any scheduled therapy or riding sessions.

The riding sessions took place for 1 hour almost every Saturday over the course of 8 weeks. Classes were cancelled once in the 8 weeks. Participants in the riding

group were tested before riding in the first week and again before riding in the eighth week. Participants in the nonriding group were tested on a Monday the first week and on a Wednesday on the final week.

Because of the small sample size, I was unable to generate inferential statistics. Therefore, the results are based on descriptive statistics. The mean reaction times of the participants in the nonriding group and in the riding group were calculated (Table 17.1). Figures 17.3 and 17.4 show the reaction times of the participants in the nonriding group in graphical form, and Figures 17.5 and 17.6 show the reaction times of the participants in the riding group in graphical form. The means shown in Table 17.1 reveal that both of the participants in the riding group had shorter reaction times in the posttest than in the pretest. In contrast, the participants in the nonriding group had slightly slower reaction times in the posttest than in the pretest. The differences between the reaction times in the riding and nonriding groups become even more evident when the means of both participants in the nonriding group are averaged together, and the means of both participants in the riding group are averaged together (Table 17.2). The nonriding group became slightly slower (0.620 seconds in the pretest and 0.655 seconds in the posttest),

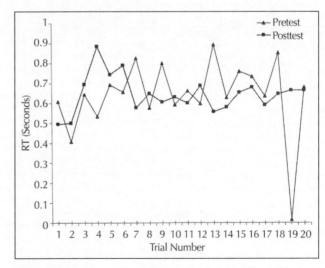

Figure 17.3. Reaction times (RT) of Nonriding Group Participant 1.

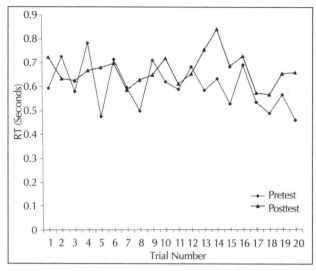

Figure 17.4. Reaction times (RT) of Nonriding Group Participant 2.

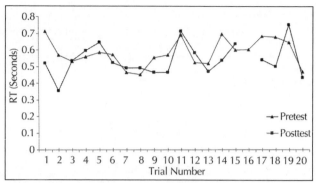

Figure 17.6. Reaction times (RT) of Riding Group Participant 2.

size* equals 1.414. According to Cohen (1988), this is a large effect size.

Sample size was calculated according to the mean difference between the difference in scores† and with an *SD* of 0.18583; using a significance level of *p* = .05 and assuming a desired power of 80%, the sample size required to reach significance was 8.

Discussion

This study measured the reaction time in children who participated in a therapeutic riding program as well as a group of children not participating in a therapeutic riding program. By measuring reaction time, it was my intent to determine whether therapeutic riding has positive effects on the child's central nervous system. By showing that the reaction time of the participants who were in the therapeutic riding program improved during the course of the study, we may be able to infer that therapeutic riding has a positive effect on the reaction time.

Although studies have shown that therapeutic riding can lead to improvements in motor control, no other studies could be found that test reaction time in the par-

and the riding group's reaction time became much faster (0.822 seconds in the pretest and 0.594 seconds in the posttest). Figure 17.7 shows the averages in graphical form.

My first hypothesis stated that a significant change in the reaction time of the children in the riding group would occur between the beginning and end of the program. As stated, I was unable to run statistical analyses because of the sample size. Both participants in the riding group did, however, show shorter reaction times in the posttest than in the pretest.

The second hypothesis stated that the reaction times of the children in the riding group would be significantly different from the reaction times of the children in the nonriding group. I was unable to draw a conclusion because of the small sample size. However, the effect

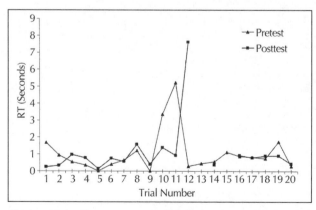

Figure 17.5. Reaction times (RT) of Riding Group Participant 1.

Table 17.2. Combined Group Mean Reaction Time and Standard Deviation

	Riding Group	**Nonriding Group**
	M (SD)	*M (SD)*
RT Pretest(s)	0.822145 (0.339707)	0.620408 (0.026974)
RT Posttest(s)	0.593981 (0.078582)	0.655055 (0.015025)

Note: RT = reaction time; *M* = mean; *SD* = standard deviation.

---

*$*d = (m_1 - m_2)/SD$, where $(m_1 - m_2)$ equals the difference of the means (0.2681), and *SD* equals the standard deviation (0.1858).
†For both groups, the difference scores equal posttest–pretest. For the riding group, the result equaled 0.228161, and for the nonriding group the result was −0.0346.

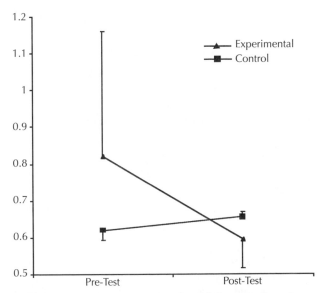

Figure 17.7. Mean reaction times of the riding and nonriding groups. The vertical lines are "error bars" showing standards

ticipants of therapeutic riding programs. Bertoti (1988), Haehl and colleagues (1999), and Land and colleagues (2001) found improvements in standing posture, postural stability and coordination, and sitting posture, respectively. Those results show that the stimulation provided from the movement of the horse can have a positive effect on the rider's posture.

Bertoti (1988), like the current study, considered children with cerebral palsy in her study. But unlike the current study, Bertoti had a population size of 11 children and studied the children's posture over the course of 10 weeks. In addition, the children in Bertoti's study had two 1-hour sessions per week, whereas the current study only had one 1-hour session per week over the course of 8 weeks. Bertoti used two pretests and a posttest, but the current study used one pretest and one posttest.

Unlike the current study, Haehl and colleagues (1999) studied postural control and coordination in two typically developing children as well as in two children with cerebral palsy. The current study compared 2 children in a riding program to 2 nonriders, but all 4 children had cerebral palsy. Haehl and associates' study took place over a 12-week period, whereas the current study took place over an 8-week period. They used a pretest–posttest method, but unlike the current study, they gave the posttest 1 week after the program ended.

Although they used a pretest–posttest design like the current study, Land and colleagues (2001) studied female riders of various ages (10, 19, and 40 years old)

and disabilities (cerebral palsy and developmental delays) in their study of sitting posture.

McGibbon and colleagues (1998) studied gait, energy expenditure, and gross motor function. They found statistically significant decreases in the energy expenditure and statistically significant increases in the GMFM scores of each participant following the riding program. There were improvements in the gaits of the children as well, but the improvements were not significant. Like the current study, all of the children had cerebral palsy, and the program lasted 8 weeks. However, the program in the McGibbon and associates study was twice-weekly for one half-hour each session. In addition, the study had a small sample size (5 children) just like the current study (4 children). Like the Bertoti (1988) study, McGibbon and colleagues took two baseline measurements and one posttest measurement. The current study took one baseline and one posttest measurement.

MacKinnon and colleagues (1995) studied gross motor control, posture, fine motor control, activities of daily living, and psychosocial changes. This study, like the current one, looked at children with cerebral palsy. The sample size of 19 was larger than the one in the current study, as was the length of the study—a 26-week riding program. Another big difference was the way in which the participants were divided. The current study had riding and nonriding groups, but MacKinnon and associates' participants were divided into four groups: mild–experimental, mild–control, moderate–experimental, and moderate–control.

Fox and colleagues (1984) and Yack and colleagues (1997) also found positive results in their research in therapeutic riding, including improvements in the balance of their participants. Fox and colleagues' study studied 19 children, which was a much larger sample size than the current study. In addition, although the study did have participants with cerebral palsy, some participants also had spina bifida, learning disabilities, and mental retardation. Unlike the current study, their riding sessions lasted 2 hours, and the program lasted 6 weeks. Improvements included increases in balance and coordination, arm strength, and leg strength. Fox and colleagues also tested participants before and after each session. Yack and colleagues (1997) studied standing and walking balance. Their sample size only contained two participants, a 9-year-old boy with attention deficit disorder and mild cerebral palsy and a 10-year-old boy with attention deficit hyperactivity disorder. Improvements were seen in scores of the P–CTSIB and BOTMP in both participants, and one participant showed improvements in the smoothness of his walking. Although their program only lasted 4 weeks, participants rode for 1 hour three times per week. The current study had four participants with cerebral palsy, and the program was held for 1 hour per week for 8 weeks. Unlike the current study, Yack and colleagues (1997) tested the balance of their participants twice a week prior to the start of the program and, thereafter, during the program. In addition, the current study had a riding group and nonriding group. In both Fox and colleagues (1984) and Yack and colleagues (1997), all participants participated in the riding program.

This study did have some limitations. The first was the sample size. Because it had only 4 participants, I was unable to do inferential statistical analyses. Another limitation was the length of the therapeutic riding program. Generally, sessions last 10 weeks at this facility, but because of scheduling problems, they were reduced to 8. In addition, class was cancelled during one of the weeks, dropping the number of weeks the participants rode to 7. A third limitation was the time of testing. The riding group was tested at the same time and day of the week during pretest and posttest (Saturday morning). The participants in the nonriding group were tested on a Monday morning for the pretest, but because of an unforeseen circumstance, they unfortunately only were able to schedule a Wednesday evening for the posttest. The time of day may have affected the participants during testing. Finally, the participants in the non-riding group were a set of twins. This may account for the low variance seen between these two.

Conclusion

As stated earlier, therapeutic riding is occupational in nature. In addition, it is a fun and motivating therapy for the riders. With the small sample size in this study, however, inferential statistics could not be used to determine whether the results were significant. However, it appears that therapeutic riding did affect the reaction time of the participants. Although occupational therapy has continued to get more involved in therapeutic riding, there is still much more potential for occupational therapy to contribute to rehabilitation of children and adults with a variety of mental, physical, and emotional difficulties.

Acknowledgments

Thank you to the children who helped so much by participating in the study and to their parents for all of their help, whether arriving early to riding or making a special trip for data collection. I also thank the staff, instructors, and volunteers at Vail Meadows Therapeutic Riding Center, especially Sandy Mauter and Robyn Shinaver, for their help with the recruitment of the participants. Thanks also go to the SON/SAH Research Support Committee for the SON/SAH Research Support Award, which was of great assistance to the project. Finally, special thanks are given to my advisor, Martin Rice, PhD, OTR/L, for his guidance and help.

The reaction time study was performed while the researcher was at the Medical College of Ohio at Toledo.

References

All, A. C., Loving, G. L., & Crane, L. L. (1999). Animals, horseback riding, and implications for rehabilitation therapy. *Journal of Rehabilitation, 65,* 49–57

Bertoti, D. B. (1988). Effect of therapeutic horseback riding on posture in children with cerebral palsy. *Physical Therapy, 68,* 1505–1512.

Bliss, B. (1997). Therapeutic horseback riding? *RN, 60,* 69–70.

Bracher, M. (2000). Therapeutic horse riding: What has this to do with occupational therapists? *British Journal of Occupational Therapy, 63,* 277–282.

Cohen, J. (1988). *Statistical power analysis for the behavioral sciences.* Hillsdale, NJ: Lawrence Erlbaum.

Drobny, M., & Kurca, E. (2000). Possible extrapyramidal system degradation in Parkinson's disease. *Brain Research Bulletin, 53,* 425–430.

Encheff, L. L. (2002). *Comparison of muscular activity of the trunk and lower extremity muscles during normal ambulation versus horseback riding.* Unpublished master's thesis, University of Toledo, OH.

Engel, B. T. (1992a). Traits of the therapeutic riding horse. In B. T. Engel (Ed.), *Therapeutic riding programs: Instruction and rehabilitation* (pp. 82–83). Durango, CO: Barbara Engel Therapy Services.

Engel, B. T. (1992b). The selection of the correct horse for a specific rider. In B. T. Engel (Ed.), *Therapeutic riding programs: Instruction and rehabilitation* (p. 92). Durango, CO: Barbara Engel Therapy Services.

Fox, V. M., Lawlor, V. A., & Luttges, M. W. (1984). Pilot study of novel test Therapeutic Riding instrumentation to evaluate therapeutic horseback riding. *Adapted Physical Activity Quarterly, 1,* 30–36.

Haehl, V., Giuliani, C., & Lewis, C. (1999). Influence of hippotherapy on the kinematics and functional performance of two children with cerebral palsy. *Pediatric Physical Therapy, 11,* 89–101.

Heine, B. (1997). Introduction to hippotherapy. *NARHA Strides, 3,* 10–13.

Kellon, E. (1992). Conformation affects rider comfort. In B. T. Engel (Ed.), *Therapeutic riding programs: Instruction and rehabilitation* (pp. 84–85). Durango, CO: Barbara Engel Therapy Services.

Land, G., Errington-Povalac, E., & Paul, S. (2001). The effects of therapeutic riding on sitting posture in individuals with disabilities. *Occupational Therapy in Health Care, 14,* 1–12.

Lane, R. (n.d.). *Riding for the disabled association: Highland group.* Unpublished manuscript.

MacKinnon, L. R., Noh, S., Lariviere, L., MacPhail, A., Allan, D. E., & Laliberte, D. (1995). A study of therapeutic effects of horseback riding for children with cerebral palsy. *Physical and Occupational Therapy in Pediatrics, 15,* 17–34.

McGibbon, N. H., Andrade, C.-K., Widener, G., & Cintas, H. L. (1998). Effect of an equine-movement therapy program on gait, energy expenditure, and motor function in children with spastic cerebral palsy: A pilot study. *Developmental Medicine and Child Neurology, 40,* 754–762.

Morin, C., & Carrasco, R. (1994). Sensory motor treatment in a therapeutic riding program. In P. A. Eaton (Ed.), *The Eighth International Therapeutic Riding Congress: The complete papers* (pp. 56–61). Levin, New Zealand: RDA Monograph.

Nelson, D. L. (1994). Occupation form, occupational performance, and therapeutic occupation. In C. B. Royeen (Ed.), *The practice of the future: Putting occupation back into therapy* (AOTA Self-Study Series, Lesson 2, pp. 9–48). Rockville, MD: American Occupational Therapy Association.

Newman, J. (1995). Thalamic contributions to attention and consciousness. *Consciousness and Cognition, 4,* 172–193.

Ottenbacher, K. J. (1986). *Evaluating clinical change: Strategies for occupational and physical therapists.* Baltimore: Williams & Wilkins.

Pennock, K. (1999). *Rescuing brain-injured children.* London: Ashgrove.

Rosenbaum, D. A. (1991). *Human motor control.* San Diego: Academic.

Salman, M. S. (2002). The cerebellum: It's about time! But timing is not everything—New insights into the role of the cerebellum in timing motor and cognitive tasks. *Journal of Child Neurology, 17,* 1–9.

Sayler, P. L. (1992). Selecting the hippotherapy horse. In B. T. Engel (Ed.), *Therapeutic riding programs: Instruction and rehabilitation* (pp. 86–87). Durango, CO: Barbara Engel Therapy Services.

Schmidt, R. A., & Lee, T. D. (1999). *Motor control and learning: A behavioral emphasis* (3rd ed.). Champaign, IL: Human Kinetics.

Schultz, M. (1994). Psychomotor aspects of movement and developmental riding evaluated on a case-study of an autistic child. In P. A. Eaton (Ed.), *The Eighth International Therapeutic Riding Congress: The complete papers* (pp. 105–107). Levin, New Zealand: RDA Monograph.

Schultz, M. (1999). Remedial and psychomotor aspects of the human movement and its development—A theoretical approach to developmental riding. *Scientific and Educational Journal of Therapeutic Riding, 5,* 44–57.

Stockmeyer, S. A. (1967). An interpretation of the approach of Rood to the treatment of neuromuscular dysfunction. *American Journal of Physical Medicine, 46,* 900–961.

Tortora, G. J. (1999). *Principles of human anatomy* (8th ed.). Menlo Park, CA: Benjamin/Cummings Science.

Wu, C., Wong, M., Lin, K., & Chen, H. (2001). Effects of task goal and personal preference on seated reaching kinematics after stroke. *Stroke, 32,* 70–76.

Yack, H. L., Bartels, C., Irlmeier, J., Lehan, A., Voyles, H., Haladay, K., et al. (1997). The effects of therapeutic horseback riding on the quality of balance control in children with attention disorders. *Scientific Journal of Therapeutic Riding, 3,* 3–9.

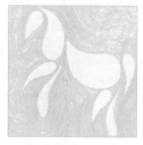

*In training the horse,
one trains oneself.*
—Antoine De Pluvinet

CHAPTER 18

Effect of Hippotherapy on Physical Capacity in Parkinson's Disease: A Single-Case Study

Rebecca Cook, OTR, HPCS

Willard and Spackman's Occupational Therapy (Hopkins & Smith, 1983) has defined *Parkinson's disease* as a slowly progressive, degenerative disorder of the central nervous system. According to the *Quick Reference to Occupational Therapy* (Reed, 1991), treatment models for Parkinson's disease are based on sensorimotor activities and sensory integration. Because Parkinson's disease is a progressive disorder, therapy can slow the degree of disability, but not the course of the disease. Turnbull (1999) proposed a model paradigm of treatment that supports the following progression: first, therapy to enhance skills; then, as the disease advances, to maintain those skills; next, adaptations to disability; and in the last stages, palliative care. He suggested that occupational therapists consider "pre-habilitative" treatment, which is proactive for functional management, rather than rehabilitative treatment, which aims to bring back lost function. Hippotherapy provides a strong sensorimotor and sensory-integrative component and thus is an appropriate occupational therapy intervention for the enhancement and maintenance stages of Parkinson's disease. Therapy for those stages focuses on decreasing secondary motor complications (soft-tissue adaptation, deconditioning, muscle imbalance, and weakness) and slowing deterioration of function (gait, posture, balance, and activities of daily living [ADLs]). Upon investigation, however, no studies were found that used hippotherapy strategies with the diagnosis of Parkinson's disease, although information about hippotherapy and other neurological disorders was discovered in Engel (1997). Thus, this lack of research created the genesis to follow the effect of hippotherapy on this client with Parkinson's disease.

This study set out to answer the following questions:
- Will hippotherapy affect long-term physical capacity of people diagnosed with Parkinson's disease, a progressively debilitating disease?
- Will hippotherapy affect short-term physical capacity of people diagnosed with Parkinson's disease?
- What effect does stopping hippotherapy have on physical capacity?
- What is the effect of reinitiating hippotherapy treatment after a 1-month discharge?

Investigation Methods

This study focused on a 42-year-old man ("Jim") diagnosed 11 years previously with Parkinson's disease. He received occupational therapy treatment involving 30-minute weekly hippotherapy sessions for 1 year, with a 1-month hiatus between the 9th and 10th months of treatment. During the study period, Jim received prescribed medication (carbidopa–levodopa, selegiline, pramipexole, diphenhydramine, amantadine, Percolace [a stool softener], and folic acid) and botulinum toxin injections in the lower left extremity every 3 months and completed a recreational home swim program that was initiated during the treatment hiatus. Hippotherapy was the only form of therapy received during the study time. Hippotherapy was consistently scheduled on Thursdays from 10:30 to 11:00 a.m., and the assessments were completed as outlined in the following parameters.

Assessment Parameters

Gait analysis and dynamometer grip strength testing were chosen to measure physical capacity because of their consistency and reliability, ease and efficiency of administration in the clinical setting, ability to permit comparison of results, and functional significance. Gait analysis relates to function in the following areas:

- The more severe the pathology is, the slower the walking speed is.
- Both poor balance and muscle spasticity result in a shorter stride length and decreased stride time.
- Relative speed is an important safety measure for community activities such as crossing a street at a crosswalk, which is generally set at normal relative speed of 0.8 to 1.0 statures per second.

Grip strength is functionally related to completion of ADLs such as zipping, dressing, eating, and bathing. It also is related to community living skills such as opening doors, carrying items, and cleaning (Adams, 1990).

Gait Analysis

Gait analysis was conduced using side-view videotapes of Jim's walk. The initial assessment was completed with 1-person assist in the clinic because he was able to ambulate only 3 of 13 meters before becoming fatigued and requiring rest in a wheelchair. The remaining gait scores were completed with 1-person assist on the 13-meter cement walkway to and from the barn parking area. Jim's ambulation from the car to the walkway was 2 meters and from the walkway to the arena was 2 meters; thus, the total ambulation was 17 meters, and the middle 13 meters were scored. The pretreatment videos were taken immediately prior to therapy, and posttreatment videos were taken within 5 minutes of dismounting the horse.

- Stride length in meters (m), right heel contact to the next right heel contact, was calculated from the number of strides walked divided by the distance traveled.
- Stride time in seconds (sec) was averaged by dividing the amount of time (measured by a multifunction stopwatch) into the number of strides taken.
- Walking speed was determined by average stride length (m) divided by stride time (sec).
- Relative speed was calculated by walking speed (m/sec) divided by height (m), which equals statures per second (st/sec). Jim's height is 1.71 m.

Grip Strength

Jim was seated in a high-back, armless chair for each testing session; his feet were on the floor, his arm at his side, and elbow at 90°. Two trials were completed on the right and left using Jamar hand grip dynamometer readings. Trials were taken immediately before and after treatment; the highest reading for each hand was

recorded (to the nearest kilogram) and a combined left and right hand score was tallied.

Hippotherapy Intervention

Jim's treatment plan read,

Patient will be seen once a week for individualized occupational therapy treatment. His session will be based on the neurodevelopmental, human occupation, and sensory integration treatment approaches, with an emphasis on improving balance reactions, increasing strength and coordination, exploring various exercise activities, and expanding self-esteem. Hippotherapy, treatment with the use of the horse, will be incorporated to provide graded tactile, proprioceptive, and vestibular input and to facilitate dynamic postural reactions.

Each hippotherapy treatment was facilitated by an occupational therapist with a clinical specialty in hippotherapy. Sessions used a three-step mounting block; a 15-hand, medium-build Morgan horse; a Natural Ride bareback saddle with peacock safety stirrups; a Western-style safety helmet; and a professional horse handler using a halter and lead rope. Jim sat astride facing forward; the horse handler led from the near side; and the therapist walked at Jim's knee on the off side, requesting speed and direction changes and verbally (or physically, if needed) prompting balance, symmetry, posture, weight shifts, and breathing exercises for Jim. Initially, only a fast walk was used, which produced rotation in Jim's pelvis and assisted in decreasing muscle spasticity. Treatment progressed to figure eights and serpentines with walk–halt transitions in both directions, then to activities that promoted arm extension and abduction, and finally to use of the stirrups for sit–stand–sit transitions at the walk. Other exercises completed on the horse included walking with eyes closed and counting the number of steps taken, deep breathing for relaxation, an occasional trot, and sometimes assisting with unbuckling the girth after the session was over.

Results of the Study

From the initial evaluation to the 1-year evaluation, gait analysis demonstrated the following changes (Table 18.1):

- Increased stride length of 78%, which indicated improved balance and range of motion as well as reduction in spasticity or rigidity.
- A 16% slower stride time. (Parkinson's patients tend to take short and fast shuffling steps, so a slower stride time can be indicative of improvement.)

Table 18.1. Results of Gait Analysis

Gait Analysis Date	Stride Length (m)	Stride Time (seconds [s])	Walking Speed (m/s)	Relative Speed (statures/s [st/s])
Nondisabled average comparison	1.5	1.0	1.5	0.8–1.0 st/s
9/29: initial evaluation, Year 1 (% of normal)	0.203 (14%)	0.86 (86%)	0.236 (16%)	0.14 st/s (18%)
6/08 Year 2 pretest	0.81	0.90	0.90	0.53
6/08 posttest	0.93	1.03	0.90	0.53
6/15 pretest	0.93	1.09	0.85	0.50
6/15 posttest	1.08	1.25	0.86	0.50
7/13 pretest	0.47	1.08	0.44	0.26
7/13 posttest	0.65	1.03	0.58	0.34
7/20 pretest	0.72	1.08	0.67	0.39
7/20 posttest	0.87	1.12	0.78	0.45
10/19: annual evaluation, Year 2 (% of normal)	0.93 (62%)	1.03 (103%)	0.90 (60%)	0.53 (66%)
Total change	48%	17%	44%	48%

Note. Relative nondisabled average speed: Slow walking = 0.4 to 0.6 st/s and fast walking = 1.2 to 1.4 st/s.

- A 74% increase in walking speed. (The more severe the pathology is, the slower is the walking speed; thus, an increase in walking speed would correlate to a decrease in pathology.)
- An improvement of 74% in relative speed. (Relative speed is an important safety measure for community activities such as crossing a street at a crosswalk; Jim's relative speed, although improved, remained in the slow category, confirming the appropriateness of a handicapped parking sticker and possibly a wheelchair for community outings to increase safety and decrease fatigue.)

Comparisons of most pre- and post-treatment measures on any given date indicated immediate short-term gains following treatment in all areas of the gait analysis. During the 1-month hiatus in hippotherapy, Jim experienced a significant decrease in function (approximately 50%) in all areas of the gait analysis (compare scores from June 15 and July 13 in Table 18.1). After only two treatment sessions, gait analysis scores improved nearly to prehiatus levels, and after 3 months the scores had stabilized and equaled those recorded prior to the month without treatment.

From the initial evaluation to the 1-year evaluation grip strength showed an increase of 17% on the right, no decrease or increase on the left, and a combined score increase in strength of 9% (Table 18.2). Comparisons of pre- and posttreatment scores reveal mixed results regarding immediate short-term gains. On June 8 and June 15, posttreatment improvements were noted. The scores for July 13 and July 20, immediately after the hiatus, showed a slight decrease in strength posttreatment.

Subsequent to the 1-month hiatus in hippotherapy, grip strength scores were higher than those preceding the break. Possible explanations are the variability of strength from day to day in Parkinson's disease or effects of medication; it also may be that hippotherapy, for this client, had a diverse impact on grip strength.

Discussion

This study has the following limitations:
- It does not take into account the stages of Parkinson's and Jim's stage at the time.
- It does not address the question of when discharge from hippotherapy is appropriate.
- It did not consider the daily changes in function that could affect a particular test date.
- It has questionable applicability of the results to other people with Parkinson's disease because it involves only one participant.

Future research should compile the results of hippotherapy completed with several people diagnosed with Parkinson's disease over any 3-month period using the Webster Parkinson's Disease Scale (Webster, 1968) to classify the stage of Parkinson's disease, pre- and post-therapy gait analysis, and grip strength dynamometer readings as used in this study.

Conclusions

Results of this single-case study indicate that occupational therapy using hippotherapy had a positive effect

Table 18.2. Results of Dynamometer Testing

Dynamometer Readings	Right (kg)	Left (kg)	Combined Right and Left (kg)
Nondisabled average comparison	54 (dominant)	48	102
11/29: initial evaluation (% of normal)	19 (35%)	20 (42%)	39 (38%)
Following year pretest	26	22	48
6/08 posttest	27	25	52
6/15 pretest	26	24	50
6/15 posttest	25	24	49
7/20 pretest	29	23	52
7/20 posttest	28	23	51
10/19: annual evaluation, Year 2 (% of normal)	23 (43%)	20 (42%)	43 (42%)
Total Change	8%	0%	4%

on both short- and long-term physical function. Improved strength, endurance, balance, and range of motion was demonstrated by improved stride length, stride time, walking speed, and relative speed as well as, perhaps, by grip strength dynamometer testing. Stopping hippotherapy treatment for a 1-month period had a significant negative impact on gait analysis scores and a negligible impact on grip strength scores. Gait analysis scores showed improvement within two treatment sessions of initiating hippotherapy again and regained prehiatus levels within a 3-month time period.

On an endnote, Jim now ambulates for short community outings and successfully navigated an airplane aisle for a flight to visit relatives in another state. At this writing, he had begun a stationary bicycling program at home, and he was planning on swimming in the summer.

References

Adams, G. M. (1990). *Exercise physiology laboratory manual. Hand grip strength norms for males and females of different ages.* Dubuque, IA: Wm. C. Brown.

Engel, B. T. (1997). *Rehabilitation with the aid of a horse: A collection of studies.* Durango, CO: Barbara Engel Therapy Services.

Hopkins, H. L., & Smith, H. D. (1983). Parkinson's disease. In *Willard and Spackman's occupational therapy* (6th ed., pp. 405–407). New York: J. B. Lippincott.

Reed, K. L. (1991). Nervous system disorders. In *Quick reference to occupational therapy* (pp. 170–175). Rockville, MD: Aspen.

Turnbull, G. I. (1999). *Course manual on stroke and Parkinson's: Physical therapy management of chronic neurological disability.* Alpharetta, GA: Dogwood Institute.

Webster, D. D. (1968). Clinical analysis of the disability on Parkinson's disease. *Modern Treatment, 5,* 257–262.

Resources

A 1999 physician interview about Parkinson's disease: www.findarticles.com/m2578/10_54/56535594/p1/article.jhtml

American Academy of Family Physicians: www.aafp.org/afp/, search on Parkinson's for a list of symptoms

American Parkinson Disease Association: www.apdaparkinson.com

The Michael J. Fox Foundation for Parkinson's Research: www.michaeljfox.org/

National Institute of Neurological Disorders and Stroke—Parkinson's Disease: www.ninds.nih.gov/health_and_medical/pubs/parkinson_disease_htm

National Institute of Neurological Disorders and Stroke—Research Topics: www.ninds.nih.gov/health_and_medical/research.htm#p

National Library of Medicine, National Institutes for Health, PubMed: www.ncbi.nlm.nih.gov, search on Parkinson's

National Parkinson Foundation: www.parkinson.org/newnews.htm

The Parkinson's Institute: www.parkinsonsinstitute.org

Rehabilitation R&D Progress Reports: Section 9, Neurological and Vascular Disorders—*Muscle Strength and Functional Performance in Parkinson's Disease: A Pilot Study:* www.vard.org/prog/98/98prch09.htm

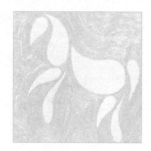

The horse is God's gift to mankind.
—*Arabian Proverb*

CHAPTER 19

What Is the State of Hippotherapy Research, and Where Should We Go From Here?

Joyce R. MacKinnon, PhD, OT(C), OTR

To determine the status and development of hippotherapy research and where the field should go from here, it is necessary to include the umbrella field of therapeutic horseback riding. If one were to consider only hippotherapy, this chapter would be limited in space, content, and benefit to readers. Including the larger body of literature regarding therapeutic riding provides additional relevant material to analyze and determine future directions.

The purpose, then, of this chapter is to examine the research that has been generated in recent years, critically analyze it, and comment on its benefits and limitations. To undertake this exercise, it was reasonable to look to a body responsible for the leadership and generation of research in this domain. Although other sources exist, it was appropriate, valuable, and manageable to review all the research articles published in the *Scientific and Educational Journal of Therapeutic Riding,* an international journal on riding for the disabled population. From the analysis of those writings, a pathway can be created along which hippotherapy researchers may direct their energies.

It was my impression that the 1997 publication of this journal was the inaugural one, but according to the editorial note in the 1997 volume of the *Scientific and Educational Journal of Therapeutic Riding,* that volume is the third annual scientific compilation of articles. The journal is published once a year, so the data include journals from 1997 to 2003. Other valuable sources of information include hippotherapy research, including the 10 conference proceedings from the International Congresses of Therapeutic

Riding. A few master's and doctoral theses focus on therapeutic riding and hippotherapy, and mainstream professional journals occasionally include an article on the subject. The rationale for limiting analyses to the *Scientific and Educational Journal of Therapeutic Riding* is that its mandate is scientific research in this area.

The articles in the journal were placed in the following categories: *Research, Programs, Horses, Theory, Training,* and *Other.* The two most difficult categories to define were Research and Other, because some articles were directly related to research but the authors had not collected any of the data that were analyzed. Although data analyzed or reviewed from other sources is legitimately considered research, those articles have been omitted here so that readers can understand the problems experienced by researchers in hippotherapy and therapeutic riding. After considerable deliberation, it was decided that for an article to be placed in the Research category, it had to directly involve the collection of data, regardless of the quality of the research.

The Other category included articles that did not fit clearly within the remaining five categories. The two articles that provided the greatest dilemma for the author are Pauw (1999) and Buck (2001), both of which offer information on the research process. The articles are well written and worth the reader's attention.

Analyses

To analyze the articles, two tables were created. Table 19.1 is a simple categorization of the types of articles so that one can see whether the amount or type of research has increased over time. Table 19.2 includes only articles with a focus on research. The table lists the author; the popu-

Adapted with permission by the Federation of Riding for the Disabled. Original version of appendix appeared in the *Scientific and Educational Journal of Therapeutic Riding* (2005), pp. 65–89.

Table 19.1. Categories of Articles From the *Scientific and Educational Journal of Therapeutic Riding,* 1997–2003

Year	Research	Programs	Horses	Theory	Training	Other
1997	Yack et al. Basile		Barrey	Klüwer		
1998	Heine & Rosensweig Longden Would		Miller (1998a) Miller (1998b) Miller (1998c)		Brown Hatton-Hall & Claridge Riffkin	
1999	Graham		Miller (1999a) Miller (1999b)	Schulz Hornacek	Brown & Tebay	Pauw
2000	Mattila-Rautiainen Freire			Allori & Pasquinelli	Murano, Allori, Pasquinelli, & Biagini	Graves
2001	Ionatamishvili, Tsverava, & Avaliani Pasquinelli, Allori, Mencaroni, & DiStefano Rufus	Burja, Zadnikar, & Lavric Silva & Freire Solt				Auvinet Claridge Buck
2002	MacKinnon & Ferreira MacKinnon & Wong Wiger Kreutzer-Brett Burgon	Boon-Thiel				
2003	Wiger Neves Juguin & Tessiot Leitao					Hauser

lation involved in the research; the condition or conditions of the population under study; the measures used; the research design specified by the authors (or perceived by the author of this chapter); the outcomes of the research; and, last, the study's limitations as determined by the author of this chapter.

Analysis of Table 19.1

During the period 1997 to 2003, a total of 45 articles were published. Of all the articles, 40% (18 articles) were research articles, which involved data collection. The remaining 60% were spread across the categories as follows: Programs, 8.9%; Horses, 13.3%; Theory, 8.9%; Training, 13.3%; and Other, 15.6%. The proportion of research articles has clearly grown; in 1997, 50% of articles were devoted to research (although it must be pointed out that only 4 articles were published). In 1998, 11.1% of the articles were research articles; in 1999, the proportion grew to 14.3%, and it continued to grow as follows: 2000, 40.0%; 2001, 33.3%; 2002, 83.3%; and 2003, 80.0%. Certainly, publication of research-based articles appears to be gaining momentum in this journal with research taking a primary seat over training and education. This increase in numbers and types of research are very positive signs, which bode well for the future for both therapeutic horseback riding and hippotherapy.

Analyses of Table 19.2

This section examines each of the eight columns in Table 19.2 in turn.

Objectives

The most interesting feature in this column is the various uses of terms to describe therapeutic riding. Only 3 of the 18 research articles (16.7%) involve the use of hippotherapy. The articles' subject matter falls within the traditional restrictive label of hippotherapy, but others terms closely resembling hippotherapy are used in the articles. The other terms used as often or more frequently than therapeutic riding are *therapeutic riding* (5 instances, 27.8%), *riding therapy* (3 instances, 16.7%), *equine therapy* (3 instances, 16.7%), and *other (vaulting, psycho-educational riding)*, and 1 not known (4 instances, 22.2%).

Population

In the 18 studies examined, the number of participants ranges from 1 to 40. In the 3 involving hippotherapy, the samples included 1, 2, and 7 participants. Seven studies (38.9%) using fewer than 5 participants, 8 (44.4%) used between 5 and 10 participants, and 3 (16.7%) had more than 10 participants.

Table 19.2. Analysis of Research Articles in *Scientific and Educational Journal of Therapeutic Riding,* 1997–2003

Author/Year	Objective	Population	Age Range	Condition	Measures	Design	Outcome	Limitations
Yack et al. (1997)	To measure the effect of therapeutic horseback riding (THR) program on balance	2	9–10	Attention deficit hyperactivity disorder (ADHD)	BOTMP P–CTSIB Walking balance	Case study	Standing balance with eyes open in support-surface condition was most improved. P–CTSIB showed variable results. BOTMP scores were close to normal. Walking balance improved for 1 child.	High-level sample was studied who obtained scores within normal range. Instrument lacked sensitivity. Frequency of testing may have resulted in learning effect in the testing procedure.
Basile (1997)	To describe the psychological effect of equine-facilitated physical therapy (PT) on self-esteem	13	9–14	ADHD	Child Behavior Checklist Coppersmith Self-Esteem Inventory	Pretest-posttest	No difference in pretest and post-test scores on either measure.	Participants dropped out, reducing sample to 7. No control group as planned. Number of classes reduced from 12 to 2. Measuring tools were not sensitive to change.
Would (1998)	To improve gait during hippotherapy	2	5 and 10	Cerebral palsy (CP) Diplegia Hemiplegia	Baseline skills were determined for each child and assessed after each session	Case study	Improved balance weight bearing, and postural awareness. Moved from walker to elbow crutches. Symmetrical sitting without associated reactions during walk and trot on either rein. Ability to right self on the horse.	No objective measuring tools were used. Sample size was small. It was difficult to tell progress in hippotherapy from Bobath treatment and interaction effects of PT on hippotherapy.

Study	Purpose	N	Age	Diagnosis	Measure	Design	Results	Comments
Graham (2000)	To determine the psychological and physical benefits of equine therapy (ET) List centers in Northern California	8	35–58	Multiple sclerosis	Questionnaire on psychological and physical benefits	Qualitative: survey questionnaire	Improved strength. Improved endurance. Positive outlook. More recreation, self esteem, and self-confidence. Improved overall health. Obtained information on northern California centers.	Study does not provide measurements of ET results. There is a risk of flawed evidence because results could be exaggerated. This is not a pure qualitative as author suggests; structured questions are more quantitative in design.
Freire (2000)	To evaluate ET as a tool in treatment of autistic children	7		Autistic and atypical autistic	Behavioral observation Evaluation card that reports assessments on 10 variables	Case study	Significant changes in postural tone.	Difference between autistic and atypical were not discussed. Reliability and validity of measurements are unknown. The sample size was small for the number of variables.
Rufus (2001)	To determine the value of riding therapy (RT) on the self-concept of children with learning disability (LD)	24	7–10	LD	Piers–Harris Self-Concept Scale Researcher-developed in-depth measure of riding skills using principles of classic equitation	Quasi-experimental, A-B-A design	Experimental and control groups improved on self-concept. No difference between groups and no correlations for riding and self-concept could be determined. RT's values lies in its "adjunctive nature."	No information was given on principles of classical equitation or in-depth measurement of riding skills. No information was given on what the control group did, if anything. It is unclear what "the value of RT lies in its adjunctive nature means."

(continued)

Table 19.2. Analysis of Research Articles in *Scientific and Educational Journal of Therapeutic Riding, 1997–2003 (Cont.)*

Author/Year	Objective	Population	Age Range	Condition	Measures	Design	Outcome	Limitations
Pasquinelli et al. (2001)	To test an evaluation tool in therapeutic riding (TR), focusing on time required to meet riding objectives	10	10–57	Extrapyramidal disorders (ED) CP (7 participants)	Initial assessment by neuro-psychiatrist, who gave a disability rating Dystonia Movement Scale ED protocol developed by Centre for Extrapyramidal Disorders	Qualitative: observation	Improvement was noted for all 10 riders after 12 months, with some variability. No further improvement was noted in TR riders after 40 and 60 months. Functional competencies retained after riding varied from 6 to 36 months.	Several concepts were unclear: • The meaning of TR on the horse and TR on the ground • Where neurological competencies on the horse and on the ground originate • The meaning of "consensus mechanisms" • Whether all 10 riders were involved in 60 months of riding. Language in this article is problematic (e.g., "excellent," "good," and "mild" are not defined).
Ionata-mishvili et al. (2001)	To assess the influence of RT on motor function in CP	40	6–12	CP	6-point system developed to measure hyperkinesias Memory test based on 35 objects in environment (1 point per object) Knowledge-of-horse test consisting of naming parts of horse	3 comparison groups: 2 groups of children with CP who received either RT (Group 1) or Bobath treatment (Group 2); 1 group of children without disabilities	Intensity of hyperkinesia was most reduced in Group 1. Treatment produced significant memory improvement across all groups. Knowledge of horse: significant effect across all groups.	No reliability and validity measures were developed. No time frame was identified as to when posttreatment measures were taken. Each child received 5 to 6 minutes of riding per week, yet dramatic changes were noted.

Study	Aim	N	Diagnosis	Age	Intervention/Measure	Design	Results	Comments
Ionata-mishvili et al. (2001) (Cont.)								No information was given as to what the children in Group 1 and 2 were doing when they were not riding.
MacKinnon & Ferreira (2002)	To identify key and important concepts in THR	7	CP	8–12	Measure of 10 variables from the literature that are related to 3 important concepts: social, personal, and sport	Quantitative: questionnaire	Riders found the social aspects of riding most meaningful, followed by personal aspects (especially sense of control and mastery) and sport.	Study used small sample size. Issues of meaning may be better addressed using qualitative methodology. Questionnaire was not tested for reliability or validity, and some questions were not clearly linked to the construct they were measuring. All questions were worded positively, increasing likelihood of acquiescence bias. Consistent order of yes–no questions may have influenced response to open-ended question. Reading comprehension skills may have affected the validity of children's responses.
Kreutzer-Brett (2002)	To improve social, physical, and psychological	1	Athetoid CP Insulin-dependent diabetes	Not given	Behavioral management compliance or no riding	Single-case study	Improvement in social, physical, and psychological functioning were noted.	Writing style makes the meaning unclear at times.

(continued)

Table 19.2. Analysis of Research Articles in *Scientific and Educational Journal of Therapeutic Riding, 1997–2003 (Cont.)*

Author/Year	Objective	Population	Age Range	Condition	Measures	Design	Outcome	Limitations
Kreutzer-Brett (2002) (*Cont.*)				Behavioral problems				Clinical advice in the report is not always supported by evidence within the case. Areas of improvement are outlined, but not attributed to specific aspects of the program. No references were provided.
Burgon (2002)	To determine the effects of riding on a group of adult clients with mental illness	6	30–40	Depression Schizophrenia Psychosis Stroke	Participant observation questionnaire Semi-unstructured interviews	Qualitative case study of a group of riders	Increase in riders' confidence was the most consistent finding, attributed to the horse as the motivating factor and the environment being perceived as safe and nonjudgmental. The new skill translated into confidence into other social situations.	This is an excellent example of documentation and of using theory to guide research and support findings. Weaknesses of the study are that the reader is not provided with the details of the source of data, and insufficient detail is provided on the data analysis process.
Wiger (2002)	To document development of participants, produce a video to confirm changes, and identify areas for further study	4	5–11	Physical Psychosocial	Videotaping Journal notes	Qualitative: questionnaire	Children and parents had different goals: Children had riding goals, whereas parents had therapy goals. No difference was found in perceptions of riding competence.	This study used a small sample size with a wide age discrepancy. A copy of the questions that the parents, school, and health professional were asked would have provided clarity.

Author (year)	n	Age	Diagnosis	Purpose	Measure	Design	Results	Comments
MacKinnon & Wong (2002)	8 (4 children, 4 parents)	7–13	CP	To determine whether riders set the same goals as parents; To examine perceptions of parents and children on riding competence	Canadian Occupational Performance Measure (COPM)	Qualitative: descriptive interview	Children and parents had different goals: Children had riding goals, whereas parents had therapy goals. No difference was found in perceptions of riding competence.	This quantitative study used a small sample with a wide age discrepancy. One child was unable to identify any goals, further reducing the child-generated data. The method involved in gathering data with the COPM was not detailed, making replication difficult. Qualitative design might have been more useful with such a small sample.
Wiger (2003)	4	5–11	Congenital lower-extremity skeletal deformity Turner syndrome Prenatal drug exposure	To document the effects of an adapted vaulting course for children with disabilities; To clarify the value of horseback riding to uninformed audiences	Participant observation (videotape) Questionnaire	Qualitative: parent-completed questionnaire regarding changes in child's status	All children were reported to show improvement in some areas. Parents of 2 children attributed the improvements to the program.	Only 14 of 25 questionnaires regarding child's status were returned. The small sample size makes the results difficult to interpret. No control group was used for comparison. No measurement or assessment tools were used, so it is difficult to quantify or qualify the amount of success. The hypothesis stated that positive gains would be made, but author did not specify the areas of expected gains.

(continued)

Table 19.2. Analysis of Research Articles in *Scientific and Educational Journal of Therapeutic Riding, 1997–2003 (Cont.)*

Author/Year	Objective	Population	Age Range	Condition	Measures	Design	Outcome	Limitations
Neves (2003)	To observe communication behavior in the context of hippotherapy sessions	7	4–16	Language acquisition and development difficulties A variety of intellectual, affective, and motor control issues	Participant observation Questionnaire	Quantitative design: content analysis of children's communication preferences and patterns	Children used gestural communication most frequently.	Researchers reported difficulty recording children's activities and interaction when horse was moving. Small sample size (15% of children attended the center with language limitation) and lack of detail on data gathering and analysis process make replication difficult. Research design is limited because there is no comparison group or before–after measurement; it is more of a status report than a research study.
Juguin & Tessiot (2003)	To determine the effects of hippotherapy on physical and cognitive deficits	1	16	5 years after traumatic brain injury; residual cognitive deficits and hemiplegia	Participant observation (documented via dictated field notes) Photographs, film	Case study	Child improved in understanding of safety, and began to develop concentration and pelvic positioning.	Researchers reported that sessions attempted to make too much progress too quickly. Final results are difficult to interpret because of client's agitation at the final session.

166

	Purpose	N	Age	Diagnosis	Measures	Design	Results	
Juguin & Tessiot (2003) (*Cont.*)								Lack of reported baseline and subjective measurement of results make it difficult to verify findings. No research design was used; this is more of a case report then research project.
Leitao (2003)	To determine the effects of psychoeduca-tional riding on behavior and develop-ment of chil-dren with autism	5	5–10	Autism	Participant observation (field notes, Observational Grid and video) Psycho-educational Profile–Revised Autism Treatment of Evaluation Checklist (ATEC)	Pretest–posttest	All children showed an increase in developmental age, increased eye contact with others, better response to physical contact with others, and cessation in aggression toward others. Many other improvements were shown by some partici-pants.	Results are diffi-cult to attribute to the program, because some participants were engaged in other inter-ventions during the study. The study was completed with a small sample. ATEC results may be biased be-cause parents completed it. The study ran for 16 weeks, and only 1 child made more than 4 months' change in that time. It is not clear whether these are signifi-cant gains with children with autism.

Note. Hippotherapy and equine-facilitated or -assisted therapy focus on therapy goals, whereas other types of riding focus on riding skills. Vaulting may focus on psychoeducational skills when supervised by a psychologist.

Age Range

Of the 18 studies, 12 (66.7%) focused on children, 2 (11.1%) on adults, 2 (11.1%) on both, and 2 (11.1%) did not specify the age of participants. From this information, it is clear that most of the studies involved children. The 3 hippotherapy studies focused on children from ages 4 to 16 years. An interesting feature of these studies is the wide age range of children in most of them. Most, including one on hippotherapy, involved a group of children spanning 5 or more years of difference in age. Age is probably not as important in a questionnaire situation, but in looking for cognitive, social, or physical changes, large age differences among children can be a confounding factor.

Conditions

In the 18 studies, 7 (38.9%) involved participants with mixed or more than one medical condition. Four (22.2%) involved participants with cerebral palsy, 2 (11.1%) worked with people who had attention deficit hyperactivity disorder, another 2 had participants with autism (11.1%). One study (5.6%) focused on multiple sclerosis, 1 (5.6%) worked with riders who had no disabilities, and 1 (5.6%) involved participants with learning disabilities. In the 3 hippotherapy studies, 1 included children with cerebral palsy, 1 had participants with traumatic brain injury, and 1 had participants with language problems in combination with cognitive or motor difficulties.

Measures

On reflection, this heading is probably not the best one to use, because qualitative researchers almost never use measures. A more appropriate term has not been found, however. In this series of research articles, many featured measurements as part of the research process. Thus, the following results should be taken with caution.

Of the 18 articles, only 6 used a standardized measure. Eleven of the 18 articles that involved measurement of variables did not use a standardized measure, however, a design flaw that does not bode well for the reliability and validity of the results. One study did not use any measure at all. This pattern denotes a lack of scientific rigor in the quantitative studies. The use of nonstandardized measures is to be avoided and discouraged in future quantitative studies.

Unless the researcher is actually trying to create a new measure, he or she might consider using qualitative methods if standardized measurement instruments are not available. The lack of measurement in qualitative

research is quite legitimate, because they generally are exploring concepts of a more subjective or affective nature that are not easily or appropriately measured by quantitative methodology.

In summary, then, the weakness of the quantitative studies being analyzed is their lack of use of standardized measures. Admittedly, it is difficult to find measures sufficiently sensitive to measure either therapeutic riding or hippotherapy; this difficulty is one of a multitude of reasons Buck (2001) and Pauw (1999) suggested that qualitative research might be more appropriate for the field. It is difficult to design a proposal involving quantitative research design without standardized measures and a homogenous population in terms of conditions, age ranges, and intellectual development of the participants.

Some researchers have suggested a balance between quantitative and qualitative research. Although it appears that quantitative research is still the gold standard in occupational therapy, many more researchers are moving into qualitative research because it seems more suited to evidence-based practice in occupational therapy; in many instances, qualitative methodology may have more to offer hippotherapy than quantitative methods.

Design

In this section, it was difficult to tease out the studies that were quantitative, qualitative, or of a mixed design. The designs were not clearly one design or another but bits and pieces of quantitative or qualitative designs, often used incorrectly. In some instances, the researchers said they were using a particular design, yet they failed to rigorously follow the elements of that design. In other instances, the researchers stated that they were using one design or the other, yet they did not have the necessary elements to undertake that design. Finally, some studies were not research at all but simply a report of findings, as an occupational therapist would undertake in a typical treatment plan. For all of those reasons, trying to dissect and categorize each study was extremely difficult.

Outcomes

Eight of the quantitative studies reported statistically significant findings, and 1 reported nonsignificant results and gave a rationale for why the study did not find statistically significant findings. The latter study actually provided more helpful information than the studies with statistically significant findings. Many of the qualitative studies did explore and find some meaningful information, but most of the studies were superficial in nature.

Limitations

When all 18 studies are examined, it is clear that their most outstanding limitation is the design and analysis of the studies. Because most of the studies were quantitative in design, the following comments are directed toward those articles. To complicate the credibility of the data, authors were unclear about their methodology, portrayed the methodology they used inaccurately, or even did not mention the methodology they thought they were using. These difficulties make it easy for other researchers to disregard these studies as invalid research. The devastating contribution of poor research is that novice or naive researchers or clinicians may not disregard the research and instead find the results appealing and accept them as fact.

The studies had particular problems with their sample selection. In several instances, the age range of the participants was sufficiently wide to question whether the population was homogeneous. It seems unlikely that the expectations for a 9-year-old are similar to those for a 15-year-old. Similarly, the degree of disability, whether physical or mental, often was undefined, again raising concerns for a homogenous sample, which is necessary for quantitative research methods. As is frequently the case, instrumentation was a problem for many researchers. The problems involved either nonstandardized instruments or the use of standardized instruments with too small a sample to reliably report the results.

Although the above problems were found mainly with the studies using quantitative methods, the few qualitative studies also had methodological problems. The primary problem was that the authors were not sufficiently clear on what kind of qualitative research they were using. The studies that are reported here tended to use only superficial analyses and relied solely on client quotes to substantiate their claims rather than using theory or in-depth interpretation by the author. The client's words are an important element in qualitative research, but not the only one. As Popay and Williams (1998) indicated, there is a tendency for some researchers to view qualitative research as a "tool box (including focus groups, in-depth interviews, methods for developing consensus, participants' observations) devoid of epistemological salience or theoretical foundation" (p. 33) or a method that does not require an opposing perspective (Green & Britten, 1998).

The studies had smaller problems; only the larger ones have been identified here. In summary, the quantitative studies suffered from problems in design, analysis, and methodological and instrumentation issues, whereas the qualitative studies were limited because of superficial analyses.

Discussion

The foregoing analysis suggests that the research on therapeutic riding published in the *Scientific and Educational Journal of Therapeutic Horseback Riding* is significantly deficient. The situation seems dismal—but is it? In my opinion, it just means we in the therapeutic riding and hippotherapy fields have a long way to go to become strong researchers. Research has to start somewhere, and the research being reported in this journal began only in 1997. It is in its infancy, and other, stronger articles may be appearing in more established journals. Certainly, both the *American Journal of Occupational Therapy* and the *Canadian Journal of Occupational Therapy* have been publishing for at least 40 years. Research methodologies have changed as well: Qualitative research in occupational therapy is fairly new and has been published only since approximately the 1980s.

Two authors were not included in Table 19.1 as research because they did not include collected data, but they do offer guidance.

Buck (2001) pointed out that the most common types of research designs used in quantitative studies include one group pretest–posttest design; pretest–posttest design with control group; single-group repeated-measures and time-series designs; single-case design; and other experimental research designs, such as series of surveys. Although all designs have a contribution to make to quantitative methodology, Buck noted that they all have their limitations. She recommended that researchers be aware of the limitations of the design they are using.

Pauw (1999) stated that when researchers find non-statistically significant results, it often is the result of a small sample size or a nonhomogeneous sample, which decreases the power of the test to detect a clinically meaningful change as statistically significant. She suggested that researchers specify which difference is of importance (clinical or statistically significant) and power the studies to detect true differences so that meaningful changes. Pauw also suggested that larger sample sizes could be used to compensate for the lack of homogeneity.

Moving to qualitative studies, Buck (2001) made several recommendations regarding research for emotional or behavioral disorders when she stated, "To measure variables such as self-concept and behavior requires a degree of subjectivity, even when recognized, standardized assessment is used" (p. 77). Measuring psychosocial variables is not a precise science, she wrote, but requires some subjectivity. According to Buck, qualitative studies lend more flexibility to the researcher and are not limited by the strict parameters of quantitative studies. Moreover, they can rely on the data collected to develop their conclusions and not be constrained by having to begin with a hypothesis to be accepted or rejected.

DePauw (1992) stated, "Therapeutic riding research must now move from reliance upon descriptive and experimental (quasi-) research designs to more naturalistic inquiry using qualitative research paradigms" (p. 44). MacKinnon and colleagues (1995) noted,

> On the one hand, the qualitative results from parents, attending physiotherapist, and riding instructor generated highly positive, endorsing comments. . . . On the other hand, statistical analyses of the quantified measures produced results that suggest the riding program was unsuccessful in demonstrating therapeutic benefits. (p. 28)

MacKinnon and colleagues highlight the difference in results between quantitative and qualitative studies. As Green and Britten (1998) pointed out, personal experience is often characterized as "anecdotal, ungeneralisable, and a poor basis for making a scientific decisions" (p. 1230). They continue, however, by saying that it is often a "more powerful persuader than scientific publication in changing clinical practice" (p. 1230).

For readers who are unfamiliar with principles underlying quantitative and qualitative research, an ongoing conflict exists as to which paradigm can provide the "best evidence." Most writers agree that the two approaches are different and result in different information, for the most part, but they share some commonalties (Barbour, 2000; Green & Britten, 1998; Hammell, 2001; Popay & Williams, 1998). These authors agree both paradigms require rigor.

Quantitative research focuses more on outcomes, whereas qualitative research focuses more on process (Green & Britten, 1998). Quantitative research stresses the generalizabilty of results, whereas qualitative research uses the term *transferability* (Green & Britten, 1998; Popay & Williams, 1998). Sample sizes tend to be larger in quantitative studies, but in qualitative research they tend to be small, although that is not always so (Barbour, 2000; Popay & Williams, 1998). Hypothesis testing is part of the quantitative domain, whereas qualitative research seeks to explore the client's beliefs, values, and meanings (Barbour, 2000; Hammell, 2001; Popay & Williams, 1998).

Quantitative researchers are looking hard data, whereas qualitative researchers are seeking understanding of the meanings behind a phenomenon (Barbour, 2000). Bias is a topic of serious discussion in the quantitative paradigm, whereas subjective immersion into the subject matter is stressed in the qualitative domain.

Quantitative studies are designed to focus on prediction, prevalence, cause and effect, or outcomes, which qualitative studies cannot do (Barbour, 2000). Barbour pointed out that no matter how well designed or how rigorous the study is, the results are not always accepted by the clinical community. In fact, she found that clinicians relied on reinforcement of information from several sources. Hammell (2001) elaborated on this point, stating that often "research is not necessarily useful" (p. 229); she noted that a growing body of knowledge is not clinically relevant and often invalid.

Qualitative studies can examine beliefs of practitioners or clients, attitudes and preferences, and how evidence influences practice (Green & Britten, 1998). Green and Britten went on to say that qualitative research often takes on research questions that experimental methods cannot answer.

Which Paradigm Provides the Best Evidence?

Green and Britten (1998) stated that qualitative methods have the ability to pursue systematically kinds of research that are not easily answered by experimental or quantitative designs. Qualitative research can accomplish the following tasks:

- Bridge the gap between scientific and clinical practice
- Provide rigorous accounts of treatment modalities in everyday contexts
- Help understand barriers to using research results
- Create awareness that different research questions require different kinds of research
- Interpret how clients and practitioners use objective data.

In addition to these benefits, the authors make two important points. First, simply telling people's stories for dramatic effect or other reasons is not qualitative research. Research requires analyses and critical evaluation. Second, good evidence involves more than simply the results of randomized clinical trials.

Popay and Williams (1998) suggested ways in which research using qualitative methods supports quantitative studies to

- Understand why interventions work,
- Improve the accuracy and relevance of quantitative studies,

- Identify important variables to be studied from quantitative studies,
- Explain unexpected results from quantitative studies, and
- Generate hypotheses to be tested by quantitative methods.

Barbour (2000) added that the hallmark of qualitative research is that it acknowledges the importance of the context in which the data are generated and focuses on multiple views. Often it uncovers unintended consequences of service developments. Morse, Swanson, and Kuzel (2001) made a case for qualitative research by pointing out that it is systematic and produces evidence that is relevant to clinical practice. They note that in the 1970s, when the Cochrane collaboration promoted evidence-based medicine, researchers did not use qualitative methods in medicine. *Evidence,* as defined Morse and colleagues, is "art, it's experience, it's intuition, it's history, it's literature, it's many, many things" (p. 3). *Scientific evidence,* according to Upshur (2001) "is a property of data that makes us change our beliefs on how the world is working" (p. 7). The determinants of evidence in health care may arise from either qualitative or quantitative grounds. Excellent evidence, Upshur indicated, is not derived from qualitative or quantitative methods but rather by determining how reasonable it is to apply the results in a particular context. Evidence is only part of what makes a course of action reasonable, and evidence varies with the context. The goal of evidence-based practice is to integrate research with practice.

In summary, determining which paradigm is most useful appears to depend on the evidence and what use one wants to make of it. Being aware of the benefits and the problems of each approach is the best way to determine which method of inquiry to use in any given situation.

Which Paradigm Do Occupational Therapists Support, and Which Is Best for Hippotherapy?

Savin-Baden and Taylor (2001) stated that qualitative research has not yet received global acceptance. Hammell (2001), an occupational therapy researcher, makes several important points about qualitative research as it relates to occupational therapy:

- There is a need to ensure that measurements occupational therapists use are relevant to the client's needs, not just that a score improved, which may not be relevant.

- Occupational therapists need to look beyond muscles and joints to improve the understanding of interplay between impairments and the client's various contexts.
- Occupational therapists hoping to use research to inform client-centered practice must ask research questions that are congruent with that philosophy.
- Qualitative research is helpful in generating new research questions by identifying the limitations or inconsistencies of current knowledge and theory.
- Qualitative inquiry can establish the foundation for subsequent quantitative analyses.
- Therapists should include the client at every step of the research process; occupational therapists who determine their own research agendas and use research methods that exclude the perspectives of the clients will generate evidence that is determined by the therapist's values, assumptions, priorities, and objectives, not the client's.
- Qualitative methods are compatible with client centeredness and therefore enable researchers to identify ways in which intervention and delivery of service can be improved.

Having been primarily a quantitative researcher for more than 20 years, it appears to me that qualitative research has much to offer not only occupational therapy but also hippotherapy in studies that have small numbers, in situations in which context and client perspective are important, and when researchers want to extend the theory base. In addition, it is critical that whatever research in which occupational therapists engage be relevant to practice. Once we have validated our practice more, it can be expanded into areas that may not be as clinically relevant. Occupational therapy cannot afford to stick solely to one methodology; rather, methodologies appropriate to answer the research question should be selected. Hippotherapy is so specialized that qualitative research may be most appropriate to it.

Law and colleagues (n.d.) provide help in the form of a Web site that can be of real benefit to therapists engaging in research. Their materials include a quantitative review form, quantitative review guidelines, a qualitative review form, and qualitative review guidelines. The guidelines are especially useful for any occupational therapy researcher because they provide an overview of critical components for each methodology. If all occupational therapy researchers were to follow those guidelines and review forms, the research in the field of therapeutic riding would develop into a solid body of work.

Acknowledgments

It is with deep gratitude that I acknowledge the assistance of my graduate research assistant, Kathleen Gahagan, who diligently edited numerous versions of this chapter. She found many of the sources for this chapter and copied them for me. Her great care and attentiveness to detail helped greatly.

References

Allori, P., & Pasquinelli, A. (2000). Therapeutic riding as a model of integrated rehabilitation. *Scientific and Educational Journal of Therapeutic Riding, 6,* 46–52.

Auvinet, B. (2001). Medicine and equestrian activities: The paradox of lumbodynia. *Scientific and Educational Journal of Therapeutic Riding, 7,* 44–56.

Barbour, R. S. (2000). The role of qualitative research in broadening the "evidence base" for clinical practice. *Journal of Evaluation in Clinical Practice, 6,* 155–163.

Barrey, J. (1997). The horse and its spaces. *Scientific Journal of Therapeutic Riding, 3,* 31–48.

Basile, R. B. (1997). The psychological effects of equine-facilitated psychotherapy on behavior and self-esteem in children with attention deficit/hyperactivity disorder (ADHD). *Scientific Journal of Therapeutic Riding, 3,* 10–15.

Boon-Thiel, U. (2002). The horse as equine intermediary during the healing process in psycho-motor therapeutic vaulting (PMTV). *Scientific and Educational Journal of Therapeutic Riding, 8,* 31–42.

Brown, O. (1998). Educating future therapeutic riding specialists. *Scientific and Educational Journal of Therapeutic Riding, 4,* 10–17.

Brown, O., & Tebay, J. (1999). Therapeutic riding education: Professional issues. *Scientific and Educational Journal of Therapeutic Riding, 5.*

Buck, W. (2001). Therapeutic riding for children with emotional or behavioral disorders: Recommendations for research. *Scientific and Educational Journal of Therapeutic Riding, 7,* 76–90.

Burgon, H. (2002). Case study of a group of adult users of a mental health team receiving riding therapy. *Scientific and Educational Journal of Therapeutic Riding, 8,* 55–68.

Burja, C., Zadnikar, M., & Lavric, A. (2001). Therapeutic riding in Slovenia: A story of achievement. *Scientific and Educational Journal of Therapeutic Riding, 7,* 15–17.

Claridge, A. (2001). The association of chartered physiotherapists in therapeutic riding. *Scientific and Educational Journal of Therapeutic Riding, 7,* 69–75.

DePauw, K. P. (1992). How does therapeutic riding work? Review of research in therapeutic riding. In B. T. Engel (Ed.), *Therapeutic riding programs instruction and rehabilitation: A handbook for instructors and therapists* (pp. 43–45). Durango, CO: Barbara Engel Therapy Services.

Freire, H. B. G. (2000). Equine therapy as a therapeutic recourse in the treatment of autistic children. *Scientific and Educational Journal of Therapeutic Riding, 6,* 77–82.

Graham, S. (1999). Equine therapy for the adult with multiple sclerosis. *Scientific and Educational Journal of Therapeutic Riding, 5,* 17–43.

Graves, P. (2000). Atlantoaxial instability in people with Down syndrome. *Scientific and Educational Journal of Therapeutic Riding, 6,* 1–8.

Green, J., & Britten, N. (1998). Education and debate: Qualitative and evidence-based medicine. *British Medical Journal, 316,* 1230–1232.

Hammell, K. W. (2001). Using qualitative research to inform the client-centered evidence-based practice of occupational therapy. *British Journal of Occupational Therapy, 64,* 228–234.

Hatton-Hall, C., & Claridge, A. (1998). Volunteer and professional training and qualifications for riding therapists in the UK: Partnership or conflict? *Scientific and Educational Journal of Therapeutic Riding, 4,* 18–32.

Hauser, G. (2003). Systemic counseling with the aid of the horse. *Scientific and Educational Journal of Therapeutic Riding, 9,* 9–16.

Heine, B., & Rosensweig, M. (1998). Use of strain and counterstrain to maximize the benefits of hippotherapy and therapeutic riding. *Scientific and Educational Journal of Therapeutic Riding, 4,* 36–43.

Hornacek, K. (1999). Supposed bioenergy informational processes during therapeutic riding. *Scientific and Educational Journal of Therapeutic Riding, 5,* 58–64.

Ionatamishvili, N., Tsverava, D., & Avaliani, L. (2001). Riding therapy rehabilitation methods of child cerebral palsy. *Scientific and Educational Journal of Therapeutic Riding, 7,* 7–14.

Juguin, J., & Tessiot, C. (2003). Therapeutic horseback riding: An example of use for an adolescent girl with head injury. *Scientific and Educational Journal of Therapeutic Riding, 9,* 28–32.

Klüwer, C. (1997). Presumptions for psychotherapy with the horse. *Scientific and Educational Journal of Therapeutic Riding, 3,* 16–30.

Kreutzer-Brett, S. (2002). A report of one person's experience. *Scientific and Educational Journal of Therapeutic Riding, 8,* 51–54.

Law, M., Stewart, D., Pollock, N., Letts, L., Bosch, J., Westmoreland, M., et al. (n.d.). *Occupational therapy evidence-based practice.* Retrieved December 12, 2004, from http://www.fhs.mcmaster.ca/rehab/ebp/.

Leitao, L. (2003). Psycho-educational riding (PER) and autism: An exploratory study. *Scientific and Educational Journal of Therapeutic Riding, 9,* 33–64.

Longden, M. (1998). Enhancement of self-esteem and affect through changes of perception in spinal cord injured patients: A consideration of key variables. *Scientific and Educational Journal of Therapeutic Riding, 4,* 44–50.

MacKinnon, J. R., & Ferreira, J. R. (2002). The meaning of therapeutic horseback riding for children with cerebral palsy. An exploratory study. *Scientific and Educational Journal of Therapeutic Riding, 8,* 1–15.

MacKinnon, J. R., Noh, S., Lariviere, J., MacPhail, A., Allan, D. E., & Laliberte, D. (1995). A study of therapeutic effects of horseback riding with children with cerebral palsy. *Physical and Occupational Therapy in Pediatrics, 15,* 17–34.

MacKinnon, J. R., & Wong, C. (2002). Goals and performance of children with cerebral palsy participating in therapeutic horseback riding (THR). *Scientific and Educational Journal of Therapeutic Riding, 8,* 16–30.

Mattila-Rautiainen, S. (2000). Biomechanical aspects to study riders' lumbar and spinal area movements in therapeutic riding. *Scientific and Educational Journal of Therapeutic Riding, 6,* 61–76.

Miller, R. (1998a). The senses of the horse. *Scientific and Educational Journal of Therapeutic Riding, 4.*

Miller, R. (1998b). The ten behavioral characteristics unique to the horse. *Scientific and Educational Journal of Therapeutic Riding, 4.*

Miller, R. (1998c). The unique perceptivity of the horse. *Scientific and Educational Journal of Therapeutic Riding, 4,* 64–67.

Miller, R. (1999a). Desensitization to frightening stimuli. *Scientific and Educational Journal of Therapeutic Riding, 5,* 74–77.

Miller, R. (1999b). The horse's response time—A physiological adaptation. *Scientific and Educational Journal of Therapeutic Riding, 5,* 71–73.

Morse, J. M., Swanson, J. M., & Kuzel, A. J. (2001). *The nature of qualitative evidence.* Thousand Oaks, CA: Sage.

Murano, A. C., Allori, P., Pasquinelli, A., & Biagini, B. (2000). Role of the child neuropsychiatrist in the therapeutic riding team. *Scientific and Education Journal of Therapeutic Riding, 6,* 53–60.

Neves, A. (2003). Aspects of the communicative profile of children with special needs referred for hippotherapy. *Scientific and Educational Journal of Therapeutic Riding, 9,* 17–27.

Pasquinelli, A., Allori, P., Mencaroni, M., & DiStefano, M. (2001). Focus on some basic criteria for an objective therapeutic riding evaluation: Application and results in subjects affected by extrapyramidal disorders. *Scientific and Educational Journal of Therapeutic Riding, 7,* 18–37.

Pauw, J. (1999). Data analytical problems experienced in therapeutic riding research and a statistical explanation to some of the problems. *Scientific and Educational Journal of Therapeutic Riding, 5,* 65–70.

Popay, J., & Williams, G. (1998). Qualitative research and evidence-based health care. *Journal of the Royal Society of Medicine, 91*(Suppl. 35), 32–37.

Riffkin, J. (1998). Risk-taking amongst RDA coaches: A proposed study. *Scientific and Educational Journal of Therapeutic Riding, 4,* 33–35.

Rufus, S. (2001). The effects of horse riding therapy on the self-concept of learning disabled children. *Scientific and Educational Journal of Therapeutic Riding, 7,* 57–63.

Savin-Baden, M., & Taylor, C. (2001). Evidence-based practice forum: Conference report: Qualitative evidence-based practice. *American Journal of Occupational Therapy, 55,* 230–232.

Schulz, M. (1999). Remedial and psychomotor aspects of the human movement and its development—A theoretical approach to developmental riding. *Scientific and Educational Journal of Therapeutic Riding, 5,* 44–57.

Silva, C., & Freire, H. B. G. (2001). Equinotherapy for blind children. *Scientific and Educational Journal of Therapeutic Riding, 7,* 38–42.

Solt, J. (2001). From therapy to competition, it is the horse that makes the difference. *Scientific and Educational Journal of Therapeutic Riding, 7,* 64–68.

Upshur, R. E. G. (2001). The status of qualitative research as evidence. In J. M. Morse, J. M. Swanson, & A. J. Kuzel (Eds.), *The nature of qualitative evidence* (pp. 5–26). Thousand Oaks, CA: Sage.

Wiger, N. (2002). Can a short course in adapted vaulting have a positive effect on physically and mentally challenged children? *Scientific and Educational Journal of Therapeutic Riding, 8,* 43–50.

Wiger, N. (2003). Can a short course in adapted vaulting have a positive effect on physically and mentally challenged children? *Scientific and Educational Journal of Therapeutic Riding, 9,* 1–8.

Would, J. (1998). Improved gait in two children with cerebral palsy after hippotherapy: Two case reports. *Scientific and Educational Journal of Therapeutic Riding, 4,* 51–58.

Yack, H. J., Bartels, C., Irlmeier, J., Lehan, A., Voyles, H., Haladay, K., et al. (1997). The effects of therapeutic horseback riding on the quality of balance control in children with attention deficit disorders. *Scientific Journal of Therapeutic Riding, 3,* 3–9.

PART III

Evaluation and Treatment Planning

Man has learned to share the horse's harmonious movements pattern with the horse.
Achieving harmony with the horse is considered the greatest joy,
whether at a quiet walk, a sustained trot, or a speedy gallop.
—Ingrid Strauss, 1991

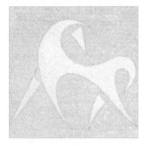

*To practice equestrian art is
to establish a conversation
on a higher level with the horse;
a dialogue of courtesy and finesse.*
—Nuno Oliveira

CHAPTER 20

Treatment Guide: A Tool for Organizing and Documenting a Hippotherapy Session

Roberta S. Devery, MS, OTR/L

Occupational therapy is based on the belief that purposeful activity (i.e., occupation), including its interpersonal and environmental components, may be used to mediate dysfunction and to elicit maximum adaptation (American Occupational Therapy Association [AOTA], 1979). Activity, as used by the occupational therapist, includes both an intrinsic and a therapeutic purpose. Active engagement in a variety of pleasurable and meaningful activities promotes health, well-being, and life satisfaction (AOTA, 2004). The World Health Organization (WHO), in a 1986 paper on health promotion, addressed the needs of elderly, homebound, or otherwise challenged people and reported that without goal-oriented activities to promote physical, cognitive, and emotional well-being, people fall into a state of malaise and eventual dysfunction (WHO, 1986). Occupational therapy serves as a foundation upon which practitioners can design a system of intervention that uses purposeful and meaningful activity to enhance functional performance of our patients in their everyday lives (AOTA, 2002).

Incorporating hippotherapy into occupational therapy practice provides therapists with a unique environment in which to challenge their clients' adaptation skills, sensory processing capabilities, and fundamental movement patterns through meaningful and purposeful activity to maximize their potential for independence. Participating in a hippotherapy program provides clients with opportunities to challenge themselves, gain skills, accomplish goals, and gain self-confidence (American Hippotherapy Association, 1993).

Designing and carrying out a well-organized occupational therapy treatment session incorporating hippotherapy presents many challenges. It is essential that everyone involved in the hippotherapy session be aware of the goals and objectives of the session and how the therapist plans to use the horse's movement to achieve specific outcomes.

The Guide

The working copy of a treatment guide is written out on an index card and reviewed with the support staff (including the instructor, horse handler, volunteer, and, at times, a family member) before each hippotherapy session so all members of the team have an understanding of the goals and objectives the session. The therapist retains the treatment guide for reference. Following the hippotherapy session, the therapist reviews the client's progress and completes a report for the next session. Figures 20.1 and 20.2 illustrate blank and completed treatment guides.

Conclusion

The treatment guide is an effective means of communication and education for everyone involved in a hippotherapy session. Primary care providers gain a better understanding of hippotherapy because the guide clearly states the activity to be done and the therapeutic objective of the activity. Specific hippotherapy activities can be referenced when explaining the importance of positioning, movement patterns, and home programs to augment therapeutic gains. Riding instructors, horse handlers, and volunteers refine their handling and support skills when they review and understand the cause-and-effect relationship of the horse's movement to the desired therapeutic outcome.

Writing out detailed hippotherapy session treatment guides serves many purposes. Of primary importance,

Goal: Objectives:		
Therapeutic Activity	**Clinical Rationale**	**Clinical Observations and Comments**

Figure 20.1. A detailed treatment guide (blank) for an occupational therapy session incorporating hippotherapy.

the treatment guide directs particular activities with specific professionally based therapeutic goals and objectives. When goals and objectives are clearly established and outcomes are measured according to one's professional training, there can be no doubt that a hippotherapy session is occupational therapy rather than physical or speech therapy.

References

American Hippotherapy Association. (1993). *Introduction to hippotherapy: Classic principles and applications. Workshop manual.* Denver, CO: Author.

American Occupational Therapy Association. (1979). Philosophical base of occupational therapy. *American Journal of Occupational Therapy, 33,* 785.

American Occupational Therapy Association. (2002). Occupational therapy practice framework: Domain and process. *American Journal of Occupational Therapy, 56,* 609–639.

American Occupational Therapy Association. (2004). Scope of practice. *American Journal of Occupational Therapy, 58,* 673–677.

World Health Organization. (1986). A discussion document of the principles of health promotion. *Health Promotion, 1,* 73–76.

Goal: Child will develop diagonal reach using dominant right hand.

Objectives: Child will reach for a desired object placed on the left side at waist height in 4 of 5 trials.

Therapeutic Activity	Clinical Rationale	Clinical Observations and Comments
Mounting	Motor planning: Left–right dissociation throughout the body and limbs.	Required maximum hands-on support to mount safely. Placed right hand on wither with emerging trunk rotation.
Walk to the right 3 times around the arena. I often allow the horse to set the comfortable pace in this phase. The horse will often slow down or pick up as the child settles into the seating system (this could be a saddle, bareback pad, or a suede pad built up to help provide pelvic stability).	Acclimate child to movement. Let child become comfortable on the horse. Allow horse's movement to provide rotation into the "system."	Initially very kyphotic. Began to relax and feel the motion on the third pass.
Stand	Give the child a moment to process what he has just experienced.	Grip on handle softened. Shoulders are relaxed. Movement noted in both hips and shoulders.
Touch red targets placed about the arena using dominant right hand. Placement is at waist level when child is mounted.	Provide child with opportunity to develop muscle co-contraction and motor planning to exhibit consistent diagonal approach skills before the complex component of reaching, hand shaping, and grasping are incorporated into the skill.	Initial attempts resulted in a tipping to the left to reach the target. Maximum support at the pelvis was required to keep pelvis from lifting off the seating surface. Following several repetitions, support at pelvis was reduced to moderate, and the child was able to successfully touch the red target in 10 of 10 trials incorporating trunk rotation.

Figure 20.2. A detailed treatment guide for an occupational therapy session incorporating hippotherapy. Notations in the clinical rationale column provide a teaching tool for new staff and volunteers and document the therapeutic value of hippotherapy as a treatment strategy.

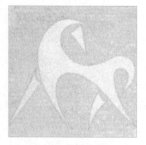

*It is only by rational and calm methods
which are never brutal that the horse may
become obedient and well balanced.*
—Nuno Oliveira

CHAPTER 21

Integrating Hippotherapy Into Mainstream Rehabilitation: The Collaboration of a Private Practice With a Hospital Rehabilitation Center

Marie Dawson, MA, OTR/L, HPCS

Using the movement of a horse as a treatment strategy (hippotherapy) in occupational therapy can improve a client's balance, postural alignment, proximal stability, sensory processing, and much more (Wham, 1992). The environment and purposeful activities that can be incorporated into the occupational therapy sessions offer limitless possibilities for achieving client goals in a natural environment in which client motivation is likely to be high. For hippotherapy to be part of "mainstream" occupational therapy, it must be incorporated into traditional rehabilitation services. Currently in the United States, some occupational therapists are registered with the North American Riding for the Handicapped Association (NARHA), but only a few have taken the American Hippotherapy Association (AHA) exam for a clinical specialty in hippotherapy. Many areas of the United States have no hippotherapy services available.

This chapter explores a model that has expanded occupational therapy services using hippotherapy in the north Atlanta, Georgia, area. In this model, a private occupational therapy practice that specializes in hippotherapy has collaborated with a hospital system. The model may not be able to be exactly replicated in other parts of the country or world, but ideally, this chapter will provide occupational therapists will some ideas on how to expand quality occupational therapy services using hippotherapy.

Program Model

The private occupational therapy practice specializes in pediatric hippotherapy. It employs four occupational therapists and three physical therapists, all of whom are

registered with their respective professional associations and with NARHA, a national nonprofit organization that promotes the benefit of the horse for people with or without physical, emotional, and learning disabilities (NARHA, n.d.). NARHA has developed standards for riding centers and riding instructors, and it maintains a registry for therapists. Two therapists in this private practice are certified hippotherapy–clinical specialists, a designation of occupational therapists, physical therapists, and speech–language pathologists in the United States who have taken an examination to show that they have advanced knowledge and experience in hippotherapy. At a minimum, they have been practicing 3 years in their profession, have 100 hours of hippotherapy practice, and have passed the AHA multiple-choice examination (AHA, n.d.). Approximately 90 occupational therapy and physical therapy sessions using hippotherapy are facilitated each week at one of four NARHA-accredited or NARHA-member centers in the area.

The hospital system with which the private occupational therapy practice is affiliated is one of the country's largest pediatric health care systems: It has two hospitals (totaling 430 licensed beds); an in-client rehabilitation unit; and 10 satellite clinics offering occupational therapy, physical therapy, and speech pathology services.

The private practice has a fee-for-service contract with the hospital system; that is, the private practice provides occupational therapy services using hippotherapy to hospital clients for a fixed fee. The hospital processes the referral, acquires physician prescriptions, verifies insurance, and performs billing. The private practice follows the hospital's guidelines for documentation and all other policies and procedures. The private practice has contracts with NARHA riding centers, which are responsible for following NARHA standards and supply the horses, volunteers, and safe environment.

The occupational therapy private practice's collaboration with a hospital system and NARHA centers has been beneficial for all parties. The client has access to services provided by therapists who specialize in this unique treatment strategy, continues to have all the available services of the hospital, and is more likely to have improved insurance coverage. The private practice has an increased volume of clients, reduced administrative work of processing and billing, the status of being associated with a dynamic hospital setting, and opportunities for clinical collaboration with a variety of specialists in the hospital setting. The hospital system has the opportunity to offer quality hippotherapy services, decreased overhead (private practice is not paid unless the client has been seen), and client and family satisfaction with outcomes. The NARHA center has the opportunity to provide services to a larger number of clients, increased revenue, increased referrals, and the status of association with both the private practice and the hospital system.

The challenges of a private practice collaborating with a hospital system and NARHA centers also are great. Many hours are spent coordinating, scheduling, and communicating to all the participants. The overhead is greater because the cost of maintaining horses and a horse facility are greater than a clinic or home health. Cancellation rates are high in inclement weather. The outcomes, however, are great, and the challenges are worthwhile in light of the many children who benefit from the services.

Conclusion

This model of collaboration is just one possibility. Occupational therapists are encouraged to be creative in developing models that facilitate quality occupational therapy services using hippotherapy to increase the available services for our clients.

References

American Hippotherapy Association. (n.d.). *Hippotherapy clinical specialist (HPCS)*. Retrieved December 15, 2006, from www.americanhippotherapyassociation.org.

North American Riding for the Handicapped Association. (n.d.). *About NARHA*. Retrieved December 15, 2006, from www.narha.org/WhoIsNARHA/About.asp.

Wham, J. (1992). Rhythmic facilitation: A method of treating neuromotor disorders using rhythm and the movement of the horse. In B. T. Engel (Ed.). *Therapeutic riding programs: Instruction and rehabilitation*. Durango, CO: Barbara Engel Therapy Services.

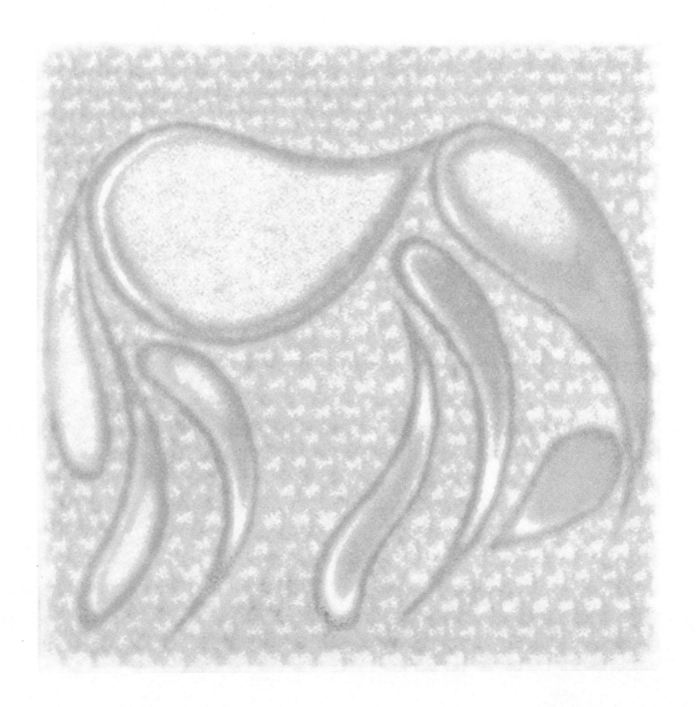

PART IV

Practice Techniques

*What a horse does under compulsion is done without understanding,
and there is not beauty in it either, any more than if one should whip or spur a dancer.*
—*Xenophon*

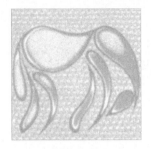

It is through our activities that we are connected with life and with other human [and animal] beings. Through the activities in which we engage, we learn about the world.
— Kenneth Ottenbach

CHAPTER 22

Occupational Activity Analysis Process: A Preparation for Treatment

Barbara T. Engel, MEd, OTR

As the profession of occupational therapy has expanded and grown, it has become more client centered than in the past, and clients are equal partners as the treatment team works together to develop an intervention approach. The person, the environment, and the occupation all must match for therapy to be effective. Therefore, the history of the client, the environment in which the client spends his or her daily life, and the client's interests and occupations must be determined. Additionally, the client's view of occupational therapy, the therapy environment, and the client's goals must be considered. Another important factor to consider in formulating the intervention plan is what the client brings to the occupational therapy session, both assets and impairments. These areas are important in the appropriate selection of activities or tasks to be incorporated in the intervention session. The client needs to understand the value of various options for progressing toward his or her goals, and he or she must be a partner in selecting activities toward these goals. Hippotherapy and equine-assisted occupational therapy offer an unusual assortment of activities, both on and off the horse, to address physical, neurological, cognitive, temporal, and psychosocial problems and to expand the client's skills.

Few people come to occupational therapy with only one problem. Someone with a neurological dysfunction caused by an auto accident also may have cognitive problems and psychosocial problems related to dealing with the change in his or her lifestyle; fortunately, the equine environment can be adapted to meet many different needs, and the practitioner (in conjunction with the client and his or her family) will make decisions to meet the client's occupational therapy goals and needs, including the client's psychosocial issues. For example,

neurological and cognitive dysfunction may be addressed while astride the horse, and the psychosocial issues may be addressed through a bonding and nurturing environment that includes interaction with a horse.

Being able to choose one's activity is an expression of motivation (Christiansen & Baum, 1997), and motivation tends to improve the end result of a task. The equine environment is quite different from the traditional school, clinic, and home environment and tends to present the client with a leisure atmosphere in which intervention can be viewed as pleasurable and as meeting some of the family's social needs (Case-Smith, 2005). Activities and tasks have unique meaning and purpose for each person. Practitioners in the field of hippotherapy can identify the special meaning that riding has for equestrians and have seen the meaningful results and joy that riding brings to occupational therapy clients.

Practitioners must have a well-developed and precise knowledge of activities and tasks because they are the tools of occupational therapy. This chapter discusses activity, task analysis, and occupation, in addition to other major components of the occupational therapy session. Through the analysis of tasks, activities, occupation, and environment, the equine environment and the horse can help the client develop transferable skills for everyday living.

History

The American Occupational Therapy Association was founded in 1917 for the "advancement of occupation as a therapeutic measure" (Nelson, 1996, p. 775). Occupation may include work, play, and leisure; has been associated with healthfulness; and has been recognized as a healing element for both body and mind (Breines, 1995).

Ensuring clients' occupation with purposeful and *meaningful* activities is the historic foundation of occupational therapy practice (Fidler & Velde, 1999). The meaning of any given activity derives from the person pursuing that activity; not all activities are meaningful to all people. A 3-year-old child may find meaning in stacking blocks to make a large tower, but a 58-year-old businessman may find that task to be dull and meaningless, regardless of the practitioner's interpretation of its coordination value.

For a person to be actively involved in an activity, he or she must be manipulating something with purpose. For example, while a client is on a horse, he or she must be involved in some way in the horse's action or movement. Fidler and Fidler (1978) pointed out that purposeful activity is action that is directed toward an expected goal. The ability *to do* and to adapt to the environment involves the integration of a person's internal skill (Baum & Law, 1997). The action in occupational therapy involves the integration of the senses; the primary senses of sight, sound, smell; and the sensorimotor, cognitive, temporal, and psychosocial systems. "In doing, the person has the opportunity to adapt, to gain experience, and to test out one's capacities," wrote Fidler and Fidler (1978, p. 305). Moreover, Fidler and Fidler believed that, through the feedback one receives from interacting with people, animals, the environment, and objects, a person gains an understanding of oneself and one's potential and limitations. This understanding is especially necessary for communication in an environment with meaningful challenges, but in which activities can be graded downward to meet a person's abilities and upward as the person increases his or her skills. For people with recent disabilities and children with developmental disabilities, it is especially important that they gain an understanding of themselves, their role in society, the possibility of developing new skills, their limitations, and the need to develop adaptive approaches to compensate for limitations.

Activity Analysis

Fidler and Velde (1999) postulated that "the purpose of activity analysis is to arrive at an understanding of the activity's inherent qualities and characteristics, its meaning, in and of itself, irrespectively of the performer" (p. 47). The analysis of activities is grounded in the practice of occupational therapy (Fidler & Fidler, 1978). Moyers (2005) stated,

Activity analysis is a process whereby the therapy practitioner determines the performance

demands of the activity by first understanding the activity as a whole and then breaking the activity down into component parts. . . . Occupational therapy practitioners analyze each task in terms of its performance, contextual, temporal, psychological, social, cultural, and meaning dimensions. (p. 224, italics added)

The practitioner and the occupational therapy assistant must have a decisive understanding of the remedial and therapeutic uses of the activities in which their clients will engage (Exhibit 22.1). Activity analysis identifies complex components or parts of activities (Kramer & Hinojosa, 1999). By analyzing activities, the occupational therapy practitioner can determine their value for intervention. Kramer and Hinojosa pointed out that activity analysis, by providing a clear understanding of its tasks and component parts, can help the practitioner teach an activity. Observing how a client reacts and interacts with a task can provide the practitioner with information on how to adapt, grade, or mix tasks (Kramer & Hinojosa, 1999). If, for example, a child does not know how to run-up the stirrups on a saddle, the practitioner can break down the activity into parts: "First, grasp the stirrup iron with the right hand and slide the stirrup iron up the leather toward the saddle. With the left hand, grasp the end of the leather and put it through the stirrup iron, then pull the leather through the iron." As the practitioner observes the client's interaction with the activity, he or she can determine the performance skill that may be missing or is weak. If the client has trouble reaching up, an adaptation can be made by having the child stand on a block so that his or her reach is within the skill limit. Or the practitioner may choose a problem-solving approach by

---

Exhibit 22.1.
Occupational Therapy Intervention Process

- Understand how the activity or task is performed by actual experience.
- Understand the values of activities and their tasks by age and skill groups.
- Understand the client, including his or her history, needs, desires, attributes, and exceptional skills.
- Understand the environment and its influence on the client.
- Understand how intervention influences the life skills and meaning of a client.
- Understand activity analysis in relationship to outcome.

asking the client what one might do so that he or she can reach the saddle. If the problem involves bilateral coordination, the practitioner can then alter the activity or choose different activities to address that problem and not have the client frustrated with a task that he or she does not have the basic skills to do.

Clark and Allen (1985) addressed activity analysis by dissecting the activity itself into three major components: (1) description of the activity, (2) its properties, and (3) performance requirements. Subsections under the three major headings include equipment, techniques, and materials required; steps to perform the tasks; role relationship to occupation; human–object relationship; and functional components necessary to perform the activity. As in the case of adjusting the stirrups, the practitioner must be familiar with the saddle and its parts, the parts of the stirrup, and the reason for adjusting the stirrups, and he or she must have performed this instruction skillfully for both right- and left-handed people.

Watson and Wilson (2003) presented a different perspective on activity analysis. They related activity to occupation and stated that *task analysis* is the process of analyzing the dynamic interaction among a person, his or her environment, and selected tasks (a subset of occupation). Breines (1995) wrote that practitioners should have a large repertoire of activities from which to choose and that it is advisable to obtain experience by performing each activity that they will use with a client, then analyzing the activity's components, therapeutic values, and potential for achieving the desired outcome. In hippotherapy, this approach is not only advisable but necessary for practitioners who are not seasoned equestrians and are unfamiliar with all aspects of the extensive equine environment. Because a large animal is involved, one must understand the field of horsemanship before working with people in hippotherapy and equine-assisted occupational therapy. Many tasks may be second nature to experienced riders, but to a child or a person in a wheelchair, they will appear complicated; therefore, even people who have ridden for many years need to examine components of the activities they will be doing. If a practitioner is to be effective in the field of hippotherapy and equine-assisted therapy, riding and horsemanship skills are essential; it is not enough to have an instructor handle the horsemanship aspects.

Breines (1995) divided activity analysis into three categories:

1. *Egocentric elements* include perception, cognition, motivation, dynamic states, temporality, spirituality, the body, motor components, and sensory components.

2. *Exocentric elements* include objects that can be manipulated, spatial environment, and temporal environment.

3. *Consensual elements* include dyadic relationships, small-group relationships, social interactions, social responsibility, and societal inferences (pp. 29–30).

Each category has 4 to 24 subcategories to guide a person through the complete process of breaking down what a client needs. Breines observed the activity itself, then looked at the skills needed to perform each task making up the activity. Last, she analyzed the communication involved.

This chapter uses Fidler and Velde's (1999) definition of activity analysis and views the analysis of an activity's integral qualities and characteristics separately from analysis of the client. The environment and the interactive components are taken into account later.

An activity analysis allows practitioners to understand the dimensions and impact of an activity and interpret the information so the client can carefully select activities that are appropriate to his or her goals. After the practitioner has performed a full analysis of the chosen activity, he or she must decide whether the process of performing the activity needs modification, whether the activity needs to be modified or adapted, or whether the client can execute the activity as is; such decisions involve task analysis.

Task Analysis

Tasks are combinations of actions that are involved in an activity; they are a piece or unit of an activity, not the activity itself (Velde & Fidler, 2002). By analyzing the tasks involved in the activity, the practitioner can tailor the activity to meet the specific needs of the person and predict the outcome of the intervention without much difficulty. Preparing the horse for riding is an activity; grooming the horse is a task or part of the activity of preparing the horse for riding. It also can be a separate activity for someone whose job only is to groom horses. Grooming might include brushing, washing, and drying the horse, cleaning the hoofs, untangle and braiding the mane, and putting the horse back into his stall.

For example, "Joe" developed a weakness of the right upper extremity after a work-related injury and came to hippotherapy to develop functional use. Grooming the horse from the top of the back to the belly increases range of motion, strength, and coordination of the right upper extremity; therefore, the occupational therapist determined that grooming would help Joe improve his function so that he could perform his self-care skills and return to work. From past experience, the therapist could say that Joe would be able to use his right upper extremity effectively for self-care after 1 month of three-times weekly therapy sessions. In 4 months, Joe will have gained enough strength to return to work. Joe especially likes the horse and enjoys grooming her in a worklike situation, thus increasing his motivation. He therefore puts special effort into the activity of grooming the mare, who responds well to him. This motivation helps the therapy process and affects the recovery of the function of his right arm. Note that Joe finds the activity meaningful, enjoyable, and functional. By separating an activity into tasks, such as currying and brushing, the practitioner can see the dimensions and requirements of one aspect of an activity and, in this way, learn more about the benefits of each task as well as of that activity.

Occupation

The term *occupation* refers to all life activities and tasks that are unique and meaningful (American Occupational Therapy Association [AOTA], 2002) to people across the life span. "[Occupation] is the process of being occupied, being engaged in an activity or doing something meaningful" (Velde & Fidler, 2002). Occupations are the ordinary things people do, including social interaction, play, self-care, education, work, recreation, and leisure activities (Christensen & Baum, 1997).

Occupation and activity are two distinct concepts and are not interchangeable (Fidler & Velde, 1999; Pierce, 2001). A person's history of activities and occupations describes the essence of who that person is. Occupations may consist of many different activities. Not all occupations are necessarily pleasurable, but they contribute to a person's health, maintenance, stability, social status, comfort, and identity (AOTA, 2002). For example, cleaning a horse's stall may be a dreaded chore to a person who has three small children to take care of but a relaxing, pleasurable experience to another after a hard day at a computer job. The occupational therapy practitioner's role is to help direct the client to perform meaningful occupations that, in turn, will affect the client's quality of life, health, and well-being (AOTA, 2002). In the equine setting, for example, the client who has difficulty maintaining focus will be helped by the practitioner to find the right saddle pad, saddle, girth, and bridle. Then the client must recall the order in which the equipment is put on the horse. While on the horse, the client is encouraged to recall the trail course that he or she is to ride. The focus

always remains on the goal to be accomplished, never on the skill of riding.

Nelson (1996) described *therapeutic occupation* as a special form of occupation. He explained that the practitioner develops an occupational synthesis or analytical reasoning "to advance therapeutic assessment or achieve a therapeutic goal" and provide the client with an accurate challenge to achieve the desired goal (Nelson, 1996, p. 777). Nelson reasoned that the occupational synthesis promotes therapeutic occupation. The client learns about him- or herself from the feedback received as he or she interacts with the human, animal, and nonhuman environment.

In the equine setting, the human interaction is provided by the occupational therapy practitioner, the riding instructor, other people, and family. The horses generously provide the animal interaction. Special horses—those who are person oriented—are selected to be therapy partners. Their sensitivity allows them to respond to humans in a unique way (Scanlan, 1998). The horse is a herd animal and will accept a human as a partner, will respond to the human's temperament, and will bond and take care of the rider in unusual situations and ways (Scanlan, 1998).

The nonhuman environment—the farmlike surrounding, the arena, horse tack, stalls, cleaning equipment, and possibly a horse trail through the woods—provides a rich milieu. Feedback from this environment offers opportunities for accomplishments and for accepting or going beyond one's limitations in a way that gives one a sense of worth (Fidler & Fidler, 1978).

The occupational therapy practitioner, working with the client or significant others, selects and uses the environment, the horse, and the activities to develop therapeutic occupation to achieve the client's goals. The client evaluation may include appropriate measurements and observations, but most important is the interview in which the client describes his or her interests, past and present daily activities, and desired goals.

The uniqueness of this nonclinical setting may help motivate the client. For example, a child with cerebral palsy who has had many years of clinic therapy will find this "treatment" setting refreshing and motivating. Motivation can increase a person's participation in activities. Velde and Fidler (2002) stated that motivation is when something known through the senses leads to human behavior and is triggered when agreement occurs between the characteristic of the person and the characteristics of the activity. Moyers (2005) indicated that a person being able to engage in activities of his or her choice, regardless of the impairment or disease, is the ultimate measure of health; thus, providing them a healthy balance of meaningful and nurturing occupations in a stimulating and health environment is important.

Purposeful Activity

Purposeful activities are those that have a special meaning to the person who is interacting with the non-human environment, either alone or with others. Challenges that are meaningful and within the person's skill, ability, and interest levels provide a positive experience. If a client is receiving hippotherapy or equine-assisted occupational therapy, he or she (or the caregiver) has made a selection of their own accord; therefore, the equine activities are more likely than those in a traditional occupational therapy setting to increase motivation and positive results.

Purposeful activities for toddlers mainly involve play, which may mimic parental activities. For children of school age, schoolwork, social interaction with classmates, and home chores make up the bulk of purposeful activities. Luebben, Hinojosa, and Kramer (1999) commented that children's activities focus on sensorimotor play, constructional play, imaginary play, social play, and exploratory play. In the equine setting, the practitioner can provide age-appropriate play activities both on and off the horse, and those activities can be initiated by the child in purposeful play. Most children love horses, and horses respond well to them. To be involved with horses brings joy to their lives.

"Jean" found purpose in her occupational therapy. She grew up on the family cattle ranch in the Dakotas, where she learned to ride as a young child. She continued to run the cattle ranch and ride until, in her 40s, she left for Africa to be a Vista Volunteer. There, she contracted a viral disease that caused partial paralysis involving her entire body. After basic rehabilitation in a primary hospital, she chose to complete her rehabilitation through hippotherapy. Jean loved horses and was comfortable with them. Her level of ability allowed her to sit on the horse, but with marginal balance and strength. The occupational therapy practitioner explained that Jean would be carefully monitored in her ability to maintain her balance and to stay safe and that she should say when she began to feel tired.

This method was chosen over giving her direct occupational support to encourage Jean to develop a sense of inner self. She was closely monitored by the spotters, who were close by. The horse chosen for intervention had the ability to sense his rider's level of ability and could determine when the rider was getting tired by her moving less and feeling heavier or unbalanced. The goal for Jean at first was to increase balance, strength, and awareness of her skills. As she improved in those areas, basic riding skills were added to increase her ability to control her body and increase coordination and cognition. The horse sensed her increased ability and slowly demanded more from her.

Therapy focused not on Jean's ability to ride but on regaining skills in an environment that was familiar to Jean. The activity gave Jean a sense of self-esteem and a feeling of total involvement in her therapy. She felt good to be back on a horse independently. Hippotherapy addressed physical, cognitive, sensory, coordination, and psychosocial skills. When the challenge became too great, Jean would say that she was tired, the horse would slow down, or the practitioner would note that Jean was beginning to slump; at that point, therapy would stop for the day. Jean's therapy was a collaborative experience among her, the occupational therapy practitioner, the horse, and spotters in a comfortable environment that brought positive results and enjoyment.

Occupational Performance Used During Treatment

To create a match between activity and person, the practitioner uses activity analysis and synthesis, as described by Nelson (1996). People come to occupational therapy with a variety of limitations. Some are temporary, in which case occupational therapy will focus on recovery. Clients who have permanent limitations generally have goals of improvement, adaptation, and development of new skills that lead to decreased dependency and independent lives and job opportunities. Practitioners must ask (and answer) the following questions, among others, to properly match the person, environment, and occupation:

- What assessment and problem re-education will be necessary?
- What frame of reference is most suitable to this client's problem?
- How can this frame of reference be used in practice?
- What movements are required by the client to perform the activity, and what movement does he or she require?
- What cognitive, coordination, and sensory components shall be developed?
- How much sensory input is needed to perform the chosen activity?
- Can the activity be subdivided into tasks that can be adapted, graded, or sequenced to meet the client's ability?

- Are the chosen activities appropriate for the age and gender of the client?
- How can the horse be used to provide necessary input?
- What horse-related activities will provide needed stimuli?
- Is there evidence to support this intervention?

The client's positive perception of this unique non-clinical setting may help him or her become comfortable with the horse and the equine environment, thereby increasing motivation to participate in the activities available. Moyers (2005) made the point that the uniqueness of occupational therapy is that the practitioner understands all aspects of occupational performance and that this understanding helps the client engage in sought after and healthful occupations within his or her environment.

Occupational practitioners "are concerned with both observable aspects of performance as well as the more subjective aspects of performance" (Moyers, 2005, p. 222). Information from and perceptions of other professionals that have had contact with the client are of great value and should be sought.

To begin the process of planning an occupational therapy intervention for a client, the practitioner must first have a definitive understanding of every activity that is available in the therapy setting (i.e., an activity analysis). Fidler and Velde (1999) said that the intent of an activity analysis is to reason out and understand the activity's inherent qualities and characteristics, its meaning separate from the person who may perform the activity. Breaking the activity into tasks gives the practitioner a closer look at its components. Moreover, an activity is viewed as encompassing form, structure, and action. In addition, properties, outcomes, and realistic and symbolic meanings and inferences are within each of the five elements and in the total activity (Fidler & Velde, 1999).

By making an accurate and conclusive activity analysis, the practitioner must identify each task within the activity and recognize its value for meeting therapeutic needs. The activity may need to be adapted to benefit the client's level of function in the areas of cognition, physical and sensory ability, and interests.

For instance, riding a horse is an activity that can be divided into two parts: the preparation of the horse for riding and riding astride the horse. The preparation of the horse involves many tasks, including finding the horse; putting on its halter; leading it to the tie-rack, where it is groomed, saddled, and bridled; then taking it to the mounting block. The riding activity involves the rider mounting the horse and performing riding skills as directed. Riding skills can be broken down into the tasks that are required to become a beginning or skillful rider. During a therapy session, a rider can be involved in tasks that involve sensorimotor, perceptual, cognitive, or psychosocial objectives.

This process requires the practitioner to have a full understanding of the activity, which is gained by riding the horse and learning its conformation, way of going, communication methods, mannerisms, and method of obtaining its submission to people riding or handling it. Activities off the horse also must be analyzed, because some may involve the horse, whereas others will involve barn and arena management skills and games.

Client Involvement in Therapy

How does an activity analysis relate to the treatment and needs of a client? "Ally," a woman in her late 40s, is receiving hippotherapy from a team of practitioners. The physical therapist is on the left side using a hands-on approach of neurodevelopmental treatment to encourage body alignment, and the occupational therapist sidewalks on the right side to provide support for balance and solicit cognitive reactions from Ally. The speech pathologist observes the session and waits to work with Ally as she becomes more active. The riding instructor is leading the horse, who appears subdued. Ally is sitting on the horse slouched forward, is nonverbal, and appears withdrawn. She shows no response to the practitioner's intervention or to the people around her. What is wrong? The problem appears to be one of a person who is disconnected with the therapy session. Is she depressed, or is she uninterested? Little progress in any area is likely to occur unless the client can become alert and involved. Moreover, sitting slouched forward on the horse causes the horse's weight to be on his forehand (front) and prohibits rhythmic forward motion.

Had an additional interview occurred before beginning treatment, in addition to the normal evaluation process, the client would have understood why she was on the horse. She would have participated in the choice of activity and would be a full member of the treatment team. An activity analysis would have given Ally an understanding of what was to be gained in this type of therapy, and she would be able to cooperate with her desired goals.

One of the therapists suggested that the client become involved in the session by having the riding instructor take charge. He gave Ally the reins and asked her to ask the horse to move forward. He gave Ally some basic riding instructions, and she seemed to listen to him. She took the reins and asked the horse to walk on. As she moved the horse forward, she became more alert, sat up, and moved a little with the horse. The horse picked up his pace because the heavy weight of Ally on his back began to shift and became lighter, allowing him to become active. Ally began to talk, and the speech pathologist could work with her. The physical therapist provided verbal input to Ally with limited hands-on assistance to help her strengthen her weaker side, and the occupational therapy practitioner gave Ally an obstacle course to guide the horse around. Ally is now an active part of the therapy session, and the whole picture has changed. The practitioners can interact with her, and she has become a motivated participant in her therapy. She appears to enjoy what she is doing; the activity and approach have become person-centered, making Ally a true partner in *her therapy*.

This vignette demonstrates the need for the client to understand the activity and why it is being used by the practitioner. Moreover, the client's history, needs, interests, motivations, and involvement in treatment need to be understood. By understanding the client and her needs, therapy time will not be wasted figuring out what method to use for intervention or applying techniques that will not show effective results.

References

American Occupational Therapy Association. (2002). Occupational therapy practice framework: Domain and process. *American Journal of Occupational Therapy, 56,* 609–639.

Baum, C. M., & Law, M. (1997). Occupational therapy practice: Focusing on occupational therapy performance. *American Journal of Occupational Therapy, 51,* 277–288.

Breines, E. B. (1995). *Occupational therapy activities from clay to computers: Theory and practice.* Philadelphia: F. A. Davis.

Case-Smith, J. (2005). *Occupational therapy for children* (5th ed.). St. Louis, MO: Elsevier Mosby.

Christiansen, C., & Baum, C. (Eds). (1997). *Occupational therapy: Enabling function and well-being* (2nd ed.). Thorofare, NJ: Slack.

Clark, P. N., & Allen, A. S. (1985). *Occupational therapy for children.* St. Louis, MO: C. V. Mosby.

Fidler, J. W., & Fidler, G. S. (1978). Doing and becoming: Purposeful action and self-actualization. *American Journal of Occupational Therapy, 32,* 305–310.

Fidler, G. S., & Velde, B. P. (1999). *Activities, reality and symbol.* Thorofare, NJ: Slack.

Kramer, P., & Hinojosa, J. (1999). *Frame of reference for pediatric occupational therapy* (2nd ed.). Philadelphia: Lippincott Williams & Wilkins.

Luebben, A. J., Hinojosa, J., & Kramer, P. (1999). In P. Kramer and A. J. Hinojosa (Eds.), *Frame of reference for pediatric occupational therapy* (2nd ed.). Philadelphia: Lippincott Williams & Wilkins.

Moyers, P. (2005). Introduction to occupation-based practice. In C. Christiansen & C. Baum (Eds.), *Occupational therapy performance, participation, and well-being* (3rd ed., pp. 220–241). Thorofare, NJ: Slack.

Nelson, D. L. (1996). Therapeutic occupation: A definition. *American Journal of Occupational Therapy, 50,* 775–778.

Pierce, D. (2001). Untangling occupation and activities. *American Journal of Occupational Therapy, 55,* 138–146.

Scanlan, L. (1998). *Wild about horses.* New York: HarperCollins.

Velde, B., & Fidler, G. S. (2002). *Lifestyle performance.* Thorofare, NJ: Slack.

Watson, D. E., & Wilson, S. A. (2003). *Task analysis: An individual and population approach* (2nd ed.). Bethesda, MD: AOTA Press.

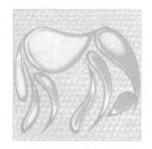

*Contact with the horse is the most important
basic requirement for making learning possible.
A good inner direct line to the horse
dismantles fear and creates...mutual trust.*
—Susanne von Dietz

CHAPTER 23

Treatment of Hypotonia

Colleen M. Zanin, MS, OTR

For years now, we have witnessed the results of the horse's three-dimensional movement and its effect on relaxing spastic or hypertonic muscles. Typically, we can observe a rider with restricted movement in the pelvis or legs struggle to abduct the legs to straddle the horse. Almost magically, the rider sits upright and astride after 15 to 20 minutes of sensory input supplied through the horse's back muscles. Along with the improvement noted in the rider's balance, this relaxation of muscle tone, particularly noted in the lower extremities, has helped to put the horse in the same arena as the therapy ball or bolster as an aid in the treatment of children with movement disorders resulting from central nervous system damage or dysfunction.

This chapter discusses another aspect of neuro-motor disorders: *hypotonia*, or low muscle tone—the flip side of hypertonus. Because the characteristics of hypotonia often are less obvious than hypertonus, they frequently are overlooked. As occupational therapists with expanding caseloads of children with Asperger syndrome, Down syndrome, fragile X syndrome, and a host of developmental disabilities, it is important to be aware of the impact of the horse's movement and the child's position on the horse when treating low muscle tone, which is often associated with these diagnoses.

Definition of Hypotonus

The term *hypotonus* is frequently misused or used interchangeably with words such as *flaccidity, flaccid paralysis, paresis,* or *weakness.* This chapter uses the term according to the definition given by Carr and Shepherd (1980), who described hypotonus as "decreased postural or muscle tone caused by a lesion or lesions in a part of the brain which results in difficulty or inability to move, to sustain a posture against gravity, or to support functional movement (p. 170)." Hypotonus is not

the result of injury to the spinal cord resulting in paraplegia or quadriplegia and is sometimes confused with weakness (Kramer & Hinojosa, 1999). The quality of the muscle tone is associated with postural limpness or a feeling of heaviness when the limb is moved passively by the clinician. Definite head lag occurs when the head is lifted against gravity (Boehme, 1987). Hypotonia frequently is seen in diagnoses such as athetoid or ataxic cerebral palsy, Down syndrome, and various developmental disorders. Ayres's (1972) early research in sensory integration stressed the importance of the vestibular system and the effects of this system on the function of the muscle spindle and the centrality of its role in maintaining muscle tone. Ayres stated,

> A number of children with sensory integrative deficits have reduced muscle tone, a condition which may hold considerable significance. . . . The brain of a hypotonic child is receiving less sensory input than it would if tone were normal. (p. 85)

Characteristics of the Hypotonic Child

The hypotonic child may have difficulty interacting with the environment because of a limited ability to maintain a secure posture. The limbs and trunk appear to sink into gravity. The child lacks joint stability, particularly in the proximal musculature and throughout the midline, which limits dynamic postural stability or graded movement. Hypotonic children may appear passive or unmotivated to move (Boehme, 1987). The lack of movement is likely due to the amount of energy that they must expend to move their heavy, limp limbs. The child has difficulty with shifting weight and has an inability to bear weight through the limbs in normal alignment (Bobath, 1980). Because of decreased sensory awareness, the hypotonic child or adult usually has a high threshold for pain and decreased perception of body awareness (Boehme, 1989). Endurance for anti-gravity activities is usually poor, and coordination may be impaired due to poor sensory feedback. Postural insecurity or fear of movement also may be seen in children with hypotonia (Bundy, Lane, & Murray, 2002). Respiration often is shallow and noisy and may not be sufficient to support the development of vocalizations and functional communication. Weak oral–motor musculature may be seen, resulting in drooling and poor sucking and chewing patterns.

Treatment of the Child With Hypotonia

The treatment of the child with hypotonia is based on the principles of neurodevelopmental treatment, an approach developed by the late Karl and Berta Bobath (Bobath, 1980), and the principles of sensory integration developed by A. Jean Ayres (Bundy et al., 2002). Several techniques are used to gain joint stability and to improve the quality of the movement patterns:

- Weight-bearing or joint compression is used to increase joint co-activation and improve proximal stability.
- The facilitation of weight shift and balance reactions is stressed during the treatment to improve movement transitions.
- Proper biomechanical alignment of the joints is monitored and facilitated. Training the child to place and hold a limb against gravity is encouraged to promote strength and joint stability.
- Application of external sensory input, such as tapping or vibration, may be used to help activate the muscles.
- Graded movement and vestibular stimulation are provided to increase level of alertness and motivation.

In addition to these therapeutic techniques, the therapist's use of speech is important. Frequently, the correct phrase to trigger a motor response must be found. A child may not respond to a request when it is phrased one way but may respond when it is phrased differently. For example, "push" may not get a response, but "reach toward the sky" may get the desired reaction. The child may want to use his or her own speech while doing a movement. This often is an effective way to reinforce movement because it helps the rider concentrate and regulate the movement through auditory feedback. Specific oral–motor activities (e.g., blowing bubbles, using whistles, articulation drills) may be included in the treatment session and can set the stage for a well-integrated co-treatment session with a speech–language pathologist.

Visual stimulation is an effective teaching tool. The child can be encouraged to look at the part of the body he or she is trying to move. A mirror can give the rider an opportunity to "check" his own posture and to provide a visual picture of what correct postural alignment in the saddle looks and feels like. The child can stand in his stirrups, play Simon Says, or perform exercises while visually monitoring his own position. This feedback helps the child concentrate his or her attention on movements of the limbs and reinforces kinesthetic awareness. Incorporating games and activities on the horse that use weighted toys, vibrating toys, and objects can be an effective way to increase proprioceptive input and tactile stimulation. Such activities also provide opportunities for language development and motor planning.

The beautiful and athletic conformation of a therapy horse has firm muscles and gentle contours, enveloped by a warm soft coat; the horse provides a dynamic treatment environment for enhancing weight-bearing activities, graded joint compression, and improved equilibrium reactions. The free-moving walk can be slowed for riders who cannot tolerate too much movement. A slight jog can be incorporated for those needing short bursts of intermittent activity or for longer periods of time for those who are demonstrating increased postural control. Changes of direction, school figures, halts, half-halts, and walks all can be used by a skilled occupational therapist to challenge postural alignment and balance.

Throughout the treatment session, the occupational therapist uses ongoing clinical assessments of the child to monitor and facilitate proper biomechanical alignment of the joints to prepare the child for a functional task. In his book, *Physiotherapy on the Horse,* Riede (1986/1988) stressed the importance of pelvic alignment when addressing postural dysfunction. Depending on the postural control of the child, a variety of exercises can be incorporated into the treatment session. The following exercises are initiated with the child positioned astride the horse in the typical balanced seat facing forward:

- Start all exercises with the "ideal sitting posture" on the horse: The pelvis is in an upright position, the heels are pointed downward, and the abdominal and gluteal muscles are tightened.
- The neck is lengthened through an "occipital lift." While this posture is maintained, a straightening of the thoracic spine occurs during maximum exhalation (Riede, 1986/1988, p. 102).
- From the ideal sitting posture on the horse, the child leans forward and strokes or pats the horse without losing pelvic correction and occipital lift (Riede, 1986/1988).

- At the walk, the child learns to accommodate to the rhythm of the horse's movements without losing correct pelvic alignment of thoracic extension.
- Gradually encourage the child to let go of any hand holds and prop hands on the withers of the horse; eventually encourage him or her to rest his or her hands on his or her thighs while maintaining postural control (Riede, 1986/1988).
- Facilitate weight shift and balance reactions through straight and curved lines. Reposition hands so that the inside hand is forward and the outside hand is backward during weight shift activities to the inside (Riede, 1986/1988).
- Continue training of equilibrium reactions through alternating halt and walking activities over varied terrain.
- As the child's posture and balance become more stable, activities can progress to trunk rotation while propping one hand on the croup, arm- and leg-swinging activities, and the use of the sidesaddle.

As the occupational therapist assesses the hippotherapy milieu, he or she draws on his or her knowledge of occupational science by analyzing the environment, the activity, and the physical and social–emotional needs of the child to establish treatment goals and intervention priorities. The trained therapist will determine whether a saddle with a deep seat will provide a more secure base of support and whether stirrups are to be incorporated for weight-bearing activities. Conversely, the child may require active handling and supportive positioning, in which case a pad and surcingle may be the equipment of choice. Depending on the child's needs, the therapist may want to introduce pre-riding activities (e.g., grooming the horse, lifting the saddle onto the horse's back, using barn tools to sweep the floor and remove the manure).

The farm setting is ripe with natural therapeutic activities that can be individualized for children with low muscle tone. It is the occupational therapist's responsibility to capitalize on the assets of this environment to optimize the results of intervention.

Precautions for the Child With Hypotonia

The child with hypotonia may have more subtle movement problems than the child with hypertonicity, but he or she is just as much at risk for improper handling while on the horse. Unlike the hypertonic child or adult who has a limited range of motion because of restrictions in muscles range, the hypotonic child or adult is "hypermobile" and has an excessive range of limb excursions because the person lacks ligament, muscle, and tissue resistance toward extreme movement ranges. According to Boehme (1987), repetitive use of positions in this extreme movement range may cause immobility in the opposing joint range. For example, consistent use of the hip abduction, flexion, and external rotation (the riding position) may create a lack of joint range into hip adduction, extension, and internal rotation. Hip dislocation also may occur when this position is used excessively or when hip ligaments are excessively weak (Boehme, 1987). Scoliosis may result from postural asymmetries and the effects of gravity on the low-tone trunk (Scherzer & Tscharnuter, 1990).

A good clinical eye for normal movement and proper alignment on and off the horse is important. To provide a safe and effective therapeutic ride, immediate alterations of improper alignment are vital when abnormalities are observed. Finally, selecting the appropriate therapy horse is of paramount importance. Because the hypotonic child has ample range in abduction, it may be tempting to put him on a nice round pony. Doing so, however, may affect the integrity of the hips and the proper position of the pelvis. A therapy mount with an active walk may be good for a child with mildly low tone but may tax the stability and the endurance of the child with severe hypotonicity. Children with cerebral palsy may have mixed tone (high-tone extremities, low-tone trunk, and poor head control). Those riders must be carefully evaluated to determine if they have sufficient postural tone and head and neck stability to tolerate the repetitive undulations created by the horse's back. Adaptive equipment and alternative positions may be used if it is determined that the rider is a candidate for using the horse as an occupational therapy strategy. A shortened treatment time on the horse should be used so that the child has enough endurance to participate in activities off the horse as well.

Conclusion

Occupational therapists who choose to incorporate hippotherapy into their treatment for children with hypotonia have a brave new world opened up to them. The unique use of the horse and its "home environment" is gaining popularity because of the results that have been achieved. Continued research in the field is needed to validate hippotherapy's efficacy, and careful controls and standards must be maintained to ensure that quality and safety are never compromised.

Although hippotherapy has been used in the United States only since the 1980s, the motivating and functional use of the horse in medicine has been known for centuries. According to Riede (1986/1988), Tussot (a famous French physician in the 1700s) viewed rehabilitation in the following way:

> In all cases of therapeutic exercise one should choose, as much as possible, the method that the patient likes best. Then it can lift his spirits as soon as he sets his body in motion. According to Plato "the union of body and soul does not permit the body to function without the soul nor the soul without the body." (p. 44)

It is that spirit-lifting movement and charisma of the horse that keeps our children coming back. We owe it to them to do it right!

References

Ayres, A. J. (1972). *Sensory integration and learning disorders.* Los Angeles: Western Psychological Services.

Bobath, K. (1980). *A neurophysiological basis for the treatment of cerebral palsy.* London: William Heinemann Books.

Boehme, R. (1987). *The hypotonic child: Treatment of postural control, endurance, strength, and sensory organization.* Milwaukee, WI: Boehme Workshop.

Bundy, A., Lane, S., & Murray, E. (2002). *Sensory integration theory and practice* (2nd ed.). Philadelphia: F. A. Davis.

Carr, J., & Shepherd, R. D. (1980). *Physiotherapy in disorders of the brain.* London: William Heinemann Books.

Kramer, P., & Hinojosa, J. (1999). *Frames of reference for pediatric occupational therapy.* Philadelphia: Lippincott Williams & Wilkins.

Riede, D. (1988). *Physiotherapy on the horse* (P. A. Dusenbury, Trans.). Riderwood, MD: Therapeutic Riding Services. (Original work published 1986)

Scherzer, A., & Tscharnuter, I. (1990). *Early diagnoses and therapy in cerebral palsy: A primer on infant developmental problems* (2nd ed.). New York: Marcel Dekker.

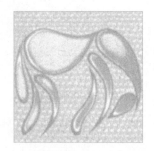

Only the teacher who has himself mastered what he is teaching will know better and never ask more of his pupil than he is able to do.
— *Alois Podhajsky*

CHAPTER 24

Developmental Sequence on Horseback

Colleen M. Zanin, MS, OTR

The term *developmental sequence* is commonly accepted as describing the typical sensorimotor progression of development in the first few years of life. *Neuromotor development* is concerned with this maturation of the nervous system and the parallel acquisition of control over the muscular system (Banus, Kent, Norton, & Sukiennicki, 1979). Four principles govern "anatomical directions of development." First, maturation begins in the head region and proceeds toward the feet (the cephalocaudal direction). Control of the joints closest to the central axis of the body occurs before control of the joints farther away from the body (proximal joints develop before distal joints; the shoulder joints develop before hand control). Maturation proceeds from the front surfaces of the body to the back (ventral to dorsal). Finally, control spreads from near the midline in the anatomical position outward, or in the ulnar to radial directions (Banus et al, 1979). Neuromotor maturation can be regarded as the acquisition of postural control against gravity and balance, which seems to follow a definite sequence relative to the planes of the body (e.g., sagittal, frontal, transverse; Scherzer & Tscharnuter, 1990). These stages of neuromotor development generally occur in a smooth and overlapping fashion.

As control over the muscular system is achieved, different postures emerge (e.g., front lying, back lying, sitting, crawling, standing, walking). Again, the anatomical direction of development is repeated in each positional level. In abnormal development (as in a child with cerebral palsy), the sequential development of postural control is arrested at the initial phase. Therefore, the smooth transition between stages of development is interrupted, and faulty movement patterns emerge that prevent control over the muscular system (Conolly & Montgomery, 1987).

Developmental Sequence on Horseback

Just as the traditional treatment of clients with movement dysfunctions has been strongly influenced by the work of the Bobaths (Bobath, 1978), the emerging field of equine-assisted therapy also draws from the treatment principles of the Bobaths' Neurodevelopmental Treatment. The scope of this chapter is not to compare the use of these techniques in the clinic to their applicability on the horse; it is to discuss how the use of developmental positioning and handling on the horse can be an effective form of assessment of and treatment for clients with movement dysfunction.

Throughout the years, several misunderstandings have arisen regarding the use of developmental positions on horseback. Occasionally, these positions are used as a "cookbook approach," and each rider is routinely moved in and out of the designated positions with limited regard to purpose, quality, or individual treatment goal. Beth Stanford, Barbara Glasow, and Jan Spink stressed in early seminars the need for an experienced therapist to assess and direct treatment for the client. This principle is reinforced today through the development of the *Hippotherapy Competency Guidelines* (Tebay & Rowley, 1990).

The goals of therapy on horseback are the same as accepted neurodevelopmental techniques used by physical and occupational therapists: reduction of spasticity; reduction of postural compensations; and subsequent facilitation of normal movement skills, such as improved posture, balance, trunk control, weight shift, rotation through the body axis, and dissociation at the shoulders and pelvis (Bertoti, 1988). The use of developmental positions, coupled with the movement provided by the horse and the *graded* handling by the therapist, helps achieve these goals.

Reprinted by permission of Barbara J. Engel from *Therapeutic Riding II: Strategies for Rehabilitation.*

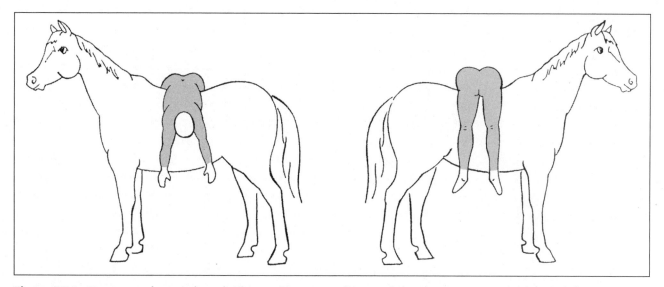

Figure 24.1. Prone over horse's barrel. This position normalizes and develops extensor control (mobility).

Client Lying Prone Over the Horse's Barrel

Lying prone over the horse's barrel may be uncomfortable for the client, and the position therefore should be used sparingly (Figure 24.1). The speed of the horse's walk and the length of stride should be carefully monitored. As long as the client is not experiencing discomfort, this position provides the therapist with an opportunity to mobilize the client's pelvis and scapulae, improve symmetry throughout the body, and promote generalized relaxation throughout the trunk and pelvis. Specific techniques of sensory stimulation, such as approximation, tapping, and vibration, can be incorporated into treatment, but they need to be applied with good judgment. All techniques should be familiar to the horse before using them with the client on the horse (Scherzer & Tscharnuter, 1982). The unique demands of the client, coupled with the skills of the therapist, will determine the precise use of intervention techniques.

Precautions

The prone position can cause dizziness in some clients as a result of the strong vestibular stimulation while the horse is walking. This position should be used only as a preparation for function at a higher level (moving from developmental sequential position to one requiring more maturity). Be aware of riders with a shunt, stomach tubes, or ileostomies, and use experienced sidewalkers, because clients have a tendency to slip in this position.

Client Lying Prone Over the Horse's Back and Sitting Backward on the Horse

The prone position over the horse's back is usually more comfortable for the client and provides greater opportunity to incorporate relaxation techniques to reduce spasticity (Figure 24.2). This position also can be used to improve symmetry and upper-extremity weight bearing in bilateral and unilateral prone positions (Figure 24.3). Improved trunk control and abdominal and extensor strength may be achieved by facilitating control of upper-body flexion and extension, lateral righting, and rotation through the body axis (Figure 24.4). The position of the client's legs around the horse's barrel promotes abduction and external rotation; also, a strong hamstring stretch frequently occurs in this position. When the

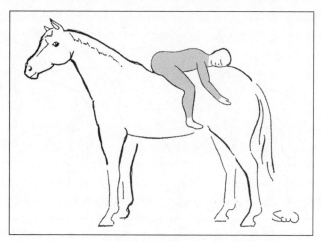

Figure 24.2. Prone on the horse's back. This position increases muscle relaxation and decreases spasticity.

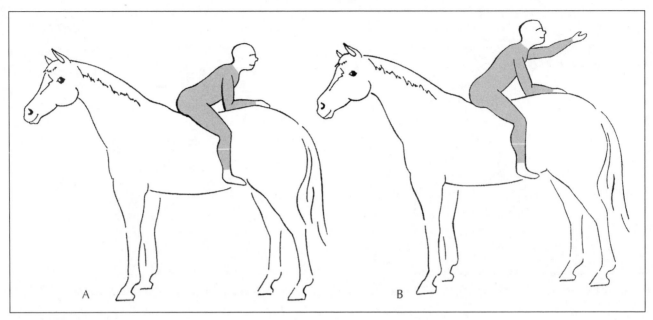

Figure 24.3. A. Symmetrical bilateral weight bearing on elbows. B. Unilateral weight bearing on elbow reaching with weight-bearing arm.

client can transition to an upright sitting position (Figure 24.4B) while facing backward, trunk extension and a neutral pelvis can be facilitated. By regulating the speed, length of stride, transitions, and direction of the horse, this dynamic treatment surface provides the opportunity to facilitate weight shift, proximal co-contraction, and equilibrium reactions (Figure 24.4A). As in all therapy sessions, good biomechanical alignment of the client, symmetry, and the reduction of compensatory movements or postures are emphasized. Occasionally, therapists prefer to ride with the client to achieve greater facilitation of normal movement.

Precautions

Some horses impart a strong anterior–posterior movement to the backward-facing client. In such cases, constant vigilance of the client's head and neck control is required. Some clients fatigue rapidly in this position, and some complain of disorientation from decreased visual input.

Client Lying Supine on Horse's Back

Like the prone position, the supine position on horseback may cause discomfort to the client (Figure 24.5),

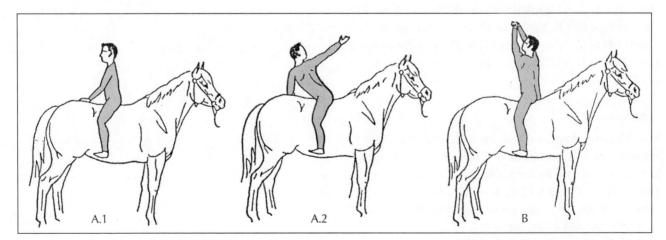

Figure 24.4. A. Sitting backward, (1) symmetrical and (2) asymmetrical. Backward positions naturally facilitate trunk extension and a neutral pelvis and are useful for riders with posterior tilt and a round back. B. Sitting backward can facilitate trunk extension and a neutral pelvis.

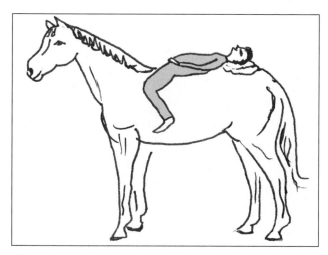

Figure 24.5. Supine position.

and proper handling and positioning are extremely important, particularly in the client's lumbar region. A pillow under the head may help reduce the strain on the back in this position. Horse selection is crucial when using this position. When the supine position is used effectively, the therapist can focus on elongation techniques for the neck and trunk, active and passive stretching of upper and lower extremities, shoulder–pelvis dissociation, and abdominal-strengthening activities. In preparation for riding astride, the client can lie supine over the horse's back with legs straddling the horse.

Activities to promote neck elongation and head control may be used in this position with extreme care. Many therapists prefer to assess the effect of this position on the client while the horse is standing still and gradually incorporate movement. A scrutinizing eye and keen observation skills are paramount to discern when the client is becoming overstressed or when the position is not therapeutic.

Precautions

Occasionally, the client becomes fearful in this position because of feelings of vulnerability and the strong effect of gravity. Specific treatment goals may be more readily achieved in other positions. A small pillow can be used under the head to decrease the hyperextension of the neck. Monitor the helmet fit carefully when in this position because the helmet has a tendency to slip. The client's legs should be supported, and his or her lower back should be monitored to avoid strain.

Client Sitting Facing Forward

This position is more difficult for many clients because the base of support and weight-bearing surface is narrower than the other positions (yet, it is more normal and easier to integrate for vestibular and visual input; Figure 24.6). As with all positions, it is the therapist's role to analyze the client's response to the horse and direct its movement (Heipertz, 1984). Treatment goals of improving the client's posture, balance, mobility, and function are continually emphasized in this position. Direct intervention by the therapist through "back-riding" techniques is most readily used with this position (Glasow, 1984). This position also is used in "classic hippotherapy" to emphasize the influences of the horse on the client. A well-trained dressage horse and a knowledgeable horse trainer with expertise in long-reining will provide the client with a variety of tactile, proprioceptive, and vestibular inputs by performing school figures on one or two tracks.

High-Level Developmental Sequences

The use of quadruped, kneeling, and standing positions in hippotherapy are similar to some of the exercises used in sports vaulting, such as flag, free kneel, and stand (Figures 24.7–24.9; Friedlaender; 1970). Because of the extreme demands on the client's balance, postural control, proximal stability, and motor

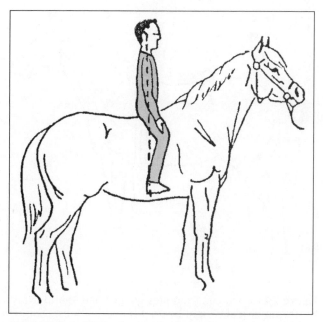

Figure 24.6. Sitting forward. This position is more difficult because the rider is sitting on a narrower base, and the horse's neck is a narrow base on which to bear weight.

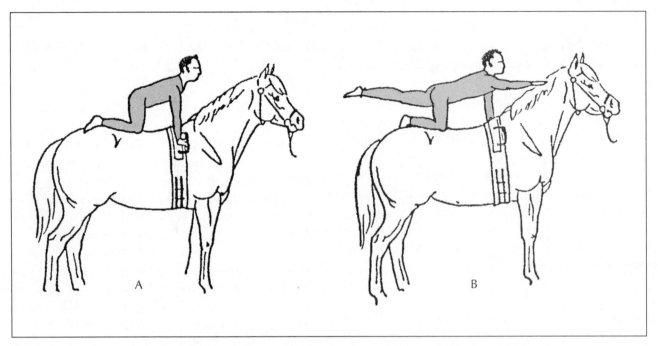

Figure 24.7. A. Symmetrical weight bearing on all four extremities. B. Asymmetrical weight bearing progressing from three extremities to a two-extremity quadruped position (hands and knees) develops pelvic and leg stability.

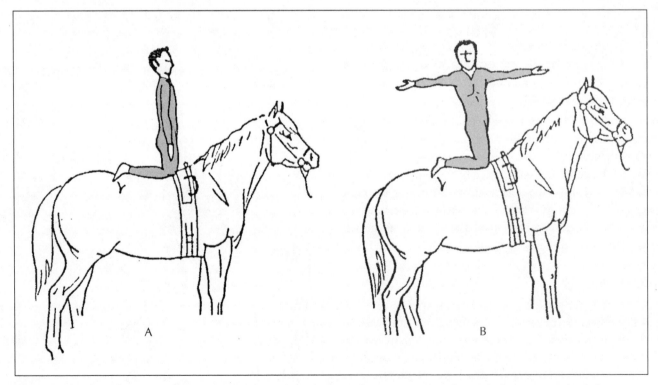

Figure 24.8. Kneeling requires greater pelvic and trunk control. A. Symmetrical weight bearing on both knees. B. Asymmetrical weight bearing on both knees, rotating and flexing the trunk, as in reaching for an object.

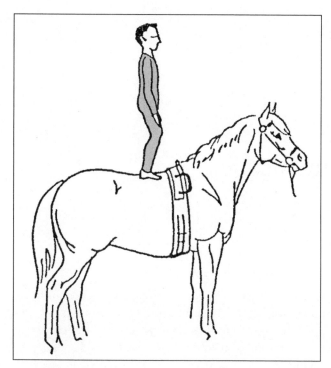

Figure 24.9. Standing requires integration of total body mobility and stability components of movement.

planning, these developmental positions are more suitable for clients with mild movement disorders, sensorimotor disorders, sensory-integrative dysfunction, perceptual–motor disorders, cognitive disorders, behavioral disorders, or language impairments. Treatment usually emphasizes movement transitions rather than postural control within a position (Tebay & Rowley, 1990).

Summary

This chapter provides a rationale for the use of developmental sequences in hippotherapy. It is strongly recommended that occupational therapists receive additional education in sequential developmental, Bobath technique, motor control, and sensory integration before experimenting with use of this dynamic treatment tool for improving the client's posture and balance.

References

Banus, B. S., Kent, C. A., Norton, Y. S., & Sukiennicki, D. R. (1979). *The developmental therapist* (2nd ed.). Thorofare, NJ: Slack.

Bertoti, D. (1988). Effect of therapeutic horseback riding on posture in children with cerebral palsy. *Physical Therapy, 68,* 1505–1512.

Bobath, B. (1978). *Adult hemiplegia: Evaluation and treatment.* London: William Clowes & Sons.

Conolly, B., & Montgomery, P. (1987). *Therapeutic exercise in developmental disabilities.* Chattanooga, TN: Chattanooga Corp.

Friedlaender, E. (1970). *Vaulting: The art of gymnastics on the moving horse.* Brattleboro, VT: Stephen Greene Press.

Glasow, B. (1984). *Hippotherapy: The horse as a therapeutic modality.* Unpublished paper.

Heipertz, W. (1984). *Therapeutic riding: Medicine, education, and sports.* Ottawa, Ontario: TROtt.

Scherzer, A., & Tscharnuter, I. (1990). *Early diagnoses and therapy in cerebral palsy: A primer on infant developmental problems* (2nd ed.). New York: Marcel Dekker.

Tebay, J., & Rowley, L. (1990). *Hippotherapy competency guidelines.* Riderwood, MD: National Hippotherapy Curriculum Committee.

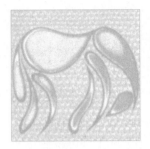

*Every time you ride,
you're either teaching or
unteaching your horse.*
—Gordon Wright

CHAPTER 25

Facilitation of Functional Communication Skills in Hippotherapy

Ann K. Viviano, MA, MS, OTR, CCC/SLP, HPCS

According to the National Institute on Deafness and Other Communication Disorders (2004), one in six Americans has a communication disorder that affects his or her ability to speak, listen, and make wants and needs understood. For a hippotherapy session to be optimal, functional communication between the rider and the occupational therapist must exist. The *Scope of Practice* of the American Occupational Therapy Association (2004) includes communication and inter-action skills as a performance skill, along with process and motor skills, which are necessary for a person to engage in everyday activities. The occupational thera-pist can enhance communication by understanding the basic developmental sequence of communication abili-ties; by implementing communication strategies when the rider has difficulty understanding instructions, expressing thoughts, and conversing; and by practicing social enactment skills to help the rider make sense of social information and develop a cognitive plan for a response.

Developmental Sequence

Shipley and McAfee (2004) offered guidelines for the normal sequence of communication development that provide background for occupational therapists to gauge the level of abilities of younger riders. A typically developing 2- to 3-year-old child's speech is 50% to 75% understandable; the child verbalizes toilet needs before needing to use the toilet, requests desired items by name, identifies several body parts, follows two-part commands, asks one- to two-part questions, responds using two- to four-word sentences, and maintains a topic over several conversational turns. A 3- to 4-year-old child's speech is 80% understandable; the child

understands opposite concepts (e.g., stop–go, in–out, big–little), follows two- and three-part commands, produces four to five words in a sentence, uses language to express emotion, and tells two events in chronologi-cal order.

A 4- to 5-year-old child produces sentences of four to eight words, uses adult-like grammar most of the time, understands most two-part questions, understands the concept of numbers up to 3, and counts to 10 by rote. A 5- to 6-year-old child follows instructions given to a group, uses past tense and future tense appropriately, exchanges information and asks questions, sings entire songs and recites nursery rhymes, accurately relays a story, and produces sentences with details.

A 6- to 7-year-old child understands most time con-cepts and directions that include left and right, uses more complex description words, engages in conversation, and uses a sentence length of approximately 6 words.

Communication Strategies

When working with a rider who has communication difficulties, the therapist may observe the rider's func-tional communication status. Vinson (2001) proposed five areas to determine the communication environment and status of a child:
1. The child's current communication abilities
2. The reasons the child communicates
3. The demands and expectations in the child's daily life
4. How the child interacts with his or her environment
5. Any differences in how the child communicates in
   one environment compared with another.
Bazaar (2005) discussed activities to facilitate speech, language, voice, and cognition improvements in riders during a hippotherapy session.

Informal checklists, such as *Language Red Flags: A Screening Checklist* (Thomas & Thorne, n.d.), *Communication Checklist for 3–5 Years* (PEEL Preschool Speech and Language Services, n.d.), and *Checklist for an Informal Assessment of Language* (Shipley & McAfee, 2004) may be helpful. The occupational therapist should find out what communication strategies are currently in place and observe the rider's comprehension and receptive and expressive language abilities. What does the rider understand? The therapist should consider the following aspects of the rider's receptive communication skills:

• Length of sentences the rider comprehends
• Number of steps in directions the rider can follow
• Vocabulary and types of words (person and object names, actions, descriptions) to which the rider responds
• Tactile or object cues that may provide additional direction or information
• Use of written words, photographs, and line drawings to supplement auditory information
• The number of conversational turns the rider can track.

In addition, the therapist should consider how the rider expresses him- or herself. What are the rider's body language and vocalizations; eye gaze and facial expressions; gestures and signs; and use of pictures and written words? What are the rider's vocabulary words and phrases? How complex are the rider's sentences, and how does he or she engage in conversation?

The following strategies for working with riders who have communication difficulties are based on principles within texts by Roth and Worthington (2001), Shipley and McAfee (2004), and Vinson (2001) and on clinical experience.

If a rider has difficulty understanding what is said, the occupational therapy practitioner can try the following strategies:

• Call the rider's name to establish attention.
• Use facial expressions, voice, and inflection to emphasize the most important key words of a sentence or direction.
• Minimize the use of indefinite words, such as *right here, this, that,* and *it.*
• Simplify one's language.
• Gradually expand the length of sentences from labels and single words to phrases and sentences.
• Start with nouns and actions and add adjectives (big, little), adverbs (slow, fast), prepositions (in, around), and temporal words (first, next).
• Use natural gestures, pantomimes, demonstrations, and signs to provide visual input to promote the rider's

understanding of directions and auditory information (e.g., moving one's hand forward while telling the rider to walk the horse).

• Check the rider's comprehension when using "Wh-" questions. For example, ask "What do you need to groom the horse?" Practitioners may need to provide a picture board of potential objects the rider could use to facilitate his or her response.
• Give the rider choices and provide vocabulary words, such as "Do you want to play with the ball or with ribbons?" while showing the objects to the rider.
• Establish a routine for the riding session. Use visual aids, such as following a schedule board with pictures of activities to be completed from the beginning to the end of the session. Mark off each activity as it is completed.
• When giving a direction, pause to allow the rider time to process the information; then repeat or rephrase the direction.
• Use short, repetitive songs to help the rider understand concepts, such as "Head, Shoulders, Knees, and Toes" when working on body parts.

If a rider is nonverbal or has speech that is not understandable, the following strategies may be of help:

• Closely observe the rider's nonverbal responses when he or she is in challenging positions that may elicit stress, pain, or fear reactions. Watch for signs of fatigue.
• Identify and label a rider's nonverbal communications. If a rider looks scared, label the emotion for him or her and put the feelings into words. Help the rider point to faces with different expressions that are on a card clipped to the surcingle.
• Create opportunities for communication. If a rider is able to use his or her voice, encourage him or her to vocalize to request a desired object. For example, provide carrots to feed the horse in a plastic bag with a zip closure. Encourage the rider to vocalize and ask for the therapist's help to open the bag. Give the rider the carrots in small pieces, so the rider has opportunities to repeat and practice requesting the carrots.

If the rider does not attempt to talk, provide hand-over-hand assistance to help the rider use natural gestures and signs to indicate actions, such as come, go, walk, and stop. Help the rider establish a system to indicate binary choices, such as "yes/no," "go/stop," and "more/done." Help the rider add meaning to differentiated vocalizations—a long sound to request "more," short sound for "stop." He or she can point to a smile face for "yes" and to a frown face for "no." The faces may be attached to the pad or surcingle. The following additional suggestions may be helpful:

- Draw a smile face on one of the rider's hands and a frown face on the other hand. Help the rider hold up his or her hand for a "yes" or "no" response. Have the rider point to a red stop sign on left side of horse's neck for "halt" and a green go sign on right side of horse's neck for "walk on." Use chalk, stickers, or tape to make the signs on the horse's neck.
- Have the rider point to one sidewalker for "yes" or "go" and the other sidewalker for "no" or "stop."
- Observe the rider's facial expressions, and interpret their meaning. A smile may represent "more" and a frown represent "done."
- Establish one eye blink for "yes" or "go" and two eye blinks for "no" or "stop."
- If the rider does not understand pictures, use miniature objects to associate with an actual object. For example, a piece of cloth may represent the horse's blanket.
- Draw activities on a marker board or use magnetic pictures attached to the arena wall. Ask the rider to point to a picture or select a magnet to indicate a choice.
- Use photographs, line drawings, or words printed on cards to provide the vocabulary that is used in the session. Put the cards on a ring that is attached to the surcingle handle, or use Velcro to attach the cards to the pad or blanket.
- Communication cards can be attached to a vest worn by the therapist or a sidewalker. The rider can point to a picture to indicate a choice.
- Use small communication boards that provide specific vocabulary words for different parts of the session, such as "colors" for a ring game and "animals" for a matching game.

If a rider uses words and needs to expand his or her vocabulary and word combinations, consider using the following techniques:

- Imitate and expand the rider's gestures, vocalizations, words, and phrases. Add new ideas and information to the rider's language. If the rider says, "Brush horse," then you can say, "Brush the horse with the red brush."
- Use a "fill-in-the-blank" approach, such as "Let's put on your helmet so you can ride the _____."
- If a rider has word-finding difficulties, provide the initial sound or syllable of the target word, such as "The horse's color is bl___."
- Rehearse a description of a sequence or event and ask the rider to restate it. Repeat a sequence and a give the rider an additional opportunity to communicate the message. For example, the therapist and rider discuss

an event during the session, then the rider repeats the event to his or her caregiver.
- Indicate when more information is needed, such as "You feed the horse because _____." Use relational terms, which include words such as *because, and, first, if, but, next, or, in,* and *beside.*
- If a rider uses incorrect words or immature grammar, restate the utterance with the correct words. If the rider says "The horse runned," then say, "The horse ran."
- Help the rider develop favorite interests and hobbies to provide topics for conversation.
- If the rider has difficulty relating events, start a riding book with pictures of the activities the rider does at hippotherapy. Have the rider practice describing the pictures to friends and family members.
- Talk about an event while it is happening and after the activity is completed to promote the rider's memory and sequencing.
- Discuss the riding session and ask "What is happening?" "What will happen next?" "What did happen?"

Asking varied questions also can help the rider enhance his or her language and cognitive skills:

- Ask "how" and "why" questions to help the rider develop problem-solving abilities.
- Ask open-ended questions to help the rider sequence ideas and formulate sentences.
- Ask "cause–effect" questions to help the rider predict the results of his or her actions.

Social Enactment Skills

Doble and Magill-Evans (1992) stated that social enactment skills are nonverbal and verbal skills that enable riders to communicate needs and intentions to others as well as to respond to the messages of others in a competent manner. The rider's ability to use social enactment skills facilitates his or her participation in the interactional aspects of functional equine activities. Social enactment skills consist of four areas of development:

1. *Acknowledgment skills* allow the rider to communicate that he or she is listening to or acknowledging the comments and actions of the communication partner. Acknowledgment skills include looking and gazing, touching, positioning, gesturing, and saying "yes."
2. *Sending skills* allow the rider to send both informational and affective messages to the communication partner. Sending skills include greeting, initiating, asking and inquiring, accepting, encouraging, refusing, revealing, and disengaging and terminating.
3. *Timing skills* allow the rider to pace his or her responses in relation to the communication partner's

responses so there are neither interruptions nor unreasonable delays in initiating a response. Timing skills include initiating without hesitation, speaking without unnecessary interruption, speaking without repeating information unnecessarily, maintaining a reasonable pace when speaking, ending messages without preservation, ending messages without stopping prematurely, and ending message after a reasonable period.

4. *Coordinating skills* allow the rider to harmonize his or her messages with the messages of the communication partner and with the expectations and demands of the environment. Coordination skills include sending message compatible with the partner's language abilities, interests, affective tone, and level of self-revelation; producing messages compatible with expectations of the physical and interpersonal situation; and using variations in message styles (i.e., alternating questions with disclosure and information provision).

The following activities have been successful in clinical situations for riders who need to develop language use in social situations:

- Model nonverbal aspects of a conversation—looking at a conversation partner, using appropriate touch to get attention, and maintaining appropriate distance from a partner.
- Develop nonverbal turn-taking skills during games with rings and balls.
- Teach verbal turn-taking skills in structured games, such as "I Spy."
- Teach conversational turn-taking. Wait for the rider to initiate a conversation, or the therapist can initiate the conversation. Signal the rider when to take a turn. Use key words, questions, descriptions, explanations, and imaginary play to stimulate conversation.
- Have the rider practice both the speaker and the listener roles in a conversation. Model a comment or question to prepare the rider for what he or she needs to say.
- Model greetings, introductions, and taking leave with other riders, sidewalkers, and staff.
- Help the rider repair a communication breakdown and restate information if a conversation partner does not understand the rider.
- To reinforce appropriate interactions, have the rider read a short story about appropriate ways to communicate, such as "I walk slowly up to the horse. I talk to the horse in a soft voice."

- Let the rider practice giving directions for tacking the horse or activities with other riders.
- Have the rider practice telling a story in which the rider takes different roles in the story.

Conclusion

Understanding communication development, using communication strategies to enhance a rider's comprehension and expression abilities, and practicing social enactment skills may facilitate communication between the occupational therapist and rider during hippotherapy. Successful use of communication strategies depends on a combination of the therapist's expertise and the rider's unique abilities, strengths, weaknesses, and level of understanding. Facilitating communication during hippotherapy will optimize the interactions during the therapy session and promote a rider's performance abilities.

References

American Occupational Therapy Association. (2004). Scope of practice. *American Journal of Occupational Therapy, 58,* 673–677.

Bazaar, M. (2005, Winter). Facilitating communication and having fun. *Hippotherapy,* p. 11.

Doble, S. E., & Magill-Evans, J. (1992). A model of social interaction to guide occupational therapy practice. *Canadian Journal of Occupational Therapy, 59,* 147.

National Institute on Deafness and Other Communication Disorders. (2004). *Strategic plan: Plain language version FY 2003–2005.* Retrieved December 23, 2006, from www.nidcd.nih.gov/about/plans/strategic/nsrp_02.asp.

PEEL Preschool Speech and Language Services. (n.d.). *Communication checklist for 3–5 years.* Halton Preschool Speech and Language Program. Retrieved December 23, 2006, from www.erinoak.org/preschoolspeech/pdf/milestones/milestones3_5.pdf.

Roth, F. P., & Worthington, C. K. (2001). *Treatment resource manual for speech-language pathology* (2nd ed.). Albany, NY: Delmar/Singular Thomson Learning.

Shipley, K. G., & McAfee, J. G. (2004). *Assessment in speech-language pathology: A resource manual* (3rd ed.). Clifton Park, NY: Delmar/Singular Thomson Learning.

Thomas, A., & Thorne, G. (n.d.). *Language red flags: A screening checklist.* Retrieved December 23, 2006, from http://www.cdl.org/resource-library/articles/red_flags.php.

Vinson, B. P. (2001). *Essentials for speech-language pathologists.* San Diego, CA: Delmar/Singular Thomson Learning.

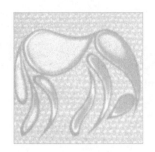

What the colt learns in youth
he continues in old age.
—French Proverb

CHAPTER 26

Grooming and Tacking-Up as Intervention

Judy Hilburn, OTR/L

This chapter is intended to demonstrate how the major frames of reference used by occupational therapists can be intricately woven into activities such as grooming and tacking-up the therapy horse. A *frame of reference* can be defined as body of hypothetical assumptions and principles that give unity and direction to practice and research. Major frames of reference referred to by occupational therapists include adaptive responses, cognition activities, dynamic systems, facilitating growth and development, human occupation, learning disabilities, occupational adaptation, occupational behavior, role acquisition, sensory integration, social cognition, and spatiotemporal adaptation (Kramer & Hinojosa, 1999).

A Therapy Experience

"Max," tall for his age, was a 4-year-old with high intelligence and advanced verbal skills. He talked excitedly and incessantly about his many superhero action figures and their grand and varied adventures. But ask Max to climb the "tower" or "leap a tall building in a single bound," and he would fail miserably. Max's big brother was excelling in school. His little brother was running circles around him, literally. Max's parents were baffled.

Then the bimonthly children's clinic came to town. During the clinic, it was discovered that this gifted child had a learning disability, with delayed gross motor and fine motor development, most likely due to hypotonia and gravitational insecurity. Max shuffled rather than ran. When he tried running, he did so with arms pinned at his sides, his shoulders fixed for extra control; even with this extra control, Max appeared to be on the verge of tumbling forward. He was fearful of climbing and could not jump down from low heights. At the playground, Max was unable to join the other

children's games (e.g., climbing on the monkey bars or playing ball).

In the classroom, Max again faced failure. Because of poor core body strength (proximal stability), his oculomotor control was poor, and his fine-motor skills were below age level. Manipulating crayons or pencils was beyond his capability. Any sense of competency he experienced came only through his above-average verbal skills. Because most boys his age relate to one another on a more visceral level, Max had trouble socializing with his classmates.

Max was admitted to a special preschool program that offered occupational therapy services. After Max had attended the program for about 6 months, a hippotherapy program was established in town. At the request of his parents, Max was enrolled in the program.

Max first was involved with grooming the horse to improve his tactile and vestibular responses, upperextremity strength, and motor-planning skills (Ayres, 1979). When Max needed to reach the horse's back while brushing him, he used a mounting block. At first, Max could tolerate only the lower step because of his gravitational insecurity. Eventually, he used the second step of the block. His interest in the horse helped him challenge his fear of movement, and soon Max began to assist in leading the horse from the stall. After about six sessions, Max found the courage to mount the horse, needing minimum assistance. Max continued to progress over the months and soon was able to ride alone in the ring. Everyone stood back and watched Max's failures slowly turn into successes.

Tacking-Up as a Component of Therapy

Before a horse can be used in a hippotherapy or equineassisted occupational therapy program, it must be regularly groomed and tacked-up. Stable staff spend many hours performing these tasks. Why not use these tasks as intervention activities for selected riders? Occupational therapists will find that horse grooming and tacking-up are easily adapted for the intervention needs of clients with disabilities.

Equipment required for such activities includes currycombs, brushes of various sizes and textures, hoof picks, halters, ropes, saddle blankets, saddles or surcingles, saddle pads, cinches or girths, and bridles. The horse to be groomed must be under the control of a riding assistant or therapist at all times, but it should be positioned so that riders of all sizes, either ambulatory or in wheelchairs, can participate fully.

Factors inherent in the activity of grooming and tacking address common client needs and enables occupational role development and performance (Case-Smith, 2005). These functions involve activities that require the client to set realistic goals and make decisions (Fidler & Fidler, 1978). Grooming and tacking-up require safety awareness and involve established routines for working around a horse and caring for him.

Grooming and tacking activities integrate the demand for various senses and skills. The areas of gross motor function, muscle tone, and co-contraction of muscles are influenced by heavy work patterns while a client carries a grooming kit, saddle blanket, or saddle (Fenton, Gagnon, & Pitts, 2003). If a platform or mounting block is used during grooming and tacking, a client has the opportunity to "practice" climbing or jumping skills. If a client is advanced enough in his or her horse skills to begin leading the horse to the grooming area, then ambulatory skills are involved. A client may walk over uneven terrain or execute stops, starts, and turns. A client must match his or her own rate, rhythm, and sequence of movement to that of the horse. In the author's experience, her mare usually changes her way of going to accommodate her client handler's gait.

A client's upper-extremity strength and range of motion are facilitated by brushing a horse because antigravity, resistive movement patterns are inherent in this activity (Fenton et al., 2003). Moreover, tightening cinch or girth straps also will increase upper-extremity strength. Bilateral upper-extremity integration and coordination are facilitated by using two grooming implements at a time. For example, a client may hold a curry comb in one hand and a body brush in the other, alternating the use of each tool as appropriate. Assisting with lacing or adjusting a cinch strap

or girth involves reciprocal, alternating, hand-over-hand movement patterns.

Similarly, grooming and tacking affect fine-motor development in many ways. For example, skills for activities of daily living are improved by the tasks involved in manipulating buckles on halters, bridles or girths; handling rein and lead-rope snaps; or brushing the mane and tail (Christiansen & Baum, 1991). Pincer grasp is facilitated while picking a horse's loose hair out of a curry comb or body brush. During combing of a mane, the client may use his fingers as the comb. Such an action is effective as an active–resistive exercise for strengthening the hands. Brushing and combing activities affect establishment of dominant and nondominant hand patterns because they are rich in spatial and sequencing patterns. One can see this establishment as a client handles the brush with his dominant hand while placing his nondominant hand on the horse's body for support. The same effect also is seen while the client adjusts a latigo cinch.

Establishment of hand dominance is facilitated while the client is leading the horse and carrying the lead rope properly (i.e., the dominant hand holds the rope near the snap end, and the nondominant hand holds the coiled, excess rope). Tactile perception for fine-motor development is enhanced because the lead rope is being held on the diagonal, against resistance.

Postural responses are facilitated whenever a client must reach high spots, either during grooming or tacking-up (i.e., standing on tip-toes to brush the horse's back or position the saddle blanket). Equilibrium responses are elicited when a client bends over to brush the horse's belly or legs, to reach under the barrel to grasp the cinch, or to assist with cleaning the horse's hooves. Leading a horse facilitates improved proximal stability. Such an activity facilitates co-contraction; trunk rotation; and separation of head, eyes, and upper extremities.

Grooming and tacking provide a high level of tactile input. Grooming implements are made of various textures: Brushes are stiff or soft, and curry combs are made of rubber, plastic, or metal. Tack includes ropes of nylon or cotton; ropes may be braided, round, or flat; reins may be of cotton webbing, rubber, or leather. The horse has myriad textures. The mane and tail are coarse; body hair can be furry or smooth; the muzzle is velvety; and hooves are hard and rough. A groomer comes in contact with all of these areas.

Development of cognitive–perceptual skills also is easily worked into the grooming and tacking activity.

Spatial terms are an integral part of those activities—brushing the horse *on top* of his back or *under* the girth area. The client can start brushing from *front* to *back*. Body scheme concepts are continually used as the client brushes *softly on the horse's face* and *carefully around his eyes and ears*. Comparison of human body parts to the horse's parts also is easily done. The horse might have a scrape on his *knee,* just like a child sometimes gets on his or her knee. While leading the horse, a client is faced with "body map" dilemmas such as where to stand, how close to stand to the horse, how fast to walk, and how to get both the horse and him- or herself safely through a gate or barn door.

Cognitive integration and performance skills are involved in the contact with the horse (Kramer & Hinojosa, 1999). Opportunities to use verbal and non-verbal communication skills are many when dealing with the horse. Simply looking for and greeting the horse encourages communication. Communication is facilitated when various verbal and body cues are used for leading or halting the horse (e.g., finding ways to praise the horse either by patting or verbalizing "good girl"). Some horses will actually seek out the client with a look or movement that might suggest "Rub me here" or "Who are you, brushing me so nicely?" And we all have seen every horse nonverbally (or verbally!) say, "Where is my carrot?" Such demonstrative body language by the horse is hard to miss, and the client usually has no choice but to respond.

Grooming can lead to enhanced tool use and motor planning. The client will realize how the rubber curry comb should be used to remove dried mud, and during tacking-up, the client will learn how to get the awkwardly shaped saddle or vaulting surcingle onto the horse properly. The activity of grooming and tacking-up easily lends itself to development of skills for following directions and solving problems. Tacking-up requires that specific sequences be followed: The saddle blanket must be placed under the saddle, and the girth must be tightened before mounting. Figuring out how to pick up the hoof for cleaning or how to keep the reins from dragging on the ground facilitates the use of problem-solving skills. Other cognitive areas, such as ideation, sequencing, and programming are enhanced when other questions arise: "In which corral is my horse?" "How will I get him out of the corral?" "Will the horse come willingly?" "What equipment will I need?"

Many benefits in the area of social and emotional development are inherent in tacking and grooming (Case-Smith, 2005). For example, the activities may arouse the client's nurturing instincts toward the horse. Needs of the horse, such as brushing away a bothersome fly, cleaning off dried mud from the girth area to prevent chafing, or removing twigs from the mane or tail, may be met. The client finds that he or she must be attentive to the horse's likes and dislikes during grooming, such as avoiding ticklish spots or taking care of an itchy spot behind the horse's ear. The client becomes aware of his or her own behavior and how it might affect the horse, such as learning that running and jumping could startle the horse or that jerking on the lead rope or hitting the horse may hurt or scare it. The client learns to understand others' behavior (the horse's) when he or she has to deal with a horse that momentarily balks or veers off course while being led. The client learns what pleases the horse (grain, hay, or carrots) and how the horse acts to get that treat. Self-esteem is enhanced when the client is successful in controlling such a large animal as the horse. The client receives approval when he or she properly prepares the horse for riding.

Finally, the caregiver of the client sees positive effects on the client. The intervention setting has usually been a clinic or hospital, in which the clients are surrounded by other people in wheelchairs, on crutches, and with walkers. In contrast, hippotherapy and equine-assisted occupational therapy involve fresh air, trees, birds, and horses. The caregiver happily sees his or her loved one as a part of an active, bustling environment in which people are busy working with their horses.

Summary

Grooming and tacking-up the horse are occupations that contain the frames of reference occupational therapists use when treating clients with decreased function and skill. During grooming and tacking activities, clients must learn policies and procedures established at the barn. They are expected to execute specific skills to adequately prepare their horse for riding. They must learn to make appropriate decisions as to the use of tools or equipment. These activities involve role acquisition, human occupation, and occupational behavior.

Clients are required to be physically active and alert throughout the activity. They must carry equipment, learn body parts of the horse, and demonstrate safety awareness. These skills facilitate growth and development, sensory integration, and cognition. Clients also are exposed to basic horse-handling techniques and horse psychology (e.g., horses are kept in fenced areas and must be led out); horses have special needs, responding to which facilitates spatiotemporal adaptation and adaptive responses.

References

Ayres, A. J. (1979). *Sensory integration and learning disorders.* Los Angeles: Western Psychological Services.

Case-Smith, J. (2005). *Occupational therapy for children* (5th ed.). St. Louis, MO: Elsevier Mosby.

Christiansen, C., & Baum, C. (1991). *Occupational therapy: Overcoming human performance deficits.* Thorofare, NJ: Slack.

Fenton, S., Gagnon, P., & Pitts, D. G. (2003). Interventions to promote participation. In E. B. Crepeu, E. S. Cohn, & B. A. Boyt Schell (Eds.), *Willard and Spackman's occupational therapy* (10th ed.). Philadelphia: Lippincott Williams & Wilkins.

Fidler, J. W., & Fidler, G. S. (1978). Doing and becoming: Purposeful action and self-actualization. *American Journal of Occupational Therapy, 32,* 305–310.

Kramer, P., & Hinojosa, J. (1999). *Frames of reference for pediatrics occupational therapy* (2nd ed.). Philadelphia: Lippincott Williams & Wilkins.

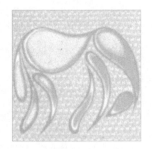

Knowledge is a function of being.
When there is a change in the being of the knower,
there is a corresponding change in the nature
and amount of knowing.
—Rudy Rucker

CHAPTER 27

Hippotherapy and Sensory Defensiveness

Melanie M. Tidman, MA, OTR/L

Sensory integration is the central nervous system's ability to organize and use sensory input in order to respond appropriately to the environment (Jacobs, 2004). *Sensory integrative dysfunction* is a general term characterizing the inability of the nervous system to organize incoming stimuli and allow a person to respond in an appropriate way to his or her environment (Ayres, 1979). When the central nervous system is unable to perform sensory integration, adaptive responses are impaired and behavioral changes occur that may result in symptoms of *sensory defensiveness.* As is the case with many sensory dysfunctions, sensory defensiveness often is misdiagnosed.

Sensory defensiveness, a concept first introduced by Knickerbocker (1980), has been defined as an imbalance in the inhibitory receptors that prevents modulation of incoming sensory information. It can affect the tactile, visual, and auditory systems and may produce symptoms of gravitational insecurity like those seen in dysfunction of the vestibular system (Fisher, Murray, & Bundy, 1991). Specifically, Fisher and colleagues described children with sensory defensiveness as being overly active, hyperverbal, and destructible and as having disorganized responses to the environment (Fisher et al., 1991). Sensory defensiveness differs from a general sensory integrative dysfunction because is it a collection of symptoms that mainly have to do with the inability to modulate incoming stimuli. Knickerbocker (1980) suggested that the problem stems from an imbalance between inhibition and excitation within the nervous system; this imbalance manifests itself as a general disorganized response to environmental demands. Parents, teachers, and professionals frequently misinterpret the symptoms of this diagnosis as a behavior problem that can be dealt with by either offering a reward for good behavior or disciplining the child for his or her inappropriate actions (Ayres, 1979).

This chapter offers insight into the world of treating sensory defensiveness through hippotherapy, therapeutic riding, and occupational therapy strategies. It begins by reviewing sensory systems and demonstrating how sensory defensiveness can affect functional responses in children. Next, the chapter discusses how hippotherapy is being used as an effective intervention to reorganize sensory systems. The chapter concludes with a case study illustrating the effects of hippotherapy intervention on the functional development of people diagnosed with sensory defensiveness.

Effects on Attention

A child with sensory defensiveness frequently has difficulty filtering and organizing incoming sensory information. It can manifest as a lack of initiation or maintenance of attention (Ayres, 1979). Experience demonstrates that a lack of attention to school-related tasks often is a reason for referral for occupational therapy services in the school setting. The author's 25 years of working in schools provided ample opportunity to observe a regular classroom and the varying amounts of stimuli that every child is exposed to throughout the day. During the school day, a child may encounter chairs banging, a teacher talking, and side conversations among peers. A child with attention problems may be unable to discern the importance of incoming stimuli or be able to filter unimportant stimuli, resulting in distractibility and poor attention to tasks. A hyperactive or defensive sensory system may, in some cases, manifest itself as inattention, as well as disobedient or disruptive behavior, which requires intervention.

Occupational therapists have had a collective interest in sensory processing throughout the history of the profession. The unique contribution of occupational therapy, not only in attaching understanding and meaning to sensory experiences but also in developing strategies to deal with the problem of inattention and disruptive behaviors, is essential in helping students to live a satisfying and functional life (Dunn, 2001). Rewards or punishments alone may be ineffective in altering behavior resulting from sensory defensiveness because these behaviors are reactions to dysfunctional processing that is occurring at a subconscious level, which illustrates the brain's processing a balance between incoming stimuli and responses.

Cognitive mechanisms, such as attention, involve a balancing of threshold demands in the central nervous system (Dunn, 2001). Genetic and environmental factors contribute to each student's degree of responding to incoming stimuli with either excitation or inhibition, the result of which affects the ability to attend to a task. Students respond to the same stimuli differently; their responses affect their daily choices and are reflected in their behavior, mood, and performance of daily tasks (Dunn, 2001). Inattention manifested as defiant or disruptive behavior from a sensory defensive child is most often misunderstood and may be, in some cases, dealt with by stern sanctions and reprimands, which may result in development of a poor self-concept (Ayres, 1979)

The ability to attend and receive sensory information is regulated largely through an area in the brain stem called the *reticular formation,* which is not a single structure and has multiple roles in central nervous system function. It is involved with a broad range of automatic or unconscious, neural functions, as well as oculomotor reflexes, postural tone, sleep–wake cycles, and autonomic function. Other parts of the reticular formation play a role in the relay of somatic and sensory information to the cerebellum. This information appears to be involved in emotional behavior (Cohen, 1999). Ayres (1979) described *reticular formations* as a "net-like structure that acts as the arousal center in our brains that either wakes us up, calms us down or excites us." Ayres further stressed the need to take both a holistic and a hierarchical approach to explaining central nervous system function. She believed that the central nervous system functions as a whole and that higher brain functions are largely dependent upon the integrity of "lower level" structures and on sensorimotor experiences (Fisher et al., 1991). The cells that form the reticular formation receive input from various hierarchical levels and systems of the brain, including cutaneous and proprioceptive signals from the sensorimotor and vestibular complex (Cohen, 1999). It is logical to assume, then, that these inputs, if not mediated at each level or properly integrated

between levels, can elicit a maladaptive response in attention when the person is confronted with the demands of his or her environment.

In communication between lower and higher level systems, the reticular formation assists in the inhibition of environmental overstimulation and permits us to attend to a singular action or shift our focus from one activity to another. Cognitive processing is optimal when a balance between internal and external information allows for task performance through the maintenance of attention (Dunn, 2001). Disorganization, either in the reticular formation or as a result of poor communication and integration between systems, may result in a complete overflow of incoming stimuli, leading to a dysfunctional physical response and inability to attend selectively to the task at hand. Ultimately, the person who has this response is unable to pay attention enough to perform an efficient, goal-directed activity (Ayres, 1979).

Tactile System

Sensory integration theory hypothesizes a relationship between the processing of certain tactile stimuli and the person's behaviors. Specifically, sensory integration theory provides explanations for abnormal behavior as it relates to the person's ability to perform tactile discrimination functions, including haptic perception, motor planning, and negative or adverse responses to tactile stimuli (i.e., tactile defensiveness). In this view, tactile aversion responses could be one manifestation of sensory defensiveness (Fisher et al., 1991).

The tactile system can be described as a two-part system that works together to integrate tactile sensations. The first part of the system, the *protective system,* begins with a series of touch receptors located throughout the body that receive sensory information from the physical environment and relay it to a network of cells located in the brain stem. This network is then responsible for deciphering incoming messages and either activating or deactivating the *sympathetic response,* which interprets the stimulus and determines whether the stimulus is hot or cold, sharp or dull, soft or hard, and so on. This process includes proprioceptive inputs and is referred to as *somatosensory processing* (Ayres, 1979). The result is either to continue to receive the specific tactile impulses or to issue a withdrawal response (Allen, Case-Smith, & Pratt, 1996). This system is responsible for the *flight–fright–fight response* (Trott, Laurel, & Windeck, 1993). The autonomic nervous system, through its parasympathetic and sympathetic branches, also regulates the ability to adapt to changes in the environment by modulating sensory functions. These branches function together for self-regulation and response to both internal and external stimuli (Schaaf, Miller, Sewall, & O'Keefe, 2003). Children with disturbances in sensory modulation may have disturbances in autonomic nervous system functioning (Schaaf et al., 2003).

The second part of the tactile system, the *discriminatory system,* involves the communication of sensory centers in the cerebral cortex with the peripheral structures through what Ayres (1979) hypothesized to be "gate" neurons in the dorsal horn of the spinal cord. These gate neurons are responsible for controlling impulses to the central nervous system and are influenced by incoming tactile inputs and by higher cortical structures (Fisher et al., 1991). Here, the cerebral cortex functions as a higher processing center (Ayres, 1979) and allows a person to determine where he or she is being touched and what is to be done in response. This response can be called *adaptive* because it allows the person to successfully meet a challenge presented in the environment; the brain has been able to efficiently organize incoming sensory information and use it as a basis for action (Parham & Mailloux, 1995).

The *limbic system* is another important influence because it interacts with the tactile system and contributes to responses in the areas of learning and memory, aggression, and self-preservation (DeGroot & Chusid, 1988). This system also has a role in modulating emotional responses (Isaacson, 1982) through its connections with the hippocampus and the hypothalamus. Thus, the limbic system is implicated in tactile defensiveness, sensory defensiveness, and sensory modulation disorders (Wilbarger & Royeen, 1987).

Effects of Sensory Defensiveness on the Tactile System

Tactile defensiveness, as one manifestation of sensory defensiveness, can be defined as an overreaction of the tactile system to a non-noxious stimulus that would otherwise not threaten an organized sensory system. In an organized system, inhibitors located within the brain stem—specifically, the nuclei of the thalamus—act as a filtering agent to sort out incoming tactile sensations and prevent overload. A disorganized tactile system may not possess an organized network of inhibitors or may lack a balance between inhibitory influences and excitatory influences; it therefore is unable to modulate incoming tactile information (Dunn, 2001).

Tactile defensiveness has a profound effect on the development of occupational behavior in a child. The child's inherent drive to engage in occupation (e.g., play) is diminished because of his or her inability to modulate sensory information. This atypical reaction to incoming sensory information has a significant impact on the quality of life and functional performance for these children and their families by limiting their active participation in their daily lives (Schaaf et al., 2003). Abnormal responsiveness may restrict interests and activities and thus affect children's play choices, which subsequently affects their development (Schaaf et al., 2003).

In the early years of life, learning is achieved through a child's exploration of his or her environment, and social relationships are formed. Humans are innately motivated toward mastery of their environment. Through participation in the challenges encountered in their environment, humans make adaptive responses, the outcomes of which provide meaning and satisfaction. The tactile system plays a role in motivation and self-direction (Fisher et al., 1991). A tactilely defensive child learns from his or her adverse tactile experiences and may ultimately avoid valuable opportunities for tactile exploration (Ayres, 1979). These exploration opportunities provide information to the child concerning spatial relations, visual perception, coordination, and other basic sensorimotor concepts (Engel, 1984). Skill acquisition in these various concept areas is necessary for the development of intelligence and organization of the central nervous system (Ayres, 1979).

Visual and Auditory Systems

Initially, the visual system receives information from the physical environment through an adequately functioning ocular system (the retinas and the optic nerves; Ayres, 1979). The information is then relayed to processing centers located in the brain stem, which issue a motor response to the corresponding muscles and joints of the body. The brain stem is responsible for automatic responses that determine the position and movements of the body in relation to the physical environment (DeGroot & Chusid, 1998). Information from the visual system also is sent to parts of the cerebral cortex and brain stem that are responsible for visual tracking, coordinating eye–hand movements, and integrating various tactile sensations (Ayres, 1979).

The auditory system receives sound waves from the physical environment through a network of receptors located within the inner ear. These receptors integrate information and then relay it to the auditory processing centers located within the brain stem. The information is organized and integrated with input from the vestibular, proprioceptive, and visual systems (Ayres, 1979). Similar to the visual system, input also is sent to higher processing centers in the cortex, brain stem, and cerebellum for coordinating and producing sensory and motor responses (Ayres, 1979).

Effects of Sensory Defensiveness on Visual and Auditory Problems

The visual system provides information about spatial localization to locate an object visually in space. The central nervous system needs information about the position of the image on the retina and the orientation of the eyes in the head (Cohen, 1999). Processing mechanisms in the visual system, such as lateral inhibition and adaptation, help maintain the quality of visual representation while minimizing or filtering the amount of information transmitted (Cohen, 1999). A person who has sensory defensiveness may be unable to filter the incoming information and may become overwhelmed by the amount of visual input.

The same may be true in the auditory system. The child with sensory defensiveness lacks the inhibitory processes necessary to modulate incoming stimuli. He or she may therefore be unable to comprehend or discern relevant from irrelevant auditory data. This problem can lead to difficulties in following instructions or formulating adaptive responses. The child with sensory defensiveness may not enjoy social engagements because of the overwhelming noise that accompanies interpersonal activities. Because a main occupation of children is to learn in academic settings, learning may be impaired because information is not processed accurately through visual or auditory systems. Additionally, the portion of the central nervous system known as the dorsal column–medial lemniscal system may play some role in organization by sorting out relevant information and directing attention (Fisher et al., 1991). Defensiveness in this system ultimately may affect all areas of daily living, including cognitive, language (both expressive and receptive; see following section on language problems), physical (both gross and fine motor skills), and social development (Ayres, 1979).

Proprioception

Proprioception is the ability to organize and integrate physical input that is received through the muscles and joints in response to an organism's own movement (Fisher et al., 1991). Information from proprioception stimuli is necessary for body awareness and is needed in the performance of smooth, coordinated movements. It

is essential for detecting the position of the body in space, the rate and timing of movement, the force of muscle exertion, and the speed and extent of muscle stretch (Fisher et al., 1991). Proprioceptive stimuli alert the body to its position in space in relationship to other objects in the environment. This input is received in muscles and joints and is relayed to the processing centers of the brain stem and cerebellum via the spinal cord (Ayres, 1979). Proprioceptive input is received constantly and functions in coordination with the vestibular system to provide the body with muscle tone necessary for an upright, vertical head and body position and for organized antigravity movement. Proprioceptive input, together with tactile input, is important in the development of body scheme and provides a basis for the development of praxis (Fisher et al., 1991).

Effects of Proprioceptive Dysfunction on Sensory Defensiveness

Proprioception can be explained as centrally generated motor commands responsible for our sense of effort to maintain movement in space (Fisher et al., 1991). A child who does not adequately integrate proprioceptive input is not receiving or organizing the input necessary for functional postural and equilibrium responses and, thus, can be observed to have difficulty maintaining posture in space or maintaining limb position against gravity (Fisher et al., 1991). Dysfunction in the vestibular–proprioceptive system often is present in people displaying hypotonic or low muscle tone. Hypotonic musculature cannot adequately receive sensory input, and it results in difficulty initiating or sustaining appropriate muscle contraction necessary for holding the body upright or active movement against gravity. When a person's vestibular–proprioceptive system is not functioning properly, he or she often will display poor righting and equilibrium responses when positioned to work against gravity (Ayres, 1979). Children who have deficits in the modulation of vestibular–proprioceptive information have decreased ability to maintain head orientation in space, inability to determine the relative position or movement of their body or body parts in space, and difficulty judging the amount of force or effort required to accomplish a task (Fisher et al., 1991). A child displaying hypotonic muscle tone often will compensate by leaning against a stable structure or using extremities to support his or her lack of stability.

People with poor vestibular–proprioceptive function often appear to be clumsy and demonstrate poor ability to plan new or novel movements; they require significant rehearsal of required movements to be successful. *Praxis* can be defined as *action based on will.* Ayres (1979) defined the concept of *developmental dyspraxia,* which has its basis in dysfunction in the vestibular–proprioceptive system. Accordingly, children with dyspraxia have deficits in motor planning that result in observable motor clumsiness (Fisher et al., 1991). Ayres also described children whose poor motor planning appeared to have a basis in poor tactile and proprioceptive processing, thus, the term *somatodyspraxia* (Fisher et al., 1991).

Vestibular System

The vestibular system can be characterized as a sensory system that detects the pull of gravity and coordinates adjustments to the movements of the head and neck. The vestibular system begins by receiving information through visual and auditory stimuli and through vestibular receptors that are located within the inner ear. Present in the inner ear are structures known as the *semicircular canals,* which are connected to the vestibulocochlear nerve. The vestibulocochlear nerve then carries the information to receptors in the brain stem and cerebellum that integrate this information to produce a desired adaptive response. The receptors operate on a subconscious level and are continuously working to counteract the constant gravitational pull. The goal of this network is to maintain equilibrium and detect head position during directional movement. Another important function of the semicircular canals has to do with the fluid-filled chambers and the cilia that line the perimeter of these canals. The cilia are tiny receptors that are activated as movement of the head and neck occurs. The information received from these receptors is crucial to counteract gravity and promote balance and stability. The vestibular system works with the tactile, proprioceptive, visual, and auditory systems to provide body awareness, visual perception, bilateral integration, position in space, and movement discrimination (Ayres, 1979).

Effects of Sensory Defensiveness on the Vestibular System

Children with sensory defensiveness often experience dysfunction in the vestibular system. Characteristics of children with disorganized vestibular systems include hypotonic muscle tone; deficits in endurance, bilateral integration, equilibrium, and postural responses; and a positive postrotary nystagmus (Ayres, 1979). Dysfunction can be observed in difficulty with visual tracking, gravitational insecurity, and an intolerance to rotational movement. Functionally, these deficits can be seen in eye–hand coordination, use of fine-motor coordination for hand-held utensils, reading, and gross-motor activities (Fisher et al., 1991). The problems children have in everyday childhood occupations lie in their inability to coordinate the mind–brain–body relationships in performing these complex motor skills (Fisher et al., 1991). The vestibular system is ultimately responsible for stabilizing the visual field to allow a person to focus on the task at hand and complete a goal-directed activity. A child with an overactive response to movement is unable to regulate his or her posture, position in space, or visual field, so the system is unable to send clear messages from the brain to control the movements of the muscles and joints effectively (Ayres, 1979).

Behavior Problems in Sensory Defensiveness

Children with sensory defensiveness often are identified by their teachers, parents, and community professionals through observation of maladaptive or stereotypic behaviors. Dunn, Smith-Myles, and Orr (2002) suggested that perhaps those behaviors serve an organizing function as their repetitiveness provides a method for assisting the child in equalizing hyporesponsiveness and hyperresponsiveness. Parents and teachers tend to be quick in disciplining children with sensory defensiveness when their behaviors are not socially acceptable, an approach that may perpetuate poorly developed self-concept.

Socialization challenges often exist with poor sensory processing. Either children cannot engage in appropriate social behaviors because they have poor sensory processing, or they have poor sensory processing because they have not been able to interact effectively with their environment or engage in the complexities of social situations (Dunn et al., 2002). Often, these children cannot assist in finding solutions to their behaviors because they themselves cannot fully understand the disorganization, which is occurring on a subconscious level. They may appear to be consistently agitated in group situations because they cannot determine what they need to regulate their systems. They also may appear to be uncomfortable around others and prefer not to engage in normal childhood activities. These deficits may make them subject to ridicule and name calling by their peers. The child with sensory defensiveness is less likely to try new experiences and is apt to display poor coping skills in new or unfamiliar situations (Ayres, 1979).

Language Problems in Sensory Defensiveness

Slowly developing language skills may be one of the first signs to parents or teachers that a child is experiencing sensory processing problems. Verbal communication is a primary means of social interaction, and people with impairment in communication are at a great disadvantage in developing necessary skills for learning (Case-Smith, 1996). Language can generally be classified as receptive and expressive. When a child has difficulties with receptive language, the brain is not able to fully integrate or comprehend incoming (receptive) information, either auditory or written, perhaps in part because of an inability to inhibit extraneous stimuli from disrupting his or her focus. Speech, or expressive language, is related directly to postural stability, including muscle strength, tone, and function; respiratory control; sensory processing and integration; motor planning; and the coordination of the speech mechanism (American Hippotherapy Association, 2000). The brain may become disorganized or overstimulated, making it difficult for the child to organize himself or herself and to concentrate (VandenBerg, 2001). Because of overwhelming incoming stimuli and the inability to filter out nonessential input, the child with sensory defensiveness is more prone to be delayed in developing speech and language skills. Communication is necessary for children to verbalize their wants, needs, and desires to their parents and others. Lack of functional communication may result in an irritable, socially inappropriate, disruptive, passive, or generally unhappy child because of an inability to get basic needs satisfied (Ayres, 1979).

Effects on Independence in Activities of Daily Living

Children who avoid age-appropriate motor and social activities may experience limited development in the areas of fine- and gross-motor strength, motor planning, eye–hand coordination, tactile perception, visual–perceptual skills, and social skills. All are foundational for development of independence in activities of daily living. Performance areas such as dressing, bathing, grooming, and feeding also are affected by sensory defensiveness (Case-Smith, Allen, & Pratt 1995).

A child with sensory defensiveness may not like the textures of food or the feel of water or certain fabrics. Activities such as painting, playing in the sand, or accidental bumps from classmates may produce a response that may appear to be severe in light of the situation. Such episodes can lead to a lack of social acceptance and perpetuation of a poorly developed self-concept (Ayres, 1979). Children diagnosed with sensory defensiveness are unlikely to initiate play with their peers or to attempt new opportunities for developmental growth. Frustrations over difficulty with everyday tasks that their peers accomplish with relative ease may increase the likelihood of decreased self-confidence (Case-Smith et al., 1996).

Benefits of Hippotherapy

People participating in a hippotherapy program experience many benefits aside from the obvious physical benefits. Hippotherapy techniques have a profound effect on sensory systems in people experiencing sensory defensiveness and can lead to increased functional independence in physical, social, and cognitive areas. The following sections describe specific benefits to sensory areas.

Vestibular System

Ayres (1979) stated that stimulation of the vestibular system is one of the most powerful means available for therapeutic remediation of sensory integrative dysfunction. The unique, rhythmic movement of the horse provides continuous vestibular stimulation throughout the activity. This movement can be graded by using a horse with a quicker, shorter gait to provide more vestibular input or a horse with a longer, slower gait to provide less input. The length of the session can be shortened or lengthened to fit the needs of the client. Change in direction of the horse or of the rider also provides a change in vestibular input.

Proprioceptive System

Hippotherapy also affects the proprioceptive system. The rider's proprioceptors are activated continuously in the session, resulting in improved proprioception (Engel, 1984). The proprioceptive input assists in the regulation and integration of all other sensory systems. Proprioceptive input can be graded by the speed of the horse, change in direction of the horse, change in direction of the rider, and length of the session.

Tactile System

Throughout the session, the rider receives a steady stream of tactile input, including deep and light touch, warmth from the horse's body, textures of the pads or other tack used, and pressure sensations to all body parts. All of these stimuli can assist in decreasing tactile defensiveness (Spink, 1993). Riding also has physical benefits, including relaxation of spastic muscles through

215

the smooth, rhythmic movement of the horse (MacKinnon, Noh, Laliberte, Lariviere, & Allan, 1995). Reductions in abnormally high muscle tone and increased relaxation have been noted (Bertoti, 1988).

Olfactory System

The *olfactory system*—the sensory tract that organizes and processes odorants—is stimulated by the many smells of a stable or ranch environment (Engel, 1984). Riders are so engaged in maintaining balance and postural control that they often are able to tolerate smells they would otherwise find noxious. As a result, sensory defensiveness to olfactory stimuli may decrease.

Visual System

During hippotherapy, riders are exposed to many visual stimuli that they must integrate and organize. Hippotherapy often takes place in a circular or oval-shaped arena, which produces somewhat repetitive visual stimulation. This repetition is helpful to people who are defensive in their visual system. Predictability of oncoming stimuli may be comforting to a rider.

Auditory System

Auditory stimuli also are present in the voices of the handler, sidewalkers, the horse's steps, other noises the horse may make (such as sneezing), and all other sounds common to an equestrian environment. As riders attempt to localize and interpret the sounds, they can learn to identify and integrate noxious sounds and sounds that calm or interest them.

Case Study

"Sarah" is a 7-year-old girl with a primary diagnosis of Down syndrome and a secondary diagnosis of cerebral palsy. This section describes Sarah's level of functioning in the areas of gross-motor, fine-motor, and self-care skills, as well as communication and sensory processing, at the time of her initial occupational therapy evaluation prior to the initiation of hippotherapy.

Presenting Strengths and Deficits

Upon initial evaluation, Sarah required moderate to maximum support to maintain balance while walking. Sarah would take steps with her mother holding both of her hands, but she fatigued after short distances of only 5 to 10 feet. When sitting and walking, Sarah demonstrated a lordotic posture of the spine secondary to lower trunk weakness; she also had weakness of the neck musculature and hypermobility of the hips and

spine. Sarah was unable to maintain sitting balance on a therapy ball for more than 10 seconds without falling forward and to the side. She exhibited the underlying hypotonicia characteristic of children with Down syndrome; extensor hypertonicity in extremities also was present. Upon examination, all other joints demonstrated normal range of motion. Sarah's attention to objects or tasks averaged 10 seconds. She did not initiate or maintain eye contact at any time during the evaluation process, nor was she reported to make or maintain eye contact at home or in the school environment.

Fine Motor Skills

Sarah participated in minimal object manipulation and used open palms to explore unfamiliar objects. She indicated tactile aversion reactions to 90% of the objects presented during the evaluation.

Self-Care Skills

Sarah's mother provided information on Sarah's level of independence with self-care. At the time of the initial evaluation, Sarah was able to cooperate and assist with dressing, but she was dependent with each task involved. Maximum assistance was required for all areas of undressing, except for removing shoes and socks, which Sarah was able to do independently. Dressing and undressing skills were scored at approximately a 1-year-old level. At the time of the evaluation, Sarah was not toilet trained.

Sensory Processing

Sarah's mother completed a questionnaire on Sarah's observed levels of function in tactile, vestibular, visual, olfactory, and auditory areas. Her mother reported that Sarah liked to initiate touch and had a strong need to touch objects and people when she initiated the interaction. In contrast, she disliked the feeling of certain clothing, rough food textures, and taking a shower. She would not initiate grasp on any object, and when objects (e.g., blocks) were placed in her hands, she would immediately throw them or randomly release them. She also had no controlled release of objects and was unable to place objects in containers or visually follow objects with her eyes. When Sarah was overstimulated, she would pull hair or scratch her therapist, parent, or teacher. She usually was easily calmed and redirected by using a tape player with her favorite musical tape. Sarah enjoyed being rocked, swung, and tossed in the air. Her mother reported that Sarah spun or "whirled" more than other children. In addition, she displayed no fear in space (e.g., fear of stairs or heights) but would lose her balance easily. Sarah had difficulty focusing on faraway objects and was distracted by visual stimuli within the environment. Her mother reported no olfactory or gustatory irregularities.

Sarah's mother reported that Sarah seemed unusually sensitive to loud sounds of certain tones. In contrast, Sarah found familiar sounds, such as certain songs, calming and pleasant, as evidenced by her swaying to the music and fixating on the radio or tape player. Sarah also was unable to understand or follow simple directions or instructions, and demonstrated a significant delay in speech development. She used only grunts and other sounds to indicate pleasure or displeasure. Sarah's father reported she was able to use some simple signs of her own creation and understood better if signs and voice were used in combination.

Treatment Techniques

Prescribed treatment goals for Sarah were as follows:
1. Normalize general muscle tone for Sarah to accomplish unsupported and independent sitting.
2. Improve ability to initiate and maintain eye contact.
3. Improve functional communication through the use of three manually signed words.
4. Improve use of bilateral upper extremities for sustained grasp, accurate placement, and volitional release of objects by either hand.
5. Improve bilateral lower-extremity strength and endurance for sustained standing for improved independence in transfers and activities of daily living.

Treatment techniques targeting Sarah's goals included a combination of sensory integration and hippotherapy within the session once per week and a daily home program to be conducted by her mother. Evaluation of progress would take place after 12 weeks of treatment. Some of the specific activities used within each treatment session are described below.

The evaluation revealed that the key to a successful treatment session for Sarah depended on first normalizing her muscle tone for her to achieve upright unsupported sitting on the horse, three instances of initiation of eye contact with the therapist, successful grasp-and-release of three objects into a designated container, and ambulation on the mounting ramp with hand-help assistance, and finishing going up and down twice without resistance or instances of suddenly sitting down. It was determined that consistency in the sequence of techniques used each session was vital to the achievement of the weekly observable responses.

In addition to weekly hippotherapy sessions, Sarah received Deep Pressure and Proprioceptive Technique, the sensory diet developed by occupational therapist and child psychologist Patricia Wilbarger, as well as joint compression to her upper and lower extremities while on the horse and at home three times daily. These activities helped increase her arousal level and activate her proprioceptive and vestibular systems as well as observably decreased her avoidance responses to tactile activities.

By stimulating her sensory system in the manner described above, Sarah was better able to visually attend to tasks involving fine-motor placement of objects in container; follow instructions to stand and walk up the ramp and participate in activities more appropriately; initiate and maintain eye contact with the therapist and assistants when instructed "Look at me"; and use her tactile system in a more functional way to sustain grasp on objects and manipulate them appropriately. Each session, Sarah participated in hippotherapy for 20 minutes, followed by functional activities in the clinical setting for 30 minutes. Sarah was encouraged to hold a small tape player with both hands while receiving the movement to encourage the sustained grasp of the object and the use of her trunk and pelvic muscles, rather than her upper extremities, to maintain balance. Holding the tape player also gave Sarah an opportunity to practice bilateral coordination, and the music assisted in decreasing aggressive behaviors (such as pulling the therapist's hair or scratching the assistants) when overstimulated. The therapist and volunteers sang and talked to her to encourage eye contact and increase social awareness.

Throughout each session, Sarah participated in activities on horseback that targeted her goals. Tactile activities included exploring various textures, such as shaving cream, clay, different types of cloth, carpet, sandpaper, and lotion. She also threw balls of various textures into buckets held to the side of the horse and participated in fine-motor activities such as removing clothespins from the side of a bucket or placed all around the horse and saddle pad, and by placing pegs in pegboards or blocks in containers. During these tactile and fine-motor activities, Sarah was encouraged to use her manual signs to communicate "go," "more," and "all done." Because the movement of the horse was observed to be motivational for Sarah, hippotherapy provided a great opportunity to work on decreasing her tactile defensiveness by requiring her to place her hands on the fuzzy saddle pad to indicate that she was ready to go forward.

Sarah was able to tolerate a wider variety of textures while on horseback than previously noted; various textures of cloth were rubbed briskly over her upper and lower extremities during her hippotherapy session. She was better able to tolerate the textures while on the moving horse than in the clinical setting. The increased tactile input to her system helped balance or normalize her tactile processing. After four sessions, Sarah was able to tolerate, without throwing a tantrum, the textures rubbed on her arms and legs while in the clinical setting.

Results

After 3 months of hippotherapy, Sarah made impressive gains toward many of her treatment goals. She was able to sit upright on a moving horse with minimal physical assistance (contact guard by two assistants) and moderate verbal assistance (one verbal cue to "sit up tall" every 3 minutes) 60% to 75% of the time (12–15 minutes of the 20-minute session). She also was able to engage in object manipulation for 5 minutes with intermittent moderate physical assistance to keep her positioned. She demonstrated significant increases in lower-extremity strength, as observed by her ability to maintain sustained unsupported standing for 3 minutes while accomplishing transfers on and off the horse and in and out of her car. She also experienced normalization of muscle tone as observed by her ability to maintain upright sitting on a moving horse and maintain extremities in sustained patterns of grasping objects. Her endurance during ambulation improved, as measured by her ability to walk a distance of 50 feet with one hand being held, compared with the initial evaluation of 5 to 10 feet. She exhibited fewer episodes of arms elevated in an extensor position and falling over backward on the horse when losing her balance and when throwing a tantrum.

Gains in the area of communication included the ability to sign "more" with minimal verbal cuing and no physical assistance and to initiate the signs for "go" and "finished" by placing her hands in the therapist's hands and finishing the signs with hand-over-hand assistance. Sarah demonstrated a noted decrease in tactile defensiveness; she became able to touch rough, dry textures, such as sandpaper, and initiated touch of the saddle pad with only verbal cues during hippotherapy sessions. She continued to demonstrate avoidance reactions to smooth, wet textures, but she would put lotion on her arms with moderate verbal cues and intermittent hand-over-hand assistance.

Sarah's functional mobility improved, as demonstrated by her ability to move through the developmental positions (sitting on the floor, kneeling, pull-to-stand) with moderate assistance of one person for safety. She could independently right herself to midline spontaneously when off balance in stationary sitting, either on the horse or in a chair, 50% of the time (5 of 10 observed off-balance reactions per 1-hour session). She demonstrated an apparent significant increase in social awareness by making and momentarily maintaining eye contact with the therapist 30% to 50% of the time (3–5 times out of 10 verbal cues to "look at me" per session).

Conclusion

Hippotherapy, combined with sensory integration techniques, appears to have been effective in helping Sarah improve sensory processing and decrease sensory defensive reactions. Initially, Sarah demonstrated behaviors consistent with sensory defensiveness. Hippotherapy, in combination with sensory integration techniques, helped provide the necessary sensory input and vestibular stimulation, deep pressure, tactile experiences, and environmental stimuli to assist Sarah in improving her functional adaptive responses to the environment. Her mother reported that similar improvements were observed in the home and school environments: improved eye contact, tolerance for various textures, ambulation (with hand-held assistance over greater distances), sustained standing (which assisted with transfers in and out of the bathtub at home), and communication (signing "more" during mealtimes). During the test period, hippotherapy was the only therapy Sarah received. Her mother reported that hippotherapy made the most significant difference in helping Sarah achieve her goals.

Acknowledgments

Special thanks to the following people:
- Thomas Foley, MOTS, Nova Southeastern, Fort Lauderdale, Florida
- Elizabeth Grant, OTS, Spalding University, Louisville, Kentucky
- Lauren Snepp, OTS, Eastern Kentucky University, Richmond
- Heather VanDevelde, MOTS, Nova Southeastern University, Fort Lauderdale, Florida
- Beth Woods, MOTS, University of Alabama–Birmingham.

References

Allen, A. S., Case-Smith, J., & Pratt, P. N. (1996). *Occupational therapy for children* (3rd ed.). St. Louis, MO: Mosby.

American Hippotherapy Association. (2000). *Introduction to hippotherapy: Classic principles and applications: Workshop manual.* Damascus, PA: Author.

Ayres, A. J. (1979). *Sensory integration and the child.* Los Angeles: Western Psychological Services.

Bertoti, D. B. (1988). Effect of therapeutic horseback riding on posture in children with cerebral palsy. *Physical Therapy, 68,* 1505–1512.

Cohen, H. (1999). *Neuroscience for rehabilitation* (2nd ed.). Philadelphia: Lippincott Williams & Wilkins.

DeGroot, J., & Chusid, J. G. (1998). *Correlative neuroanatomy* (12th ed.). Norwalk, CT: Appleton & Lange.

Dunn, W. (2001). The sensations of everyday life: Empirical, theoretical, and pragmatic considerations [2001 Eleanor Clarke Slagle Lecture]. *American Journal of Occupational Therapy, 55,* 608–620.

Dunn, W., Smith-Myles, B., & Orr, S. (2002). Sensory processing issues associated with Asperger syndrome: A preliminary investigation. *American Journal of Occupational Therapy, 56,* 97–102.

Engel, B. T. (1984). The horse as a modality for occupational therapy. *Occupational Therapy in Healthcare, 1,* 41–47.

Fisher, A. G., Murray, E. A., & Bundy, A. C. (1991). *Sensory integration: Theory and practice.* Philadelphia: F. A. Davis.

Isaacson, R. L. (1982). *The limbic system* (2nd ed.). New York: W. B. Saunders.

Jacobs, K. (2004). *Quick reference dictionary for occupational therapy* (4th ed.). Thorofare, NJ: Slack.

Knickerbocker, B. M. (1980). *A holistic approach to the treatment of learning disorders.* Thorofare, NJ: Slack.

MacKinnon, J. R., Noh, S., Laliberte, D., Lariviere, J., & Allan, D. E. (1995). Therapeutic horseback riding: A review of the literature. *Physical and Occupational Therapy in Pediatrics, 15,* 1–15.

Parham, L. D., & Mailloux, Z. (1995). Sensory integration and children with learning disabilities. In J. Case-Smith, P. N. Pratt, & A. S. Allen (Eds.), *Occupational therapy in children* (pp. 307–355). St. Louis, MO: Mosby.

Schaaf, R., Miller, L. J., Sewall, D., & O'Keefe, S. (2003). Children with disturbances in sensory processing: A pilot study examining the role of the parasympathetic nervous system. *American Journal of Occupational Therapy, 57,* 442–449.

Spink, M. A. (1993). *Developmental riding therapy: A team approach to assessment and treatment.* Tucson, AZ: Therapy Skill Builders.

Trott, M., Laurel M. K., & Windeck, S. L. (1993). *Sensibilities: Understanding sensory integration.* Tucson, AZ: Therapy Skill Builders.

VandenBerg, N. (2001). The use of a weighted vest to increase on-task behavior in children with attention difficulties. *American Journal of Occupational Therapy, 55,* 621–628.

Wilbarger, P., & Royeen, C. B. (1987, May). *Tactile defensiveness: Theory, applications, and treatment.* Annual Interdisciplinary Doctoral Conference. Boston University, Sargent College.

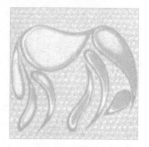

...virtue shall be bound into the hair of thy forelock...
I have given thee the power of flight without wings.
—The Koran

CHAPTER 28

Sensory Integration and Hippotherapy

Paula Hueners, MEd, OTR

Ayres (1972) defined *sensory integration* as "the neurological process that organizes sensation from one's own body and from the environment and makes it possible to use the body effectively within the environment" (p. 11). Sensory integration theory does not approach the person as a passive recipient of environmentally imposed stimuli; rather, a person not only processes sensation but also organizes and integrates it to form a meaningful outcome. A meaningful outcome occurs through what Ayres called *adaptive response*—an adjustment to environmental demands (Ayres, 1979). Implicit in the concept of the adaptive response is the active participation of the person, who actively processes and organizes responses to the changing environment. Adaptive response is, in effect, a measure of the ability to cope and successfully meet an environmental challenge. It is self-organizing, a forward drive of competence, and active rather than passive.

Kimball (1999) explained that the sensory integration frame of reference is applied when sensory system processing deficits make it difficult for appropriate adaptive responses. She identified three levels to consider when addressing sensory integration functions:

1. Sensory system modulation (underarousal–overarousal) issues include the following components:
   - Tactile, auditory, oral, olfactory, visual, proprioception arousal levels
   - Relationship to gravity
   - Movement level
   - Attention level
   - Postrotary nystagmus
   - Sensitivity to movement
   - Emotional level.
2. The functional support capabilities help integrate and modulate input from the arousal–reactivity and information–discriminative components of the sensory systems, including the following components:
   - Suck–swallow–breathe
   - Tactile discrimination
   - Co-contraction
   - Muscle tone
   - Proprioception
   - Balance and equilibrium
   - Developmental reflexes
   - Lateralization
   - Bilateral integration.
3. The end products reflect the integration of the modulation and functional support systems through appropriate adaptive responses, as follows:
   - Praxis
   - Form and space perception
   - Behavior
   - Academics (language and articulation)
   - Emotional tone activity level
   - Environmental mastery.

During treatment, occupational therapists often use a combination of frames of references to meet the needs of a client. When using any frame of reference (e.g., neurodevelopmental, motor acquisitional, sensory integration, biomechanical, psychosocial), it is important for the therapist to understand why he or she is using it and to be aware of how the approach affects the results of treatment (Kramer & Hinojosa, 1999). Motor acquisition and sensory integration are frames of reference often used within a treatment session. They can be differentiated not by the activity itself but also the reasons for using the activity and the expected outcome. For example, in a treatment session using the horse, the therapist can be "teaching" grasp and manipulative control on the reins but allowing the client to direct his or her own sensory experiences to meet individual needs through choosing developmental positions on the horse, choosing the type of games to be played, and guiding the pace and intensity of the session; in the meantime, the therapist grades the amount of stimulation to maintain organized responses. Intervention under a sensory integration frame of reference is mainly client-directed. The therapist often is nurturing and playful and is involved as an active participant in the treatment activities. Because the goal is to continually monitor the nervous system for effective adaptations to the environment, the idea is not to teach skills but to facilitate adaptive responses, both physically and emotionally.

Applying Sensory Integration to Hippotherapy

Lawton-Shirley (2002) explained that the provision of enhanced sensation is inherent to hippotherapy. Moreover, under certain circumstances (i.e., when the rider is stretching his or her abilities to respond in a more effective way than ever before), involvement and the demand for adaptive behavior also are inherent to hippotherapy. For example, a rider with sensory integrative dysfunction who moves independently into quadruped on the horse's back and remains in that position as the horse moves is likely involved in an activity that reflects the principles of sensory integration theory. When both enhanced sensation and the demand for an adaptive behavior are present, hippotherapy could be viewed as overlapping with intervention that reflects the principles of sensory integration.

Goals addressed and activities used with a particular rider, however, frequently cause hippotherapy to fall outside the traditional construct of sensory integration. For example, activities designed to reduce muscle tone and improve passive range of motion with a rider who has cerebral palsy fall outside the construct of sensory integration. Similarly, activities designed to maintain muscle strength in a rider with muscular dystrophy would not be considered to be sensory integrative in nature.

Sensory Input

Riding a horse provides constant sensory information, including tactile, visual, auditory, vestibular, and proprioceptive input. This enhanced information is derived from a number of sources. For example, grooming and maintaining sustained contact with the horse while riding provide significant tactile input. The movement that accompanies different gaits, sudden starting and stop-

ping, changing directions, and assuming different positions while riding (e.g., prone, supine, inversion) provides opportunities for enhanced vestibular sensation. Actively changing positions and independently maintaining a position as the horse moves provides intense proprioceptive sensation. Feedback from activated normalized postural movements enhances postural responses. Enhanced sensation facilitates the attainment of a number of different postural and sensorimotor adaptive responses (Lawton-Shirley, 2002). For example, many riders may do better engaging in the grooming aspect of the horse after a certain amount of input versus the traditional grooming before the ride. To attain the level of alertness and readiness for engagement, the rider may need to have sensory support during the riding, such as oral, auditory, tactile, or increased proprioceptive input throughout or at the beginning.

Sensory Integrative Framework During Hippotherapy: A Case Example

"John" has learning disabilities and is identified with poor vestibular–proprioceptive processing, with clinical observations including low proximal muscle tone and hyperextensibility of his elbows, wrists, and fingers. John is unable to assume prone extension or maintain head position in supine flexion; he also has poor postural background movements and delayed equilibrium reactions. Praxis concerns include bilateral motor coordination and sequencing; inability to complete imitative sequenced motor actions; difficulty identifying left and right body parts; and needs to visually direct the isolative control of hands, arms, and fingers. Problems with sensory modulation and tactile processing also were identified, and John's aversive responses to touch, movement, and auditory input and his somatodyspraxia dysfunction were of concern. Treatment needed to focus first on sensory modulation and aversive or defensive reactions to sensory input within home, school, and recreational environments so that the client could be attentive to the input instead of being in a flight–fright–fight mode during interactive play.

Treatment began with allowing time for John to be introduced to the various horse-related activities so that he could acquire a comfort level and understanding of the options in this new "play" environment. Once he became acclimated to the opportunities of what was available for his nervous system and his sense of self, then John and the therapist talked about how to proceed with challenges that supported his inner drive and his desire for accomplishment.

Planning and Implementing Treatment

After John became acclimated to the equestrian environment, treatment proceeded as follows:

- *Modulate sensory arousal needs.* Addressing John's defensive responses was accomplished both on and off the horse using a sensory diet along with supplemental therapy approaches prior to horse time, such as therapeutic listening, metronome, deep-touch pressure techniques, and rhythmic repetitive activities. Oral motor exercises were an option to help with modulation needs both on and off the horse.
- *Address functional support capabilities.* Once aversive responses to sensory input decreased and John was less vigilant to noxious stimuli or insecurities, then therapy focused on more mature responses. John used the developmental positions on the horse while participating in left–right games and activities, suck–blow activities, and finding small items in a pouch without use of his vision for games. All of these activities challenged his endurance.
- *Focus on end-product activities.* End-product activities required higher level adaptive responses for postural–ocular and bilateral skills. To challenge John's processing abilities, he planned and executed sequential actions that had rhythm and timing components; challenges to academic, language, and perceptual skills were incorporated into the tasks.

Summary

Hippotherapy reflects occupation. Grooming the horse represents a meaningful activity for many riders. For some people, hippotherapy provides the opportunity to develop competency in or mastery of a recreational activity or competitive sport. Interacting with the horse may lead to a special bond between the animal and the rider. Interacting with other people involved in the program provides the basis for development of friendships and opportunities to practice social skills (Lawton-Shirley, 2002).

Parham (2002) explained how sensory integration contributes to what, how, and why a person chooses particular occupations at a particular time in the life cycle and is therefore a factor in shaping life outcomes. Because occupation involves acting on environmental opportunities, can we say that engagement in occupation leads to changes in a person's sensory integrative abilities and in neurological substrates that support those abilities?

Keeping track of clients' progress well after the occupational therapist's work is finished is helpful in understanding life outcomes, impact of therapy, and occupational choices (along with successes and failures). Research in this area is significantly limited; as therapists, we can maintain a vigilant awareness of this process of understanding in our clients and the impact of occupational therapy.

References

Ayres, A. J. (1972). *Sensory integration and learning disorders.* Los Angeles: Western Psychological Services.

Ayres, A. J. (1979). *Sensory integration and the child.* Los Angeles: Western Psychological Services.

Kimball, J. G. (1999). Sensory integration frame of reference: Theoretical base, function/dysfunction continua, and guide to evaluation. In P. Kramer & J. Hinojosa (Eds.), *Frames of reference for pediatric occupational therapy* (2nd ed.). Baltimore: Lippincott Williams & Wilkins.

Kramer, P., & Hinojosa, J. (1999). *Frames of reference for pediatric occupational therapy* (2nd ed.). Baltimore: Lippincott Williams & Wilkins.

Lawton-Shirley, N. (2002). Hippotherapy. In A. C. Bundy, S. J. Lane, & E. A. Murray (Eds.), *Sensory integration theory and practice* (2nd ed., pp. 350–352). Philadelphia: F. A. Davis.

Parham, D. L. (2002). Sensory integration and occupation. In A. C. Bundy, S. J. Lane, & E. A. Murray (Eds.), *Sensory integration theory and practice* (2nd ed., pp. 413–434). Philadelphia: F. A. Davis.

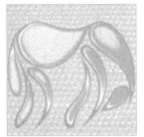

. . . I have been fearfully and wonderfully made; marvelous is thy workmanship.
—Psalm 139:14

CHAPTER 29

Improving Pediatric Cognitive Function in Equine-Assisted Occupational Therapy and Hippotherapy

Heather L. Gohmert-Dionne, MOT, OTR/L

In occupational therapy, many clients have limited or impaired cognitive function. Pediatric clients are no different, except that they may experience the most dramatic changes in cognition when appropriately treated. The unique hippotherapy and equine-assisted therapy settings can contribute to those changes and help improve cognition for young clients.

The brain weighs approximately 3 pounds, is 78% water, and has almost 1 million miles of nerve fibers (Acredolo & Goodwyn, 2000; Jensen 1998); yet, we are only beginning to discover how it works. According to Healy (1999), it is estimated that from conception to birth, more than 250,000 neurons per minute develop, resulting in approximately 100 billion neurons at birth. Moreover, by age 3 years, children have an estimated 1,000 trillion synaptic connections—about twice that of an adult.

In recent years, significant effort has been put forth in studying the developing brain of the child, and considerable emphasis has been placed on enhancing cognitive functioning during the formative years. As therapists, can we do more to improve the cognitive functioning of our pediatric clients?

According to Thompson (2004), "Healthy brain development relies on people to provide stimulation that organizes connections in the cortex for language and complex thought" (p. 17). After studying several early-development programs, Storfer, president of the Foundation for Brain Research in Douglaston, New York, stated that the quality of the intellectual environment during the first 2 years of life can have "a dramatic and lasting difference in measured intelligence" (Cornish, 1991, p. 49). Frederick Goodwin, the former director of the National Institute of Mental Health,

stated, "You can't make a 70 IQ person into a 120 IQ person, but you can change their IQ measure in different ways, perhaps as much as 20 points up or down, based on their environment" (Healy, 1999, p. 10). For some people, a change of 15 to 20 IQ points could place them in classes for the gifted; for others, it could mean remaining a special education classroom.

According to Acredolo and Goodwyn (2000), scientists until recently believed that genetics were the sole determinant of a child's cognitive potential. Scientists further concluded that the brain's "wiring," or synaptic density, was primarily attributable to heredity and physical maturation. Fortunately, those views have been dispelled. Storfer (Cornish, 1991) stated that genetics are responsible for approximately 70% of one's cognitive potential, leaving 30% to be influenced by environment. The automatic process of synaptic growth accounts for a small portion of the "1,000 trillion synaptic connections that a newborn's billions of neurons will make. That leaves hundreds of trillions of the connections to be determined by an individual's experiences" (Acredolo & Goodwyn, 2000, p. 6).

Equestrian settings offer clients enriched environments full of unique experiences. Equine-assisted therapy often is the first time a client has ever ridden a horse, reached into a bucket of oats, or smelled fresh-cut hay. Diamond (1990) documented the benefits of enriching environments by examining the quality of synaptic connections in rats. One group of rats was exposed to a variety of toys and environments, and the other group had little exposure to those things. Diamond compared the thickness of synaptic connections by measuring the cortical wall thickness in the rats. The rats raised in the enriched environment demonstrated thicker cortical walls than those raised in the impoverished environment. Moreover, her study revealed that the age of the rats placed in an enriched environment significantly affected the cortical wall thickness. Rats placed in the enriched environment later in life did not display the cortical thickness of their younger counterparts. This research implies that the cognitive functioning of pediatric clients may be enhanced through the abundance of environmental opportunities in an equestrian setting.

Recent research supports the idea that brain development is an extended process that is subtly refined throughout life in response to individual experiences (Thompson, 2004). Scientists believe that critical or sensitive periods for brain development exist, the onset and duration of which vary widely throughout the different neural systems of the brain (American Medical Association, 1999). At birth, infants have only one-tenth as many synaptic connections as adults; by age 3, they have twice the number of synapses as adults. By age 14, children have the same amount of synapses as adults (Goff, 2000; Healy, 1999). Scientists agree that in childhood, a window of opportunity exists during which our efforts to learn are most effective (Jensen, 1998). After childhood, *synaptic apoptosis,* or the atrophy and death of the infrequently used synapses, occurs. Repeatedly used synapses develop strong, stable connections, whereas others are pruned or eliminated. Pruning is necessary to allow the brain to become more efficient in its operations (Acredolo & Goodwyn, 2000; Healy, 1999). Extraneous synaptic connections have been associated with several developmental disorders, and possibly are one cause of schizophrenia (Acredolo & Goodwyn, 2000; Healy, 1999).

Creating Enriched Environments in Hippotherapy

An enriched environment is an exciting opportunity for therapists in the hippotherapy and equine-assisted therapy fields. One study found that exposure to nature has positive effects on cognitive functioning: The degree of exposure a child received to nature resulted in a subsequent improvement in cognitive functioning (Wilensky, 2002). In addition, researchers at the University of Michigan at Ann Arbor found that exposure to nature helps renew the capacity for directed attention, which allows a person to focus on a specific task while ignoring extraneous stimuli (Wilensky, 2002).

How do occupational therapists apply findings like these in a hippotherapy setting? First, we must determine what is necessary to improve cognitive function. That includes providing enriched environments, encouraging good health and nutrition, and decreasing stressful situations. Then, we may determine how best to address the specific needs of our clients while maximizing the benefits of our unique setting.

The concepts of an enriched environment and exposure to nature certainly can be applied to hippotherapy and its setting to help clients improve their functioning. In an equine-assisted therapy setting, directed attention also could be improved when small, limited distractions are permitted to occur around clients while they are working with their horses. For instance, while a client is tacking his or her horse, another horse could be led past at a safe distance. Because the distraction is meant for the client, not the horse, this maneuver should be practiced so that neither horse reacts. The length and complexity of each distraction can be safely graded as the client successfully redirects himself or herself back to the task at hand.

Physical changes in the brain occur in enriched environments. The brain structurally modifies itself on the basis of the type and amount of stimuli to which it is exposed (Green, Greenough, & Schlumpf, 1983; Healy, 1999). Studies indicate brain modification can occur within 48 hours of exposure. This transformation of the brain is both "predictable and highly significant" (Jensen, 1998). When the brain is challenged through all its sensory receptors with fresh and changing inputs, new synaptic connections grow, the cortex thickens, and dendritic branching thickens with more spines and larger cell bodies (Healy, 1999). Given these findings, hippotherapy can be an excellent strategy for improving cognitive functioning. Clients' interaction with the horse and its environment affects all sensory receptors and facilitates participation in a treatment plan reflective of individual client goals.

Greenough (1997, cited in Jensen, 1998) stated that learning must be challenging (i.e., providing new information or experiences) and that interactive feedback must be provided in the learning process. The newness of material, the degree of difficulty, and the amount of resources can determine the degree of mental challenge. Other factors include varying the length of task completion, changing the surroundings, and using different instructional strategies (Jensen, 1998). Changing the modes of delivery for instructions can challenge and vary the learning experience. Instructions to the client can be written, drawn on a map, or spoken by a peer. Directions can be offered at each obstacle or given in two- and three-step commands. In hippotherapy, the combinations of obstacles and variety of maneuvers performed are endless and quickly adapted.

Greenough (1997, cited in Jensen, 1998) stated, "[I]deal feedback involves choice: it can be generated and modified at will. If it's hard to get at, or the performance cannot be altered once feedback is received, the brain doesn't learn quickly. Immediate and self generating feedback can come from many sources. . . ." (p. 33). Encouraging clients to work through a problem can give them a basis for generalizing their learning to other environments. Allowing them to make mistakes and find alternative solutions can help teach clients problem-solving strategies help build their confidence.

A trail ride in a safe, controlled setting is a great environmental change for clients. Trail riding offers a good opportunity for clients to absorb and review new learning in a more relaxed atmosphere. According to Hobson (1994), "The association and consolidation process [of learning] can only occur during down time." Hobson's statement implies that a treatment session concluded with a relaxing activity, such a grooming a horse, can help clients develop a better understanding of what they have learned. Having a 9-year-old client develop or negotiate a trail course, either mounted or leading the horse, would be a good way to implement Jensen's (1998) concepts in the context of hippotherapy.

Enrichment and Hippotherapy

Although there are many possibilities for enrichment, those addressed in this chapter are supported by research. Enrichments include movement, language, problem solving, music, and art.

An Enriched Environment Through Movement

According to Richardson (1996), studies indicate that movement (as in hippotherapy) plays a significant role in cognitive functioning. The cerebellum plays a much larger role in cognitive functioning than simply helping to control movement; it contains more than half the brain's neurons (Richardson, 1996). The Veterans Affairs Medical Center in Syracuse has traced pathways from the cerebellum to areas of the brain associated with memory, spatial–temporal perception, and attention (Jensen, 1998; Middleton & Strick, 1994).

In a Seattle school district, third graders studied language arts concepts through dance activities. The students boosted their reading scores by 13% in 6 months, whereas the rest of the district posted a 2% decrease (Gilbert, 1977). According to Calvin (1996), one expla-

nation for improved cognitive functioning is that the prefrontal cortex and the rear two-thirds of the frontal lobes are engaged with novel movements.

Calvin's research suggests that hippotherapy and equine-assisted therapy can affect cognitive functioning. Riding a horse often is a new experience for clients. Having an engaged rider transition into a different positions to perform functional tasks increases the impact of the horse's movement as well as the degree of enrichment offered in the treatment.

An Enriched Environment Through Language

In addition to immersing children in high-quality speech, reading to them is another means of developing synaptic pathways (Jensen, 1998). Language activities can be incorporated in a number of ways in hippotherapy and equine-assisted therapy—many of which can be done while a rider is mounted. For example, nursery rhymes and poems can be recited and recorded short stories can be played while riding. Older riders may be quizzed on what they heard to challenge memory and recall. Vestibular stimulation, which occurs with movement, may assist with memory and recall; this has been the experience of the author and is supported by research (Jensen, 1998; Middleton & Strick, 1994).

Therapists can practice rhyming exercises (related to the horse), even if the child is unable to repeat them. Including nursery rhymes and rhyming books (e.g., *The Cat in the Hat;* Seuss, 1957/1985) in a child's library could help provide a foundation for practicing. Moreover, a library can be created at the riding center so that clients can "check out" books about horses or related topics.

Setting up "stations" in the arena can incorporate reading activities in the riding session. The author has found it helpful to have at least two barrels placed in opposite corners of the arena, on which the needed items, such as books or a tape recorder, can be placed. The reading activities can be performed in brief, 2 to 3-minute sessions 4 to 5 times throughout the mounted activity while standing stationary at the barrel or traversing between the barrels. For clients whose lack of head and trunk control impede academic performance, positioning them prone over the side of the horse's barrel and encouraging them to look up at flash cards or reading material can strengthen the back and neck extensors. As posture improves, the activity can be graded from static (horse still) to dynamic (horse walking). Many of the items can be placed on a clipboard to keep pieces in order. Some reading-readiness and letter recognition activities can be converted into magnetized activities by using a baking pan as the work surface and purchasing or gluing letters or words to the tops of magnets. When the client is asked to retrieve an object off the baking pan, fine-motor strengthening is incorporated into language development. Magnets can be graded for their strength.

An activity that combines many developmental components, such as reaching and grasping, with reading readiness is fishing with a clothespin "lure" tied to the end of the line to hold flash cards. A rear-facing client must grasp and remove the flash card from the clothespin to read it; the activity encourages visual tracking, bilateral integration of the upper extremities, and fine-motor strengthening. Activities such as "I Spy," scavenger hunts, and following maps and road signs can be enjoyable ways to practice reading skills while teaching *topographical orientation,* the ability to orient oneself within one's environment. Riders' developmental levels will determine appropriate levels of challenge. For instance, younger riders can try to identify letters, shapes, colors, numerals, and animals. Older riders can be given simple or detailed lists of items to find during the ride while learning to read a map. For clients who have difficulty with memory and recall, the task can be to remember the items without reviewing the list. Start with one to three items and grade the activity by increasing the number of items to remember and find. For example, riders can "dial" a phone number on horseback by riding to specified numerals.

While enjoying the gratification of helping to care for their horse, clients can follow a recipe card to prepare and feed their horse. Depending on a client's skill level, the ration could be represented as pictures of two cans of grain and one flake of hay. Or, rations could be presented with more complexity, with oral or written instructions with multiple ingredients for multiple horses; this approach requires the client to complete the task in a structured sequence.

An Enriched Environment Through Problem-Solving

Problem-solving, such as learning how to tack a horse, is considered an important activity to help create new and stronger dendritic branches and synaptic connections and thereby build a stronger brain (Jensen, 1998). Concrete problems are appropriate to introduce to children starting between ages 1 and 2. By age 11 or 12, the corpus callosum is fully developed and the brain is ready for complex, abstract problems (Hannaford, 1995). Solving a problem correctly is not necessary for

brain development; rather, it is the process of attempting to solve the problem that generates neural growth (Jensen, 1998).

Pegboard and jigsaw puzzles are problem-solving activities that can be used in treatment sessions. Puzzles may be assembled by a rider on a static or dynamic horse. They can be made with various degrees of difficulty tailored to the specific needs of each client. Pictures or postcards of horses can be cut into a selected number of pieces or shapes, laminated, magnetized (with adhesive magnetic tape), and assembled on a baking pan.

An Enriched Environment Through Music and Art

According to Acredolo and Goodwyn (2000), some experts now believe that music contributes to the development of temporal–spatial skills. Studies have shown that 3- and 4-year-olds who play the piano were "able to more easily manipulate geometrical forms in their minds, construct three-dimensional models, and generally appreciate shape, movement, and time" (Acredolo & Goodwyn, 2000, p. 151). Healy (1999) reported that passive listening to a 10-minute piano sonata "brings a more orderly and efficient pattern to the electrical impulses that pass through the higher-level processing areas [of the brain]" (p. 69). From the author's experience, having clients with diagnoses such as attention deficit disorder with hyperactivity or autism listen to soft instrumental music while lying prone on the horse, rear-facing (rather than astride), can be a good means of preparing them for the remainder of the therapy session.

Music also influences the mental state of learners by increasing relaxation or arousal. A study conducted with middle school and high school students demonstrated a substantial improvement in reading comprehension when background music was played (Giles, 1991). In addition to assisting memory and serving as a carrier for information, music can "prime" or mobilize neural pathways for clear thought and action in the midst of "neural chatter" (Jensen, 1998). Playing a song can help riders "warm up" physically and mentally. Musical games and rhymes, such as Old MacDonald and Patty Cake, are fun ways to challenge auditory memory, spatial awareness, and body scheme.

Although the "Mozart Effect" is widely recognized as supporting these findings, classical music is not the only acceptable sound for brain building (Healy, 1999). Playing a wide range of melodies and harmonies, such as those heard in the folk music of the various cultures, can be helpful in developing rhythm, sequence, and discrimination skills. The author's observations support that the diagnosis of the client is a critical factor in determining whether and what type of music is appropriate. Music can be too distracting or overstimulating for clients with sensory-related disorders. Other clients can benefit from the increased level of arousal that comes from lively music. Although there is little supporting research, anecdotal reports suggest that horses respond to music as well; faster rhythms encourage a quicker pace and animation of gait. Riders with decreased tone and arousal may benefit from faster horse movement. Just as any new addition to the treatment setting, music should be introduced to the horse before being included in the treatment.

In a study of people with brain injury, researchers discovered that the brain is able to "rewire" itself for more and stronger connections by learning and practicing art (Kolb & Whishaw, 1990). Clients can be encouraged to explore the stable for supplies and art subjects. The stable has highly tactile art supplies and tools, such as hay, grain, and rubber grooming aids. Therapists can encourage clients' artistic pursuit of stable objects. As with problem solving, the process can prove more rewarding than the results.

"Pony Painting" can be a good activity for clients who are fearful of the horse, as well as for those who have socioemotional problems or difficulty tolerating tactile input. As a client applies thinned finger paint to the horse's neck, body, and upper legs, he or she is exploring the horse's body, leading to an increased awareness. Painting the horse can develop a connection between the client and the horse. When the client has finished painting the horse and enjoyed his work, they can rinse the horse off to remove the paint and dry it.

> Allow children to use their own perceptions in developing their imaginations and intuitive skills. They begin to understand that their individuality is appreciated, and as you begin to understand that their standards are not the same as your standards, the right and left hemispheres of the brain will become integrated and creativity will flourish. (Cherry & Nielsen, 1999, p. v)

Effects of Stress on Learning

Jensen (1998) reported that emotional stress appears to take a toll on the brain, resulting in "stressed" neurons, which have fewer and shorter dendrites. Excessive emotional stress also has been linked to poor memory, decreased visual discrimination (i.e., pattern recognition), limited discernment, increased illness, and increased learned helplessness (Jensen, 1998). A study reported in Wilensky (2002) revealed that among 281 children, those with higher exposure to nature were significantly better able to deal with stressful life events than were children in "low-nature" settings. In many hippotherapy settings, clients have the opportunity to connect with nature while working with a horse in a nonstressful environment, allowing them to relax and enjoy their time with the equestrian activity. Grooming and feeding treats can facilitate more personal interactions. Often, this is best achieved with the client standing on the ground near the horse's head where he or she can pet and talk to the horse. Clients must "touch" the horse, and the horse must "touch" them so that it becomes their friend—not merely a modality or tool with which to work.

Role of Hydration on Cognitive Function

Jensen (1998) noted that the brain uses 20% of the body's energy, which is primarily supplied by the blood and circulates approximately 8 gallons of blood per hour, or 198 gallons per day. The body requires 8 to 12 glasses of water daily for optimal brain function. Dehydration is a common problem in many schools, and it is associated with impaired learning (Hannaford, 1995; Jensen, 1998).

As the percentage of water in the blood drops, blood pressure and stress rise. Researchers, using rats, discovered a marked decrease in the hormones associated with stress within 5 minutes of drinking water (Heybach & Vernikos-Danellis, 1979). This research suggests that clients should be encouraged to drink before a session begins as well as throughout the session. Drinking water is especially important because most equine-assisted therapies and hippotherapy are performed outdoors in warm weather, when dehydration is more likely. It is important to educate parents and caregivers to help ensure that clients function optimally in all settings.

One option is to have the client and horse take water breaks together. Doing so provides the therapist with an opportunity to discuss the role of proper nutrition and care of horses as well as to teach clients about their own health needs. If clients prepare feed rations, therapists can discuss and reiterate the role of food, supplements, and vitamins for maintaining a healthy horse as well as a healthy rider.

Summary

The cognitive functioning of a child is determined not only by his or her age and developmental levels but also by the activities and settings in which he or she lives, is nurtured, and performs. Research suggests that hippotherapy and equine-assisted therapy can help improve the cognitive functioning of pediatric clients by providing enriched environments through movement, language, problem-solving activities, music, and art. The horse and its environment, the therapist, and the caregivers play critical roles in ensuring that the client functions optimally in the hippotherapy setting. The caregivers help the client carry over his or her newly-acquired skills developed through hippotherapy.

References

Acredolo, L., & Goodwyn, S. (2000). *Baby minds: Brain-building games your baby will love.* New York: Bantam Books.

American Medical Association. (1999). *Implications of brain development research. Report 15 of the Council on Scientific Affairs (A-99).* Retrieved January 9, 2007, from www.ama-assn.org/ama/pub/category/13576.html.

Calvin, W. (1996). *How the brain thinks.* New York: Basic Books.

Cherry, C., & Nielsen D. M. (1999). *Creative art for the developing child* (3rd ed.). Torrance, CA: Frank Schaffer Publications.

Cornish, E. (Ed.). (1991, May/June). Smarter children in prospect. *The Futurist, 25,* 49.

Diamond, M. (1990). Morphological cortical changes as a consequence of learning and experience. In A. B. Scheibel & A. F. Wechsler (Eds.), *Neurobiology of higher cognitive function.* New York: Guilford.

Gilbert, A. G. (1977). *Teaching the three R's through movement experience.* New York: Macmillan.

Giles, M. M. (1991, November). A little background music please. *Principal Magazine,* 41–44.

Goff, K. G. (2000, June 25). Brainchild. *The Washington Times,* p. 1.

Green, E. J., Greenough, W. T., & Schlumpf, B. E. (1983). Effects of complex or isolated environments on cortical dendrites of middle-aged rats. *Brain Research, 264,* 233–240.

Hannaford, C. (1995). *Smart moves.* Arlington, VA: Great Ocean.

Healy, K. (Ed.). (1999). *Brilliant beginnings: Birth to 12 months.* Long Beach, CA: Brilliant Beginnings.

Heybach, J. P., & Vernikos-Danellis, J. (1979). Inhibition of adrenocorticotrophin secretion during deprivation-induced eating and drinking in rats. *Neuroendocrinology, 28,* 328–329.

Hobson, J. A. (1994). *Chemistry of conscious states.* Boston: Little, Brown.

Hutchinson, M. (1994). *Megabrain power.* New York: Hyperion Books.

Jensen, E. (1998). *Teaching with the brain in mind.* Alexandria, VA: Association for Supervision and Curriculum Development.

Kolb, B., & Whishaw, I. Q. (1990). *Fundamentals of human neuropsychology.* New York: W. H. Freeman.

Middleton, F., & Strick, P. (1994). Anatomical evidence for cerebellar and basal ganglia involvement in higher brain function. *Science, 226,* 458–461.

Richardson, S. (1996). Tarzan's little brain. *Discover Magazine, 17*(11), 100–102.

Seuss, Dr. (1985). *The cat in the hat.* New York: Random House. (Original work published 1957)

Thompson, R. A. (2004, November). Shaping the brains of tomorrow: What developmental science teaches about the importance of investing early in children. *American Prospect, 15.* Retrieved January 9, 2007, from www.prospect.org/web/page.ww?section=root&name=ViewPrint&articleId=8775.

Wilensky, J. (2002). Back to nature: A relationship with nature over the life course can affect our well-being, ability to manage stress, cognitive development, and social integration. *Human Ecology, 30*(3). Retrieved January 9, 2007, from www.highbeam.com/doc/1G1-120354182.html.

Suggested Reading

Acredolo, L., & Goodwyn, S. (2000). *Baby minds: Brain-building games your baby will love.* New York: Bantam Books.
Baby Minds discusses fun, creative ideas for addressing cognitive development from birth to age 3. It is parent-friendly and suggests inexpensive methods for brain-building play. The authors include support data from some of the most recent and well-respected studies.

Cherry, C., & Nielsen D. M. (1999). *Creative art for the developing child* (3rd ed.). Torrance, CA: Frank Schaffer Publications.
This book is an excellent source on how to select and evaluate art activities for early childhood. Creative ideas are presented for a variety of media. Directions are precise, and each activity lists the expected outcomes.

Healy, K. (Ed.). (1999). *Brilliant beginnings: Birth to 12 months.* Long Beach, CA: Brilliant Beginnings.
Brilliant Beginnings has numerous scholarly contributors and provides much clinical data, yet it has an easy-to-read format that includes photographs and inspiring quotes. The book offers specific advice to enhance the development of infants from birth to 12 months. It does a good job of describing developmental milestones and appropriate activities.

Jensen, E. (1998). *Teaching with the brain in mind.* Alexandria, VA: Association for Supervision and Curriculum Development.
Teaching With the Brain in Mind is an informative book on teaching strategies for the pediatric brain that are based on

research in neuroanatomy and cognitive functioning. Jensen has amassed research ranging from neuroanatomy to sensory integration. The book offers some revolutionary thinking on how to teach children and maximize their potential.

Peterson, D. (2000). *Outdoor art.* Torrance, CA: Totline Publications.

Outdoor Art contains many creative ideas that are appropriate for and bring fun to an equestrian setting. Although this book was designed for preschoolers, the ideas are adaptable for all ages.

Vitale, B. M. (1982). *Unicorns are real: A right-brained approach to learning.* Torrance, CA: Jalmar Press.

Unicorns Are Real provides insight into understanding and teaching children who function with a right-brained approach to life. The author gives simple methods for teaching these children without trying to change them. The book provides specific advice for helping them achieve academic success while being sensitive to their needs. It is useful for parents, teachers, and therapists who work with children who have learning difficulties.

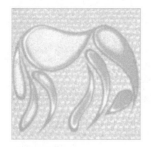

... a fine little smooth horse-colt,
should move a man as much as doth a son.
— Thomas Kyol

CHAPTER 30

Use of Hippotherapy as a Treatment Method During Occupational Therapy With Children Who Have Histories of Abuse and Neglect

Ann K. Viviano, MA, MS, OTR, CCC/SLP, HPCS

This chapter discusses the use of horses as a healing method during occupational therapy with children who have a history of abuse or neglect. Occupational therapy involves the

> therapeutic use of everyday life activities (occupations) with individuals or groups for the purpose of participation in roles and situations in home, school, workplace, community, and other settings. . . . [S]ervices are provided for the purpose of promoting health and wellness to those who have or are at risk for developing an illness, injury, disease, disorder, condition, impairment, disability, activity limitation, or participation restriction. (American Occupational Therapy Association, 2004)

Abuse and neglect may lead to profound impairments and changes in development that affect a child's ability to assume life roles and participate in daily activities at home, at school, and in the community. The horse's movement and the riding environment provide varied opportunities for purposeful goal-directed activities that can be graded across age-levels to promote growth in all developmental skill areas.

Effects of Abuse and Neglect

Child abuse and maltreatment result in a variety of problems that have been reviewed in the literature. Perry (1999a, 1999b) stated that each year in America, approximately 5 million children experience some type of trauma (e.g., physical or sexual abuse, domestic violence, natural disasters, car accidents, life-threatening medical conditions, painful procedures, exposure to community violence). An individual child's response to a traumatic event varies and may include a mixture of *fight or flight response* (e.g., hyperarousal) or an *avoidance and psychological fleeing response* (e.g., disassociation). Hyperarousal may result in hypervigilance, anxiety, reactive and alarm responses, increased heart rate, freeze, fear, flight, and panic or terror. Disassociation may result in detachment, numbness, compliance, decreased heart rate, suspension of time, derealization, minipsychosis, and fainting. Trauma may result in long-term chronic and potentially permanent changes in a child's emotions, affect, behavior, cognition, physiology, and neurophysiology.

Perry and Pollard (1997) documented that annually, more than 500,000 children are victims of neglect in the United States. Depending on the nature and extent of the neglect, these children have a much higher probability of emotional, behavioral, cognitive, social, and physical delays than children who are not neglected. Neglect of children in the first 3 years of life may change the physical growth and organization of the brain.

One study (Atchison & Viviano, 2001) found that 20 of 25 children who experienced a traumatic stress reaction (80%) demonstrated difficulty in sensory processing, as reported by caregivers who completed the Sensory Profile (Dunn, 1999). Preliminary data from the study indicated differences within sensory processing in the following 10 areas: sensory seeking, emotional reaction to stimuli, inattention and distractibility, vestibular processing, multisensory processing, modulation related to body position and movement, modulation of visual input affecting emotional responses and activity level, emotional and social responses, behavioral outcomes of sensory processing, and items indicating threshold for response. Wright (1994) completed a literature review that listed numerous references and discussed the effects of maltreatment on preschool children in four areas: developmental delay, cognitive competence, emotional development, and social development. Knutson and Sullivan (1993) reported comorbidity of abuse, developmental delays, and communication difficulties. Clearly, trauma, abuse, and neglect have a significant impact on a child's growth and development that may interfere with the child's ability to perform daily activities and develop the performance skills necessary to succeed at life occupations.

Occupational Therapy for Child Abuse and Neglect

Reed (2001) indicated six performance areas that may be affected when a child suffers abuse or neglect:

1. Self-care and activities of daily living
2. Productivity, play, and academic readiness
3. Leisure and recreation
4. Sensorimotor function (delayed developmental milestones, muscle weakness or paralysis, decreased range of motion, sensory loss, poor body image, sensory modulation and sensory integration dysfunction)
5. Cognition (learning disabilities, poor problem-solving skills)
6. Psychosocial development (poor self-image, lack of self-confidence, feelings of guilt, blunted affect, lack of self-control, feelings of helplessness, withdrawal, ill-defined role identity, lack of coping skills, delayed social skills, inadequate bonding, delayed speech and language, lack of group interaction skills).

Benefits of Hippotherapy and Equine-Assisted Activities

Gatty (2000) completed a study of 5 children who had developmental disabilities and found that participating in a therapeutic riding program resulted in an increase in self-esteem, as scored on a revised form of the Rosenberg Self-Esteem Scale (Rosenberg, 1965). The use of the horse as a co-facilitator during mounted and ground activities to affect psychosocial growth and development is discussed in *Equine-Facilitated Mental Health: A Field Guide for Practice* (Moreau & McDaniel, 1999). Other studies that documented how equine programs can affect development are listed in *Equine-Facilitated Mental Health and Learning: Annotated Bibliography* (Moga, 2003) and *AHA Bibliography* (American Hippotherapy Association [AHA], 2004).

Possible Assessments for Children With Histories of Abuse and/or Neglect

The following testing instruments may be helpful when evaluating children who have histories of abuse or neglect. Areas to be assessed and instruments used will vary depending upon a particular child's unique strengths, weaknesses, and abilities.

- Battelle Developmental Inventory (Newborg, Stock, & Wnek, 1984)
- Beery–Buktenica Developmental Test of Visual–Motor Coordination, 5th Edition (Beery, Buktenica, & Beery, 2004)
- Bruininks–Oseretsky Test of Motor Proficiency (Bruininks, 1978)
- Canadian Occupational Performance Measure [self-care, productivity, leisure] (Law et al., 1991)
- Coping Inventory (Zeitlin, 1985)
- Draw-a-Person Test (Van Hutton, 1994)
- KidCOTE [Comprehensive Occupational Therapy Evaluation] (Kunz & Brayman, 1999)
- Loewenstein Occupational Therapy Cognitive Assessment (Itzkovich, Averbuch, Elazar, & Katz, 1990)
- Miller Assessment for Preschoolers (Miller, 1988)
- Peabody Developmental Motor Scales, 2nd Edition (Folio & Fewell, 2000)
- Pediatric Early Elementary Examination–Revised (Levine, 1995a)
- Pediatric Evaluation of Disability Inventory (Harley, Coster, Ludlow, Haltiwanger, & Andrellos, 1992)
- Pediatric Examination of Educational Readiness at Middle School–Revised (Levine, 1995b)
- Pediatric Extended Examination at Three (Levine, 1982)
- Quick Neurological Screening Test–II (Mutti, Sterling, & Spalding, 1998)
- Revised Knox Preschool Play Scale (Knox, 1997)
- Rosenberg Self-Esteem Scale (Rosenberg, 1965)
- Sensory Profile (Dunn, 1999)
- Social–Emotional Pinpoint Scale, 0–96 Months (Dykes, 1980)
- Test of Playfulness (Bundy, 1997)
- Vineland Adaptive Behavior Scales–Revised (Sparrow, Balla, & Cicchetti, 1984).

Intervention Using Hippotherapy and Equine-Assisted Occupational Activities

Hippotherapy may be used as part of a child's treatment plan, depending on testing information, the child's goals, and the therapist's clinical expertise and frame of reference (AHA, 2000). I have used the activities listed in the following sections during therapeutic intervention, modifying and grading the program based on the child's response to intervention and functional outcomes. The activities are organized according to Reed's (2001) performance areas (see previous section).

Self-Care and Activities of Daily Living

- Develop arm range of motion and strength, sequencing, body awareness, spatial relationships, and grooming skills by brushing the horse.
- Develop dressing, fine-motor, and safety awareness skills by putting on and buckling the riding helmet.
- Develop sequencing, motor-planning, and fine-motor skills by placing and buckling tack.
- Develop social awareness and learn to dress for the weather by wearing appropriate riding attire.
- Develop motor planning and sequences needed to clean a house by cleaning the barn and office.
- Develop eating and meal-planning skills by preparing a drink or a snack for all the riders.
- Develop grooming skills by washing hands and face after riding.
- Develop sequencing skills by washing, feeding, and watering the horse.
- Develop toileting skills when using the restroom at the barn.
- Develop fine motor and sequencing skills by cleaning tack.

Productivity and Play

- Develop parallel play by working next to other children and adults.
- Develop associative play by completing similar activities near others.
- Develop cooperative play by working with others to complete a common goal.
- Develop pretend play by imagining different games when on the horse, such as pretending to be a kite while holding different colored ribbons.
- Develop constructional play by planning and building an obstacle course or helping to put up a fence.
- Develop spatial relationships by planning how to work in a small arena versus a large field.
- Develop the ability to follow rules by learning simple one- or two-step games versus several steps' sequences in one riding pattern.
- Develop the ability to function in a structured or unstructured situation by grading activities, such as riding in repetitive lines and circles versus free movement of the horse in the arena.

- Develop the ability for now learning by grading activities from repetitive lessons to a variety of activities learned each session.
- Develop nonverbal and linguistic skills by varying how instructions are given, such as imitation of movement, flowing picture or written directions, and verbal instructions.

Leisure and Recreation Skills

- Develop social interactions, friendships, responsibility, and leisure skills by joining a therapeutic riding or 4-H group.
- Develop responsibility and work skills by arriving on time and completing a task for a certain length of time.
- Develop leisure skills and nurturing qualities by gardening.
- Develop sharing and self-esteem by helping other riders.
- Develop creativity and a sense of contribution by making a new game.
- Develop organization, planning, and social skills by planning a picnic.
- Develop written language skills, social skills, and self-confidence by writing invitations to a riding performance.
- Develop reading as a leisure activity by going to the library and finding books about horses.
- Develop self-direction, commitment, and responsibility by setting own therapy and activity goals.
- Develop teamwork and cooperation by participation in games such as "team penning" using people in place of calves.

Sensorimotor Function

- Modulate alertness level by grading movement of the horse and type of activities, such as using slow, rhythmical brushing of the horse for calming and using fast changes in direction while riding for alertness.
- Develop balance, strength, coordination, and function—the hallmarks of hippotherapy—to influence sensorimotor performance.
- Develop the tactile system by riding bareback; choosing different blankets, riding clothes, games, and toys; and petting the horse or other animals.
- Develop the auditory system by listening to music and playing music games, such as "musical horses" or "stop and go" to music.
- Develop the vestibular system by using different positions on the horse—prone across the barrel, prone or

supine on the rump, sitting forward, backward, and sideways.

- Develop the proprioceptive system by facilitating joint compression through position, handling by sidewalkers, movement of the horse, and carrying different weights in buckets.
- Develop motor planning through sequencing movements riding the horse and manipulating objects, such as tying knots in ropes.
- Develop visual skills by playing "I Spy" or following chalk mazes in the arena.
- Develop eye–hand coordination by using balls and different-size targets, beanbag tic-tac-toe, and ring toss games.
- Develop hand skills by drawing with chalk on the horse's buttocks while riding backward, clipping clothes pins or tying ribbons to the mane, using surcingles with different handles, and opening different gates.

Cognition

- Develop problem-solving in different situations, such as what to do if a horse is tacked without prior brushing or what is the best way to walk around the back of a horse. Help the child draw inferences, predict outcomes, use contextual cues, understand "why" questions, and comprehend vocabulary.
- Develop color, number, and shape concepts through games, such as riding to different color, number, and shape cards (similar to dressage letters) placed around the arena.
- Develop the ability to follow instructions by changing the complexity of directions, such as grading instructions for a scavenger hunt.
- Develop concept worksheets, such as identifying parts of a horse and caring for a horse.
- Develop written language skills by writing a paragraph or a report about horses.
- Develop topic and supporting sentences; emphasize having an introduction, middle, and conclusion.
- Develop measuring skills by feeding the horse; learn fractions by dividing a bale of hay into sections.
- Develop letter and name recognition by learning the names of the horses written on the stalls.
- Develop time skills by determining the time the lesson starts and ends or planning how much time is left in a lesson for a particular activity.
- Develop map-reading skills by developing and reading a trail map.
- Develop written narrative skills by keeping a diary of the sessions.

Psychosocial Development

- Develop the ability to feel safe in an environment by interacting with the same horse, instructor, and sidewalkers. Then vary the horse or sidewalkers to expand the level of safety.
- Develop the ability to attach by touching, hugging, brushing, caring for, and riding the horse on a consistent basis.
- Develop social skills through interactions with the instructor and sidewalkers.
- Develop awareness of different personalities by analyzing different horses. Determine whether a particular horse is calm, excitable, fearful, or confident.
- Develop awareness of social interaction styles by watching how different horses interact; determine whether a particular horse is a leader, follower, bully, or loner.
- Develop methods to express feelings by drawing before and after a riding session.
- Develop the ability to give to others and accept responsibility for a relationship by caring for a horse.
- Develop the ability to identify emotions during the lesson, such as pointing to different pictures of faces that are clipped to the surcingle.
- Develop the ability to deal with frustration when learning skills by listing steps to a goal and checking off the steps as they are completed.
- Develop functional language skills by helping the rider comment, request, provide information, respond, discuss, protest, take turns, pick a topic for a conversation, maintain a topic, and change topics appropriately.

Summary

The horse can be an effective treatment partner in occupational therapy programs with children who have histories of abuse and neglect. The equine environment is rich in opportunities to promote self-care and activities of daily living, productivity and play, leisure and prevocational skills, sensorimotor function, cognition, and psychosocial development. When riding and interacting with horses, riders will have numerous opportunities to respond to a unique treatment that facilitates healing of their bodies, minds, and spirits.

References

American Hippotherapy Association. (2000). *Present use of hippotherapy in the United States.* Retrieved from www.americanhippotherapyassociation.org.

American Hippotherapy Association. (2004). *AHA bibliography.* Damascus, PA: Author.

American Occupational Therapy Association. (2004). *Definition of OT practice for the AOTA Model Practice Act*. Retrieved from www.aota.org/members.

Atchison, B., & Viviano, A. (2001). *The incidence of caregiver reported sensory processing disorders in children who are experiencing traumatic stress reaction*. Master's thesis, Western Michigan University, Ann Arbor.

Beery, K. E., Buktenica, N. A., & Berry, N. A. (2004). *Beery–Buktenica Developmental Test of Visual–Motor Coordination* (5th ed.). Parsippany, NJ: Modern Curriculum Press.

Bruininks, R. (1978). *Bruininks–Oseretsky Test of Motor Proficiency*. Circle Pines, MN: American Guidance Services.

Bundy, A. C. (1997). Play and playfulness: What to look for. In L. D. Parham & L. S. Fazio (Eds.), *Play in occupational therapy* (pp. 52–66). St. Louis, MO: Mosby.

Dunn, W. (1999). *Sensory Profile*. San Antonio, TX: Therapy Skill Builders.

Dykes, M. K. (1980). *Social–Emotional Pinpoint Scale (Developmental Assessment for the Severely Handicapped)*. Austin, TX: Pro-Ed.

Folio, M. R., & Fewell, R. R. (2000). *Peabody Developmental Motor Scales* (2nd ed.). Austin, TX: Pro-Ed.

Gatty, C. M. (2000). *Psychosocial impact of therapeutic riding: A pilot study*. Retrieved from www.narha.org/PDFfiles/Psychosocial_Impact.pdf.

Harley, S. M., Coster W. J., Ludlow L., Haltiwanger, J. T., & Andrellos, P. J. (1992). *Pediatric Evaluation of Disability Inventory manual*. San Antonio, TX: Therapy Skill Builders.

Itzkovich, M., Averbuch, S., Elazar, E., & Katz, N. (1990). *Loewenstein Occupational Therapy Cognitive Assessment*. Pequanock, NJ: Maddak.

Knox, S. (1997). Development and current use of the Knox preschool play scale. In L. D. Parham & L. S. Fazio (Eds.), *Play in occupational therapy* (pp. 35–51). St. Louis, MO: Mosby.

Knutson, J. K., & Sullivan, P. M. (1993). Communicative disorders as a risk factor in abuse. *Topics in Language Disorders, 13*(4), 1–14.

Kunz, K. R., & Brayman, S. J. (1999). The comprehensive occupational therapy evaluation. In B. J. Hemphill-Pearson (Ed.), *Assessments in occupational therapy mental health: An integrative approach* (pp. 266–274). Thorofare, NJ: Slack.

Law, M., Baptiste, S., Carswell-Opzoomer, A., McColl, M., Polatajko, H., & Pollack, N. (1991). *Canadian Occupational Performance Measure* (2nd ed.). Toronto: Canadian Association of Occupational Therapists.

Levine, M. D. (1982). *Pediatric Extended Examination at Three*. Cambridge, MA: Educators Publishing Services.

Levine, M. D. (1995a). *Pediatric Early Elementary Examination–Revised*. Cambridge, MA: Educators Publishing Services.

Levine, M. D. (1995b). *Pediatric Examination of Educational Readiness at Middle Childhood–Revised*. Cambridge, MA: Educators Publishing Services.

Miller, L. J. (1988). *Miller Assessment for Preschoolers*. San Antonio, TX: Therapy Skill Builders.

Moga, J. (2003). *Equine-facilitated mental health and learning: Annotated bibliography*. Denver, CO: North American Riding for the Handicapped Association, Equine-Facilitated Mental Health Association.

Moreau, L., & McDaniel, B. (1999). *Equine-facilitated mental health: A field guide for practice* (2nd ed.). Boerne, TX: Legends Equestrian Therapy.

Mutti, M., Sterling, H. M., & Spalding, N. V. (1998). *Quick Neurological Screening Test–II*. Novato, CA: Academic Therapy Publications.

Newborg, J., Stock, J. R., & Wnek, J. (1984). *Battelle Developmental Inventory*. Itasca, IL: Riverside.

Perry, B. (1999a). Effects of traumatic events on children: An introduction. *Child Trauma Academy: Interdisciplinary Education Series, 2*(3). Retrieved from www.childtrauma.org/ctamaterials/effects_I.asp.

Perry, B. (1999b). Violence and childhood: How persisting fear can alter the developing child's brain. *Child Trauma Academy*. Retrieved from www.childtrauma.org/ctamaterials/vio_child.asp.

Perry, B., & Pollard, R. (1997). Altered brain development following global neglect in early childhood. In *Proceedings From the Annual Meeting of the Society for Neuroscience, New Orleans*. Retrieved from www.childtrauma.org/CTAMATERIALS/neuros~1.asp.

Reed, K. L. (2001). *Quick reference to occupational therapy* (2nd ed). Gaithersburg, MD: Aspen.

Rosenberg, M. (1965). *The Rosenberg Self-Esteem Scale*. Retrieved from www.bsos.umd.edu/socy/grad/socpsy_rosenberg.html.

Sparrow, S. S., Balla, D. A., & Cicchetti, D. V. (1984). *Vineland Adaptive Behavior Scales–Revised*. Circle Pines, MN: American Guidance Services.

Van Hutton, V. (1994). *House-Tree-Person and Draw-a-Person as measures of abuse in children: a quantitative scoring system*. Lutz, FL: Psychological Assessment Resources.

Wright, S. A. (1994). Physical and emotional abuse and neglect of preschool children: A literature review. *Australian Occupational Therapy Journal, 41,* 55–63.

Zeitlin, S. (1985). *The Coping Inventory*. Bensonville, IL: Scholastic Testing Service.

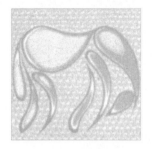

The time to understand is indispensable in establishing some basic rules between two creatures who will collaborate without the use of words.
—Michel Henriquet

CHAPTER 31

Vaulting: An Effective Therapeutic Method

Nina Wiger, MA, and J. Ashton Moore

Modern vaulting first developed in Germany as a preparatory program to improve riding skills and today is a competitive, world-class sport. Studies have shown the effectiveness of using vaulting as a psychoeducational intervention for children with behavioral problems (Kröger, 1997). Vaulting has been used in California for intervention with children and youths with physical disabilities (Spink, cited in Wiger, 2003).

In the United States, vaulting is now part of many therapeutic riding programs, and most competitive vaulting programs include people with disabilities. This chapter describes the general vaulting process, vaulting's benefits, and its versatility for therapeutic intervention.

> Some trace the origins of vaulting to Roman games, including acrobatic displays on cantering horses. Others see roots in the bull dancers of ancient Crete. In either case, people have been performing acrobatic and dance-like movements on the backs of moving horses for more than 2,000 years. . . . The present name of the sport comes from the French "La Voltige" which it acquired during the Renaissance, when it was a form of riding drill and agility exercise for knights and noblemen. (American Vaulting Association [AVA], n.d.)

Vaulting in North America can be traced specifically to 1956, when Elizabeth Searle first saw the sport practiced during a visit to Europe and brought it to the United States. Searle and Moore founded the AVA in 1966. Vaulters participated in the first international exchange in Stuttgart in Germany in 1974 with much success (AVA, n.d.).

What Is Vaulting?

Vaulting is exercises or gymnastics performed on the back of a moving, round-shaped horse. All three gaits are used: *walk,* in which the back swings three-dimensionally; *trot,* which has an invigorating springiness; and *canter,* which has powerful rocking action. The different gaits and exercises involve longitudinal, vertical, and rotational awareness and coordination.

Vaulting is an activity with the following characteristics:
• Someone other than the rider controls the horse.
• The horse is equipped with a surcingle with handles.
• The horse is longed in such a way that it has good self-carriage and moves steadily.

When the horse is used in therapy, vaulting includes the following emphases:
• The teaching methodology is not focused primarily on acquisition of vaulting or riding skills.
• Physical development, such as coordination, sensory processing, physical strength, sequencing, and coordinating movement with another, and acquisition of social skills are the main focuses.
• Enhancing developmental skills in all age groups is a focus.
• The rider can select and perform any movements that she or he desires and is comfortable with.

Vaulting is a safe activity for many reasons:
• The horse is always controlled by a longeur.
• The horse is always equipped with a surcingle with large, solid handles. The rider has something safe to hold on to.
• The degree of difficulty easily can be adapted to individual abilities within one group.

In addition, the vaulting arena has firm but resilient footing that cushions falls well. The horse is longed far from fences and other solid objects, so if the rider falls, he or she is likely to encounter few objects that could injure him or her.

In addition, adherence to certain guidelines can enhance safety. The following rules have proved successful in practice:

- Helmets are mandatory under all independent riding, even when the horse is equipped with a surcingle.
- Vaulters with strength, balance, and coordination within normal limits should not use helmets. The helmet is in the way and can even be dangerous in certain exercises.
- In doubles and triple exercises helmets should never be used. There is not much space for three riders on the back of a horse, and the bulkiness of the helmets would be a liability rather than a safety precaution.

The Horse

The horse can be of any breed or size as long as all gaits are well balanced, regular, and without tension. Personality, character, and temperament are important because vaulting horses need to tolerate movement on their back. It is not a prerequisite, although it is an advantage, to have a horse that can canter well. The horse must be healthy and well conditioned and have a strong, broad back. It must, of course, be absolutely sound physically and mentally.

Equipment

The horse is equipped with a surcingle with handles. A variety of surcingles are available, but the competition surcingle, which has half-round handles, is the most versatile, even for smaller children, because the handles are welded to the frame and do not move like some cheaper models do. Side reins always should be used. At the walk, the reins must be long enough that the horse can move its head in a natural way but short enough to keep the horse straight and to be effective in case the horse is spooked. The horse can be ridden bareback but usually wears a back pad. The therapist must balance the concern for the horse and the needs of the vaulter when selecting bareback pads.

Vaulting Exercises

Vaulting is based on seven compulsory exercises. These exercises can be modified for different skill levels.

1. *The Mount.* The rider jumps up on the horse. It requires coordination of the whole body: head, arms, trunk, and legs. It is very difficult and requires much practice, especially from the therapist, who has to learn how and when to assist.
2. *The Basic Seat.* This exercise is the same as the correct dressage seat, but the arms are stretched out to the side, and the rider holds on with the legs wrapped around the horse's belly.
3. *The Flag.* The vaulter first gets up on his or her knees while holding the handles in a four-point position. One leg is stretched and lifted, and the opposite arm is lifted forward.
4. *The Mill.* The vaulter, who sits astride, lifts one leg over the surcingle and sits in the inside side seat position. The mill has two variations: (1) The leg can be lifted back, and the other leg lifted to outside side seat, or (2) the vaulter can continue until he or she sits backward, then in outside side seat, and then forward again.
5. *Swing and Scissors.* From sitting astride, the vaulter swings the legs and body up in the air, as high as possible, and lands either sitting forward (swing) or backward (scissors). From sitting backward, the vaulter again swings the body and legs as high as possible, turns, and lands forward.
6. *Kneeling* and *Standing.* From astride, the vaulter moves to his or her knees, then stretches the arms out to the side as in basic seat. Then the vaulter lightly jumps to both feet from kneeling, then stretches the arms out to the side as in basic seat.
7. *Dismount.* An important part of learning to vault is how to get off the horse from all positions and in all gaits. In a simple dismount, the leg is lifted over the surcingle and the vaulter slides to the ground. In the *half-flank off,* the vaulter performs a swing and, at the highest point of the swing, pushes away from the horse. In the *full-flank* dismount, the vaulter performs a swing but lands in side seat. The vaulter then swings his or her whole stretched body over the horse and lands on the ground on the other side of the horse. Full flank is difficult but a great achievement for children with attention deficit hyperactivity disorder, dyslexia, or other learning disabilities.

All other exercises are called *kür,* or freestyle.

Vaulting at the Walk

Vaulting at the walk is the introduction to vaulting for everyone, regardless of ability or disability or mental, emotional, social, or other disadvantage. It is especially beneficial for children with sensory processing disorders and motor control deficits. Many children need relatively few vaulting lessons before a marked improvement is achieved (Wiger, 2003). Even very timid people dare to scoot side-to-side, lean forward and back, move a leg, and cross the hands to opposite handles. The vaulter is equally safe sitting backward, sideways, or on the horse's neck. The vaulter can find the position that affords the most sensory input about where his or her body is in relation to gravity, and he or she can safely work on balance, coordination, and orientation in space. It is, for example, scary at first to lie flat on the horse, but done sideways the rider can hold on to the handles. As courage and control increase, lying flat can be done forward or backward, on the stomach, or on one's back.

The vaulting compulsory (Fédération Equestre Internationale, 2005) and freestyle exercises provide sensory input to the entire central nervous system. Sensory processing is facilitated by the rhythmic movement of the horse and the vaulter's change of position on the horse. Balance is challenged the whole time, regardless of what task is being attempted. Even riders without disabilities of any kind must learn to reorient while on the horse. In many exercises, the head must be lower than the body, adding yet another dimension.

Vaulting at the Trot and Canter

When the rider masters vaulting at the walk, the trot can be attempted. For some vaulters, the trot will be attempted in the first lesson; other vaulters may require months. Vaulting exercises at the trot require more strength, courage, and body control than at the walk. The horse must have smooth transitions from trot to walk because a rough or unbalanced shift is difficult for the vaulter.

Canter is the preferred gait for older children "at risk" and people with social, emotional, psychological, and other nonphysical problems. The canter is a rolling, powerful gait that can give a rider a sense of freedom. At the same time, it is fast and can be frightening. The vaulter has to trust the horse to take care of him or her, even when he or she does not feel in control of the horse (Kröger, 1997).

Vaulting on the Barrel

A barrel is a great teaching asset. It consists of 1½ oil drums that are welded together and well padded, or it can be built of wood. Either fixed handles or a vaulting surcingle is attached. The barrel can be used to teach moves that will be used on the horse or as an activity in itself.

Special Aspects of Vaulting

Vaulting is unique among horse activities because it is the only equestrian activity in which control of the horse is not the issue for the participant. The horse is controlled

by another. This "other" becomes the facilitator of the contact between the person and the horse. The triad of horse, person, and longeur makes for a therapeutic setting that cannot be matched in any other sport (Kröger, 2000).

Another feature of vaulting is that everyone starts with the same exercises and progresses through stages that must be mastered before the next stage can be attempted (although this can vary in a therapy situation, depending on the needs of the client). The talented athlete might master in the first lesson what another person will require years to attain, but the two riders go through the same steps. When sitting is mastered, kneeling and standing can be attempted. When those exercises become easy, they can be done sideways or backward or at faster gaits. Thus, progression in difficulty is attained through variation of exercises, not just by refining already learned ones. The possibilities of changing the base of support, the center of gravity, and movement direction of the vaulter relative to the horse are limited only by the ability of the vaulter and the skill of the therapist.

Vaulting has "companion" activities. Before riding, both horse and vaulter must be warmed up. The warm-up routine and barrel work are multitasking, challenging activities that most children enjoy when directed by a skilled therapist. In bad weather, activities on and around the barrel, dance, gymnastic routines, and stretching games can be preferred to riding on the horse. A great advantage of the sport is that many vaulters can use the same horse and the same equipment in one lesson. Thus, the therapist needs only a limited number of horses to accommodate many clients.

Vaulting as a Therapeutic Modality

In vaulting, as in all other horse activities, the horse offers a fresh chance for development of trust. What makes vaulting different is the control the longeur has over the situation. The vaulter is free to concentrate on his or her own reactions and explore his or her own abilities and limitations without worrying about controlling the horse. Skill and mastery come rapidly. Most children without disabilities dare kneel and trot in the first lesson.

The back of the horse provides a clearly defined therapy setting. The longeur controls the situation, varying the challenge through changes in speed and gait; the longeur can move closer to the horse for added security. The children or adults are encouraged to work through a situation and stick to a task. Thus, vaulting is a great "concentration trainer." The exercises are easier when done in harmony with the horse. The horse provides the power; the vaulter both controls the exercise and gives him- or herself over to it. One cannot use force; one must learn to work with the horse.

In competitive vaulting, the horse must continue without reacting, regardless of what happens on its back. When used for therapy, the situation can be a little different, depending on the client. It can be beneficial to have a horse that gives clear, but not dangerous, signals when the vaulter does something unacceptable. The children and adults learn to trust the horse; at the same time, they develop a healthy respect for it. From respect for the horse grows respect for the longeur, who can control the big animal. They know that without the longeur, they would never dare do such difficult exercises on such a big animal. Respect for and trust in the longeur are the first steps toward healthy relationships with other people (Kröger, 1997).

Team vaulting requires use of several "stations": on the horse, behind the longeur, on the barrel, on-the-ground exercises, and ringside. This structure makes gradual introduction into a setting possible. A child can pull back a little and just watch for a while. Very active children get some training at sitting still, but they can move around as much as they want to on the horse and barrel. The vaulters must pay attention to their place and order in the group because they take turns at the various stations. They can watch and praise each other's achievements on the horse when resting between turns, or they can practice patience and self-control while waiting. A group of children with different strengths can motivate and learn from each other.

Preparing the Horse

Vaulting lessons can start with the vaulters getting the horse ready. Because one horse is used, everybody must work together. Many tasks are involved, and the vaulters can start with the ones they like best. With time, all vaulters must learn all the tasks, but they can take as much time as necessary to do so, without being noted as "the slow one." When working with children who have behavioral problems, the therapist can let the vaulters who have mastered a skill teach it to the other children and help coach them. Gradually, the instructor pulls back and intervenes only in case of conflict or when a child needs

guidance with specific tasks. The vaulters learn to work together toward a goal.

Warm-Up and Stretching

The warm-up and stretching routine is an important tool in vaulting. It can be made as simple or as complicated as desirable or necessary. The skilled therapist can develop the warm-up to engage the entire group yet address the special needs of individual clients. The warm-up is a good time to work on increasing range of motion and strengthening the shoulder girdle. Adding music to the warm-up adds rhythm and timing to motion.

Single Vaulting

Vaulting can be adjusted within the same lesson to different interests and abilities. One child may be praised for his straight legs and controlled movements, another for daring leaps off the horse. The horse can be used for individual work with two riders at a time; one rider sits forward on the neck and feels he or she is riding alone, while the other balances on the croup and figures out how and where to hold on.

Double and Triple Vaulting

As mentioned earlier, a primary way in which vaulting differs from other types of riding is that the rider does not directly control the horse. The second way in which it is different is that two or three vaulters can be on a horse at one time. The sport allows close interaction between vaulters while the longeur has full control over the situation.

The trainer can use this closeness to work on developing trust, attention, and empathy among the vaulters. Many issues can be addressed when together on the horse:

- *Physically interacting with another person.* Some people hate to touch or be touched by other people. One example of on-horse exercises is the "pattycake" game, in which only the hands touch briefly. Vaulters can work up to holding each other while helping each other get over the handles and, finally, lying on top of each other in a "sandwich."
- *Teamwork and problem-solving* (e.g., "How do I get to the horse's neck when I am sitting behind you?").
- *Working with another person to reach a common goal* (e.g., "We put our arms out and down exactly together, even when sitting back to back").
- *Helping another person* (e.g., getting on and off the horse is a challenge, and the vaulters soon find out that

they get more time on the horse when they help each other and the longeur does not have to stop the horse and come and help each time).

• *Learning responsibility.* Some clients are overprotected and seldom allowed to assume responsibilities. Sometimes they are not given as many demands as they are capable of meeting. In doubles and triples, they can take pride in being responsible for helping the other vaulters.

• *Identification with and consideration for other people.* All vaulters experience a degree of fear and uncertainty in difficult exercises. In time, they might learn to see beyond their own problems by watching others struggle with the same issues.

• *Working with people of different abilities.* People with and without disabilities can work together. A timid child can sit on the horse's neck and be strong so that someone else can hold on while doing difficult balancing exercises. Children labeled clumsy, slow, and uncoordinated can be the solid base for an impressive triple exercises. Thus, vaulting is useful for mainstreaming and integration.

It is part of the nature of team vaulting that even though vaulters might be alone on the horse at any given time, they are still part of a group that is sharing the horse. Contact within the group can be close or distant. Children who do not get along can avoid each other or be put on the horse together. The skilled instructor chooses exercises in which the two can achieve something together that would be difficult alone or with someone else. The children learn to overcome emotional, mental, or physical challenges to achieve a common goal. Their accomplishments are made possible by the authority figures—the horse and the longeur—who direct the action and cannot be ignored.

Some children and youths have problems interacting with adults and other children and have a hard time functioning in a school environment. It is easier for them to learn in closely supervised, small groups. The vaulting lesson provides a small social setting with clear rules in which the horse, not an adult, is the motivator and the authority figure. Thus, authority is easier to accept.

Who Can Benefit From Vaulting?

The immediate success that most people experience in their first lesson is perhaps one of the main reasons vaulting is such effective intervention. Most children enjoy vaulting, but it is particularly suited for the following groups:

• *Developmental delay/deficiencies.* Vaulting is well suited to young children who do not follow a normal developmental sequence and older ones who have not yet mastered certain phases. The compulsory exercises recreate most developmental stages.

• *Sensory processing and motor control deficiencies.* Being on the horse is one of the most powerful sensory experiences there is. It includes smells, much to look at, and different textures to touch and feel. The horse's rhythmic and swinging gaits challenge balance and relation to gravity. The horse offers a platform from which the child can perform many tasks with arms and hands while being moved through the whole body.

• *Physical disabilities.* Children and youths with minor cerebral palsy, perceptual disorders (e.g., sight and hearing difficulties), and other physical disabilities benefit greatly from vaulting. It is good physical training and a team sport in which the joy and success of a shared physical activity is possible. Vaulting meets physical and emotional needs. Children with tactile defensiveness can first learn to tolerate the horse; later, they can ride double and learn to touch other people.

• *Learning disabilities, dyslexia, and attention deficit hyperactivity disorder.* The complicated sequences of vaulting exercises and even more difficult combination of exercises into freestyle routines teaches concentration, persistence, and patience. The horse can be used to relax the vaulters. They calm down while lying prone backward on the croup, where they fully experience the repetitive movement of a cadenced, elastic walk. The small, close-knit group situation and the work toward a common goal teach them to moderate their behavior. The structure also fosters mutual tolerance within the group. Some children with learning disabilities have reached the highest levels of international competition.

• *Autism.* People with autistic disorders can benefit from the continuous bombardment of sensory input through and into all organs of the body. Progress in language development with sudden breakthroughs in understanding has been reported (Moore and Wiger, private communications). Much work is needed in this area because the research is minimal.

Conclusion

Vaulting is special. Something about dealing with movement and another living being at the same time seems to bring out certain operational modes that might otherwise remain dormant. It has been demonstrated in retirement homes that animals bring out positive qualities in people who otherwise seem to have lost interest in life and their surroundings. Combining animals with activity seems to generate a powerful, positive influence on perceptual and functional skills. A horse is huge and powerful but gentle and obedient. It carries the rider. As the rider's skills grow, the horse helps the rider reach even farther.

Vaulting requires learning to move in harmony with the horse, even when the vaulter moves in all directions and along all axes, alone or with other vaulters. Mastering one's own body while it is being moved leads to being able to use the horse's power to move higher and faster. Vaulting can effectively train body and mind and enhance personal development and social skills that transfer into other areas. Through vaulting, the rider acquires tools for dealing with the complicated outside world and becoming an independent person.

References

American Vaulting Association. (n.d.). *A brief history of vaulting.* West Hollywood, CA: Author. Retrieved February 26, 2007 from www.americanvaulting.org/history.shtml.

Fédération Equestre Internationale. (2005). *Rules for vaulting events.* Lausanne, Switzerland: Author. Retrieved February 26, 2007 from www.horsesport.org/PDFS/V/04_01/Vaulting Rules2005-E-updated.pdf.

Kröger, A. (1997). Using vaulting lessons as remedial education. In B. Engel (Ed.), *Therapeutic riding II: Strategies for rehabilitation.* Durango, CO: Barbara Engel Therapy Services.

Kröger, A. (2000). *Heilpadagogishes Voltigieren und Reiten.* Warendorf, Germany: Deutsches Kuratorium für Therapeutisches Reiten.

Wiger, N. (2003). Can a short adapted vaulting have a positive effect on physically and mentally challenged children? *Scientific and Educational Journal of Therapeutic Riding, 9.*

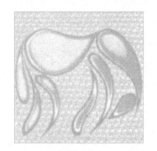

*The art [of horsemanship]
comprises three essential aspects which are
knowledge of the horse, the manner of training it,
and its care.*
—De La Guériniére

CHAPTER 32

Medical Value of Vaulting: A Review of the Literature

Barbara T. Engel, MEd, OTR

The literature on the use of vaulting as therapy for people who have disabilities is limited. Most of the research has focused on what the Germans call *Heilpaedagogik* (healing instruction; Kröger, 1997b), or vaulting that encompasses "educational, psychological, psychotherapeutic, rehabilitation and social integration aspects with the use of the horse to help individuals of all ages with various disabilities and disturbances" (Kröger, 1997b). The official German National Equestrian Federation book on vaulting was published in 1987 and translated into English (Belton, 1987). Numerous vaulting books in English are listed in the book's bibliography. Although vaulting books do not address the use of vaulting (or adaptive vaulting) for people with disabilities, they do provide the therapist with necessary basic knowledge on the sport.

This chapter briefly summarizes the research literature on the benefits of vaulting for populations with various physical and cognitive conditions.

Summary of Literature

Friedlaender (1970) stated that, although she was not an expert on vaulting, she used vaulting to increase the riding skills of the children who came to her for lessons. Dömken, Merz, and Schlobach (1978) published one of the earlier German books on vaulting, which discussed vaulting in detail, along with how to "build" a vaulter. The book covered the horse, the equipment, lunging, basic exercises, and *kürs* (freestyle dressage or vaulting set to music). The therapist must be familiar with these basic elements of vaulting in addition to the normal developmental sequence of the child. In therapy, vaulting is not used as a sport but is specifically directed toward client goals. The goals may involve aspects of developmental stages that have not been adequately developed. Basic exercises in vaulting can be used to promote devel-

opmental milestones; if one simplifies the exercises, the activity appears more like a sport than therapy, which is always a motivating factor. For example, the flag movement can be broken down to kneeling, holding on, letting go, then lifting one arm, followed by holding on and lifting one leg before putting it all together. For a child with sensory integration problems, the therapist may set a stage for the child to explore and play within it. Next, the therapist may briefly go through the basic exercises, then let the child build on them in *kürs* as she or he has motivation to do so. My practice has worked with several children who prefer just to stand on the horse as it walks.

Mehlem (2003) stated that human beings show their unconscious psyche, moods, and conflicts through body postures, in part because the body shows muscle tensions. Especially in vaulting and riding, chronic patterns show themselves and allow for diagnosis and better intervention. Vaulting requires frequent change of body position, allowing for further interpretations of patterns. Mehlem also stated that not only the therapist but also the rider can see the underlying problems. She added that the horse signals to the rider a clear resonance of his or her physical state (Mehlem, 2003).

Horvát (2003) described working with clients with autistic spectrum disorders. She stated that she focuses on the client's strengths and weaknesses, then addresses them through riding and vaulting. Horvát also described cognitive and behavioral intervention through riding and vaulting.

Schultz (1997) described the socializing influence of remedial educational vaulting on children with Asperger syndrome and high-functioning autism. The term *remedial educational vaulting/riding* came about from working with people with emotional disturbances, with whom group activity was of therapeutic value. This type of therapy addressed cognition, motor skills, and emotional behaviors. Schultz reviewed how autism differs from schizophrenia, described different types of autism, and explained how group vaulting activity addresses the behaviors of people with autism. Her literature review includes six German studies that assess the influences of vaulting on sensory integration, equilibrium, proprioception, tactile stimulation, coordination, body image, body language, movement and tension–flow, and adaptation.

Schultz (1997) also reported on her research involving children with autism, the goal of which was to determine whether vaulting would have a significant influence on their development over the course of 1 year. The conclusion stated that no child missed more than one session. Stereotypes and mannerisms were absent by the end of the year, and children were able to interact with each other. Cognitively, they were able to tack the horse and meet the horse's needs and work together to accomplish the task.

Hauser (1997) discussed the general need for integration of people with disabilities into the school system and the community. Kiphard, cited in Hauser, stated people need to acknowledge themselves in their real and personal environment and to interact with the environment in a significant way. Hauser and her assistant (a special education teacher trained in educational vaulting and riding) work with 4 children within a 10-year age range who have various problems and disabilities, along with children who have no known problems. The goals were individualized for each child with special needs. The sessions involved getting the horse, grooming and tacking the horse, vaulting, and taking care of the horse after vaulting. Hauser pointed out the influences that stimulate the children, such as the warmth of the horse, the barn, the smells, the sense of touch, and the kinaesthetic sense as the children bend and move. It is important for the children to develop individual positive behaviors and to work together and accept each other in the group. Over time, the children became an integrated working group, and the children helped and accepted each other.

Kröger (1997a) demonstrated through a video how he worked with children of average intellect who have behavioral and emotional disturbances. Kröger worked with a group of 6 children from a special education program using a large horse and vaulting sessions once a week for 2 years. Kröger's video shows the group at the beginning of 2 years in a regular school class and again after the end of the 2 years, demonstrating the positive changes in the children. The video also shows the children fighting with each other at the beginning and follows their progress as they develop trust and cooperation.

Kröger (1997b) presented a study of 6 children with social and emotional difficulties involved in remedial-education vaulting/riding. Children helped prepare the horse for vaulting, warmed up the horse and themselves, then participated in the vaulting session. After the session, the children prepared the horse for the return to stall. Kröger worked with the horse and the group without assistants; observers or "helpers" could take notes but could not interact with the group; they provided input after the participants left.

Finzgar and Schneide (1994), in an illustrated manual of vaulting exercises, divide vaulting into six levels to give both vaulters and instructors (practitioners) a guideline for skills that can be developed through vaulting. This system addresses physical, cognitive, and emotional challenges. The levels are defined as follows:

- *Level 1:* Body and spatial awareness, coordination, and balance (basic exercises)
- *Level 2:* Development of muscular endurance and flexibility
- *Level 3:* Increasing flexibility and endurance; development of body strength and coordination, dynamic and static motor control
- *Level 4:* Flexibility and strength; increased exercises requiring strength and extension, balance, and static tension and endurance
- *Level 5:* Ability to raise body part from the back of the horse and maintain equilibrium; increase endurance through more difficult kürs
- *Level 6:* Use of space in all planes; increased variety of movements, amplitude, and creativity.

References

Belton, C. (1987). *Vaulting: The official handbook of the German National Equestrian Federation* (Complete Riding and Driving System, Book 3). Boonsboro, MD: Half Halt.

Dömken, C. H., Merz, M., & Schlobach, I. (1978). *Richtlinien Für Reuteb und Fafren, Band III Volrigieren*. Warendorf, Germany: Deutsche Reiterliche Vereinigung.

Friedlaender, E. (1970). *Vaulting: The art of gymnastics on the moving horse*. Brattleboro, VT: Stephen Greene Press.

Finzgar, S., & Schneide, U. (1994). *Voltige: Progress development programme for voltigeurs with disabilities*. Guelph, Ontario: Canadian Therapeutic Riding Association.

Hauser, G. (1997). The horse—Important for every child. Vaulting as a means in integrational education. *Proceedings of the Ninth International Therapeutic Riding Congress* (pp. 180–185). Denver, CO.

Horvát, K. (2003). Main aspect of therapeutic riding and vaulting of individuals with autism. In *Proceedings of the International Congress for Therapeutic Riding* (p. 59). Budapest, Hungary.

Kröger, A. (1997a). How horses can support the educational process [videotape]. In *Proceedings of the Ninth International Therapeutic Riding Congress* (p. 235). Denver, CO.

Kröger, A. (1997b). Using vaulting lessons as remedial education. In B. Engel (Ed.), *Therapeutic riding II: Strategies for rehabilitation*. Durango, CO: Barbara Engel Therapy Services.

Mehlem, M. (2003). Body language in the therapeutic riding and vaulting—Characteristics and frequent body postures and their emotional meaning in psychotherapy with the horse. In *Proceedings of the International Congress for Therapeutic Riding* (p. 74). Budapest, Hungary.

Schultz, M. (1997). Socializing influence of remedial educational vaulting on children with autistic attitudes: Asperger-syndrome, high-function autism. In *Proceedings of the Ninth International Therapeutic Riding Congress* (pp. 67–75). Denver, CO.

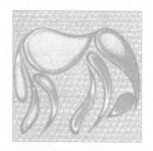

The position of the rider [ensures] maximum stability, security, and balance of the rider.
—Michel Henriquet

CHAPTER 33

A Developmental Approach to Treatment of a Child With Multiple Disabilities

Roberta S. Devery, MS, OTR/L

This case study follows "Nicholas" through his first year of hippotherapy. Nicholas was diagnosed with CHARGE syndrome when he was 14 days old. In addition, Nicholas had a secondary diagnosis of left stroke resulting in right-side weakness, right-side neglect, profound hearing loss, and respiratory complications. It is believed that Nicholas had a stroke when he was in utero. At the time of therapy, he was a delightful and engaging 1.6-year-old toddler.

Nicholas became involved with hippotherapy in the spring. His parents became interested in hippotherapy during a national CHARGE conference, where use of the horse as a treatment strategy to facilitate sensory and motor development in children with CHARGE syndrome was discussed.

What Is CHARGE Syndrome?

CHARGE syndrome is an uncommon diagnosis affecting 1 in 12,000 births with a reoccurrence rate of 1%. The diagnosis of CHARGE syndrome is based on the physical presentation of a child with a specific set of birth defects. According to the CHARGE Syndrome Foundation (n.d.), CHARGE is an acronym based on some of the most common features seen in children with CHARGE syndrome:

- *C*oloboma, a cleft or failure of the eyeball to close; includes abnormalities in the retina or optic nerve
- *C*ranial nerve damage; may result in facial palsy (cranial nerve VII), swallowing problems (cranial nerve IX/X), or sensorineural hearing loss (cranial nerve VIII)
- *H*eart defects
- *A*tresia: blockage (atresia) or narrowing (stenosis) of the choanae (the passages from the back of the nose to the throat that make it possible to breathe)

- *R*etardation of growth and development
- *G*enital and urinary abnormalities
- *E*ar abnormalities or hearing loss (conductive and/or nerve).

Children with CHARGE syndrome, as stated by the CHARGE Syndrome Foundation (n.d.), may have additional health complications, including central nervous system disorders (e.g., microcephaly, seizures, apnea, or central processing problems), pituitary abnormalities, swallowing difficulties, cleft lip or palate, and DeGeorge sequence (congenital absence of the thymos and parathyroid glands). CHARGE facial features tend to include a square-shaped face and head, flat cheekbones, facial asymmetry, a wide nose with a high bridge, and unusual ears. In addition, children with CHARGE syndrome may have omphalocele (failure of the abdominal wall to close properly around the umbilical cord, leaving intestines outside of the body), tracheo-esophageal fistula (an abnormal connection between the trachea and the esophagus), or esophageal atresia (the esophagus ends in a pouch instead of connecting to the stomach).

No laboratory tests can diagnose CHARGE syndrome. The diagnosis is made on the basis of the presence of a number of these typically unrelated anomalies. Because of the medical complexity of these varied anomalies, the diagnosis of CHARGE syndrome is best made by a team of medical specialists, including a medical geneticist who has ruled out other disorders with overlapping findings. The cause of CHARGE syndrome is not known; it is believed to be unrelated to illness, exposure to drugs, and alcohol intake during pregnancy, and it typically does not affect more than one child in a family. It is rare and cannot be determined during pregnancy (CHARGE Syndrome Foundation, n.d.).

Initial Occupational Therapy Evaluation

Nicholas came to a North American Riding for the Handicapped (NARHA) premier accredited center to receive occupational therapy, physical therapy, speech therapy, and developmental therapy. Each service was provided once a week for 60 minutes. The toddler displayed the following characteristics:

- Global low tone
- Right-side neglect secondary to a left-hemisphere stroke
- Kyphotic sitting posture
- Wide base of support needed for monitored sitting
- Compromised balance
- Limited positive interaction with his environment
- Hypersensitivities to sensory input
- A high-guard response following movement
- Compromised breathing abilities.

Initial treatment goals were as follows:

- Desensitize to motion and to diminish high-guard responses to movement
- Facilitate upright sitting posture
- Facilitate head control at midline
- Facilitate awareness of self in space
- Facilitate right-side awareness and use of right upper extremity as support to left hand function
- Facilitate independent sitting.

Treatment Plan

Nicholas was evaluated and assigned to ride a 12-hand pony. Equipment included a suede bareback riding pad and a support belt for safety. Treatment sessions included a horse handler, a NARHA-registered occupational therapist, a NARHA-certified riding instructor, and the toddler's mother to give emotional support and comfort as well as observe and learn techniques throughout the treatment session. Exercises were as follows:

- Pony walk about the arena with maximum support two times in each direction
- Pony walk about the arena with initially maximum support, grading the support down to moderate support when possible, to encourage motion in the pelvis and spine
- Pony walking with stops and starts, giving the toddler therapeutic support at the shoulders to encourage neck muscles to respond
- Pony walking with stops and starts and grading the pace of the walk
- Pony walking in a zigzag pattern between cones to encourage weight shift from left to right

- Leg-yielding the pony at a walk to the right to maximize Nicholas's weight over the right side of his body
- While on the pony, asking the toddler to reach laterally for rings of light to encourage weight shift and body awareness
- Use of plushy balls of various sizes to encourage appropriate hand grasp and shaping of the hands and to foster maintenance of body stability while playing with the balls.

First Quarter (March–May)

When placed on the pony, Nicholas required maximum trunk support for safety and stability while at the stand. He assumed a very kyphotic (bent over) sitting posture with his hands placed 12 to 15 inches in front of him to maximize his base of support. Nicholas did not like to bear weight through his upper extremities. He adjusted himself to minimize upper-extremity weight bearing without compromising his stability. When movement began, he either collapsed forward or went into a high guard posture with his hands held up like stop signs.

Following desensitization techniques and therapeutic handling, Nicholas would tolerate moderate bilateral weight bearing through his arms and hands during a slow steady walk for a distance of 100 feet. Upper-extremity weight-bearing activities required maximum assist for stability, placement, and safety. When in bilaterally weight-bearing position, Nicholas presented a concaved back and a protruding stomach, indicating lack of trunk control; lateral movement elicited a total loss of balance. When the pony stopped and started, the reaction elicited a forward or backward collapse.

Second Quarter (June–August)

Nicholas's parents reported that at home, Nicholas was ring sitting longer before he began to show signs of fatigue. His head control was improving, as noted in his ability to look at or toward an object for a few seconds without hyperextending his neck. His head came to midline sporadically. The physical therapist reported that Nicholas was moving with greater fluidity. It became easier to facilitate movements during therapeutic handling, and when movement was generated, it was more effective.

Third Quarter (September–November)

Nicholas's mother reported that he was moving around the house more than in the past. He moved faster and traveled greater distances by rolling and by scooting in

Table 33.1. Goals and Outcomes for Nicholas for 1 Year of Occupational Therapy Incorporating Hippotherapy

Goal	First Quarter	Second Quarter
Desensitize Nicholas to motion to diminish high-guard response to movement	Tolerated 18 minutes of an OT session incorporating the horse as a treatment strategy. High-guard response to movement was noted 90% of the time.	Tolerated OT session for a full 30 min. High-guard response to movement was no longer evident.
Facilitate upright sitting posture	Pelvis was in a posterior tilt with no evidence of flexibility. Maximum support was needed at the trunk to remain in an upright sitting position for safety and stability.	Could sit upright with pelvis at neutral supporting himself on extended arms leaning upon an 8″ support roll. This position was maintained for 30 min. with moderate support from therapist, supporting the involved right hand to maintain proper weight bearing positioning.
Facilitate head control at midline	Demonstrated unintentional head roll in any direction with the initiation of movement. Placed head into hyperextension for stability.	Could maintain head at midline for several (5–8) seconds following facilitation techniques and specific therapeutic handling.
Facilitate awareness of self in space	Had minimal awareness of self in space. Would tip to 40° lateral deviation before subtle awareness of loss of balance would be noted.	Could adjust self to center if he was leaning too far left or right. Lean had to be extreme (45°), but he was noting a change in his center of gravity and addressing the situation.
Facilitate right-side awareness and use of right upper extremity as support to left hand function.	Tolerance for therapeutic handling of the right arm was low. Would use right arm for weight bearing only for extreme situations by locking his elbow.	Improved arm strength. Bilateral weight bearing without elbow locking in forward and rear facing was documented for a distance of 40 feet with moderate support to maintain appropriate hand position.
Facilitate independent sitting	Required maximum support at the trunk for all sitting activities on any nonstable surface.	No longer required maximum support at the trunk for sitting activities on moveable surfaces. Moderate support was sufficient with all activities at the walk, including zigzags and stops and starts.

Note. OT = occupational therapy.

his ring walker. He was beginning to climb on playground equipment with close supervision for safety. Nicholas was beginning to climb on playground equipment with spotting for safety.

Fourth Quarter (December–February)

Nicholas's mother reported that he loved to zoom around the house in his walker. She stated that he presented good upright posture and strong hands for holding onto the walker handles. He was able to keep his head centered at midline without fixation of the shoulders. Nicholas was attempting to release one hand from the walker to reach for a toy.

Summary

Nicholas continued to be an engaged and active participant in his occupational therapy sessions incorporating hippotherapy. Upon his initial evaluation, he was totally dependent for support, balance, and stability and had a high-guard response to movement. Therapeutic handling was tolerated for a maximum of 18 minutes. At the 1-year reevaluation, Nicholas was a confident child who could sit up independently for a distance of 40 feet while the pony was walking. He used his hands for balance and reached without shoulder fixing. He assumed a four-point position on a pony and laughed with pleasure in a short-distance trot.

Table 33.1 summarizes goal progression through 1 year of occupational therapy intervention incorporating hippotherapy.

Reference

CHARGE Syndrome Foundation. (n.d.). *About CHARGE.* Columbia, MO: Author. Retrieved February 26, 2007, from www.chargesyndrome.org/about-charge.asp.

Third Quarter	Fourth Quarter
Was an active participant in OT planning sessions; often requested changes of position by motioning to mother or therapist. Tolerated forward and rear-facing prone position across the barrel and supine along the back with ease and pleasure.	Laughed out loud when trot steps were introduced. Requested additional trotting by gently rocking on the pony to mimic the motion he was craving.
Assumed rear-facing position, placing his pelvis in upright and neutral position for the straight walk, end cone circles, and serpentines. Upper extremities were weight bearing on the suede pad surface. Minimal support was used to keep the right hand in weight-bearing position.	Accepted handling and facilitation techniques to mobilize hips and spine to encourage independent upright sitting posture.
Could position himself to stabilize his shoulders over extended, weight-bearing arms to provide enough stability for him to intermittently hold his head at midline at the straight walk for a distance of 60 feet.	Could bring his head up from forward flexion to midline with shoulder support from therapist at the stand and at a slow walk for a distance of 60 feet.
Would initiate changes of position by holding therapist's hand and pushing in a desired direction or by actively motor planning to execute the desired change of position.	Was developing trunk rotation (segmental movement) with left shoulder leading with good balance. Would reach out with his left hand for lighted toys presented by his mother.
Actively turned his head to see his mother when she was positioned to his right in 3 of 5 trials.	Maintained side-sitting position (left hand on the wither) with moderate assist to maintain hand position support and to encourage cooperative independent upper-extremity weight bearing.
Could sit independently for a distance of 25 feet at a slow walk with weight bearing on extended arms for balance and support. Head position was intermittently at midline.	Could sit independently for a distance of 40 feet with the horse at a slow walk, with hands either placed on his own thighs or placed on the withers for support and balance. Hand placement was his choice and often changed positions during the slow walk. Maintained head at midline for 50% distance traveled.

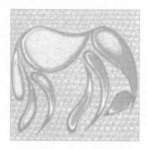

The hooves of the horses! Oh! Witching and sweet
Is the music earth steals from the iron-shod feet;
No whispers of lovers, no trilling of bird,
Can stir me as hooves of the horse have stirred.
—Will H. Ogilvie

CHAPTER 34

Visual Perception and Low-Vision Training: A Follow-Up Activity After Hippotherapy

Cynthia A. Marx, OTR/L

Visual perception is the ability to understand, process, and interpret what one sees. Vision is the key to learning, and visual–perceptual skills are dependent on visual skills, eye tracking, scanning, and convergence. The puzzles, tracings, and activities that follow were designed to promote visual–perceptual skills accessed and enhanced by hippotherapy.

Gains in visual–perceptual skills from a hippotherapy session may occur from the heightened state of awareness and alertness experienced by the client. The increased, focused vestibular input simply overflows from the close connection between the inner ear and the ocular motor muscles. The puzzles on the following pages (see Figures 34.1–34.5) may help produce visual–perceptual growth in the client, once the hippotherapy session is concluded. The puzzles are progressive and an easy way to chart gains.

> **Answers to puzzles:**
> A. Riding arena—8
> B. Horse Constellation—Pegasus
> C. Color, cut out form. Works best on index and middle fingers.
> D. Carrots and apples—5 each
> E. 81 apples in the barrel

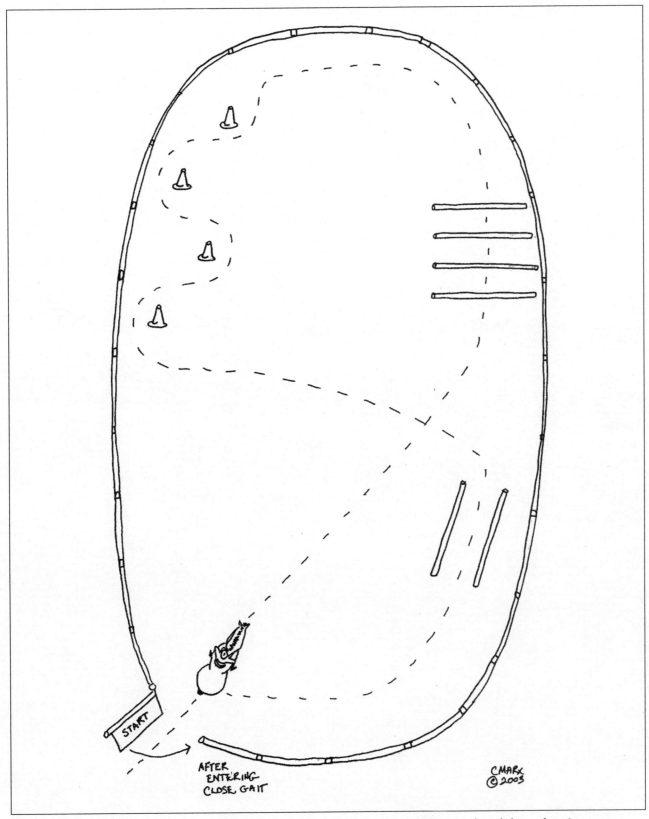

Figure 34.1. Puzzle A: Can you trace the pattern around the riding ring? What number did you form?

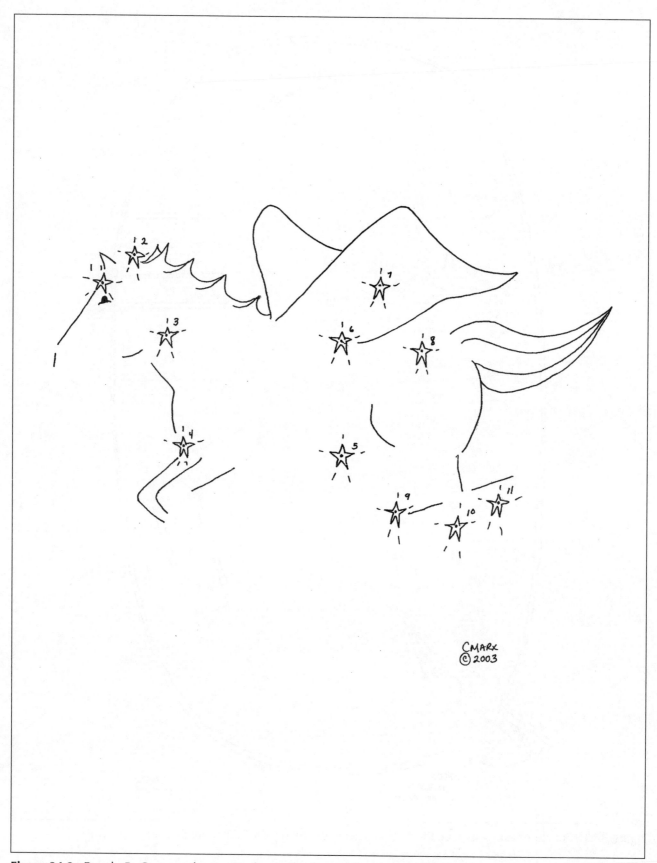

Figure 34.2. Puzzle B: Connect the stars to form what famous horse constellation?

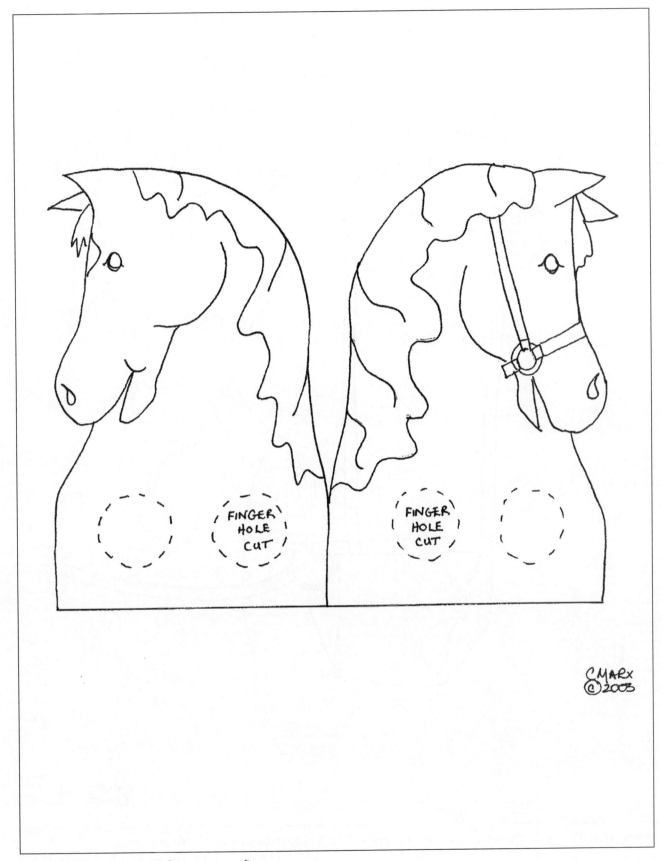

Figure 34.3. Puzzle C: Make your own finger puppets.

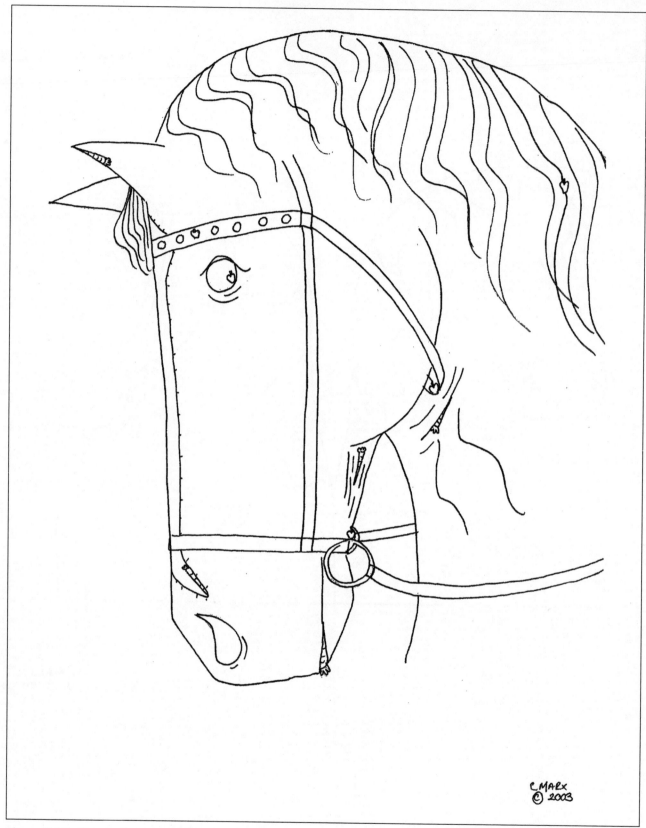

Figure 34.4. Puzzle D: Horses like carrots and apples. Find 5 of each hidden in the horse's head!

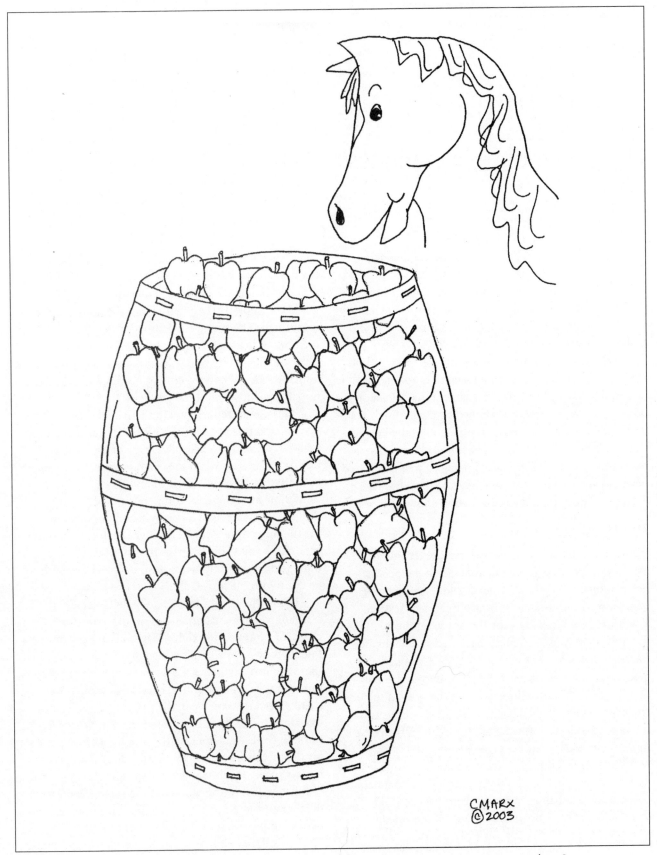

Figure 34.5. Puzzle E: Can you help the horse count the apples in the barrel? How many are there?

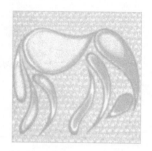

*A horse is worth
more than riches.*
—Spanish Proverb

CHAPTER 35

Horse-Handling Techniques

Jan Spink, MA

Developing a repertoire of skilled horse-handing techniques is a critical aspect of equine-assisted therapy (whether it be hippotherapy or developmental riding therapy). This chapter outlines treatment-specific methods of handling the therapy horse developed by the author during service work with clients.

Traditional horse-handling techniques, such as leading and longeing, are commonly seen in hippotherapy and equine-assisted therapy. A broader range of adapted horse-handing techniques, designed by the author, are particularly client centered and respectful of the horse's valuable contribution to the therapeutic process. These modifications in handling offer improved treatment flexibility for the therapist, and they add the advantage of decreased burnout due to routinization and work stress.

The Therapy Triangle

Figure 35.1 illustrates the therapy triangle technique. The horse, the head developmental riding therapist or occupational therapist, and the assistant, expert horse-handler form this triangle during a treatment session. The horse is controlled by the therapist and the assistant therapist by means of a light, woven canvas line approximately 6 feet long. The excess line is neatly folded and held in the outside hands of the therapist and the assistant therapist. The two lines make up the sides of the triangle and allow the therapist and the assistant therapist to make specific adjustments to the quality of the horse's movement throughout the session.

The therapist and the assistant are positioned directly at the client's sides so they are able to maintain constant physical and eye contact with the client. This three-point bond consisting of therapist, mounted

Note: This chapter was reprinted from *The Therapy Horse* with permission from Jan Spink.

client, and assistant horse-handler makes up the base of the triangle. In this arrangement, the therapist and the assistant can use their free inside hand to constantly guide and support the client within the moment of the movement. The triangle is a closed system because each member of the team can have a direct effect on every other member. When the circuitry is used appropriately, a strong sense of connectedness, both physical and emotional, develops within the group.

This connectedness is a fundamental aspect of the system, and it is used for three parallel purposes. First, it allows the team to take advantage of every moment during the session when the client is open for learning or ready for a positive shift in an objective area, such as midline awareness. In comparison, when leading, driving, or therapeutic longeing techniques are used, the therapist sometimes gets caught slightly behind the action or event. This happens mostly when the therapist must verbally communicate to someone else what is to be done with the horse.

Using the therapy triangle, the therapist and the assistant can give instantaneous input to the horse, the client, or both because they are in constant communication by touch or proximity. That crucial moment when the client is ready to learn or is prepared for a shift in function is easier to capture, because as soon as the client's need is seen or felt, the therapist can instantly offer input. The short distance to the horse's side and, through the canvas lines, to the mouth, make it possible for the therapist to instantaneously effect changes in the horse's speed, rhythm, or direction. The close proximity of the therapist to the horse and the client also allows the therapist to anticipate any needs and apply preventive or supportive measures ahead of time.

Second, the therapy triangle provides an in-hand method of handling the horse that is client centered.

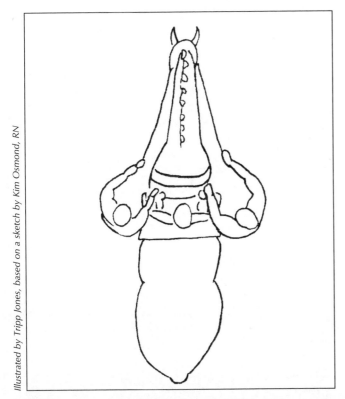

Illustrated by Tripp Jones, based on a sketch by Kim Osmond, RN

Figure 35.1. Therapy triangle technique.

The therapy horse maintains more definition in its gait and rhythm because it receives input on both sides of its body. This consistency has a direct impact on the quality of movement the client is able to experience. Also, because the client is being guided on both sides of the body, the client is able to develop even, bilateral control and can feel an added sense of security and centering.

Third, the therapy triangle requires a client-specific safety and handling protocol. This method establishes a clear hierarchy of control and safety for the client. The head therapist usually is positioned on the near side to give primary input to the horse and the client. It always must be clearly understood that this member of the team is responsible for getting the horse under control should there ever be a problem such as shying or stumbling.

The head therapist also determines how and where the horse should be moving during the therapy session. The assistant, on the off or right side of the horse, is there to support the horse's movement and offer directional changes as requested by the head therapist. In a therapeutic sense, the assistant's primary responsibility is collaborative. In terms of safety protocol, the assistant is responsible for securing, supporting, or dismounting the client if necessary in an emergency.

Generally, this safety rule is followed when the therapy triangle is used. If a client requires two side supporters for *complete* postural security on the horse, then another method of horse handling must be used. This technique was designed by the author and intended specifically for clients who have good trunk and head control, possess appropriate postural reactions in regard to upright posture on the horse with graded movement challenges, and have consistent behavior control.

Summary

The therapy triangle is an advanced and specialized method of handling the horse. It is not considered suitable for beginning practitioners, handlers of less than first-level dressage competency, or therapeutic recreational riding programs. It is especially unsuitable for programs using lay volunteers, because the horse must have the utmost consistency and specificity of handling to avoid possible confusion. That said, this technique has been my first choice for handling for 25 years. It keeps the horses very happy and allows the team maximum productivity.

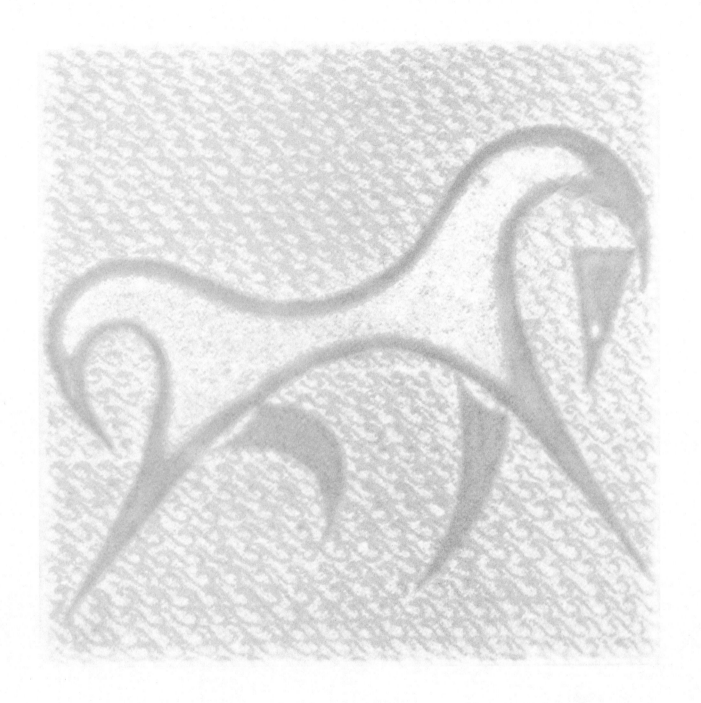

PART V

Business Management and Training Techniques

…Through his mane and tail the high winds sings,
Fanning the hairs, who wave like feather'd wings.
—William Shakespeare

A canter is a cure for every evil.
—Benjamin Disraeli

CHAPTER 36

Hospital-Based Hippotherapy Programs: Business Plan and Marketing

Teresa Tisdell, MPH, OTR

Managers of hippotherapy centers must answer many ongoing questions about overcoming challenges and expanding their program. Questions may include, How can therapeutic riding centers and hippotherapy programs cope with the challenges confronting them, which potentially threaten their existence? How do programs build on strengths and minimize weaknesses so as to better position themselves for success? This chapter addresses these and other questions and shares the experiences of one program to illustrate the importance of implementing a strong business plan.

Strategic planning can be defined as "a disciplined effort to produce fundamental decisions and actions that shape and guide what an organization is, what it does, and why it does it" (Bryson, 1995). Strategic planning requires broad and effective information gathering, exploration of strategic alternatives, and emphasis on future implications of present decisions (Bryson, 1995). It helps organizations focus on producing effective decisions and actions that further their mission (Cleveland, 1993), and it provides for directional strategies (Kaplan & Norton, 2001). A strategic plan is not useful unless it strategically improves thought and action (Bryson, 1995).

A business plan operationalizes the strategic plan; it should be concise and provide as much information as possible (Kaplan & Norton, 2001). For example, components of such a plan might include an executive summary, an organizational plan or systems change initiative, a marketing plan, financial documents, and other supporting documents (Mintzberg, 1994).

Why is it important to develop a strong plan in the world of therapeutic riding and hippotherapy? Therapeutic riding programs and hippotherapy programs

may be continually challenged to provide evidence of therapeutic effectiveness and clinical research to support their claims. Therapeutic riding and hippotherapy centers also grapple with typical nonprofit issues such as fundraising, volunteer management, board development, and marketing. Meeting these ongoing challenges, along with external threats and opportunities, requires a strong plan, support network, and broad range of resources.

The following sections describe the author's personal experience with one hippotherapy program and its struggle to survive within a health care organization during the 1990s, a time of U.S. health care reforms.

Case Report

In the mid-1990s, the rehabilitation health care market was prosperous and receptive to innovative, alternative methods of rehabilitation care. It was a time of fee-for-service reimbursement; that is, the higher costs of services allowed for higher reimbursement rates from Medicare. It was the perfect opportunity to propose hippotherapy as a program within the rehabilitation hospital, and that was exactly what happened in the case of the Rehab A* program.

Rehab A is a 130-bed rehabilitation hospital comprising five inpatient rehabilitation floors, multiple outpatient centers, and a home health agency. Rehab A's corporate objectives included being recognized as one of the top rehabilitation centers in the nation. Innovative programs were quickly emerging within the

---

*The name of the program has been changed to protect the privacy of its staff and patients.

organization to provide excellent services and maximize patients' outcomes. This environment provided the perfect opportunity for a hospital-based rehabilitation program.

Hippotherapy was quickly embraced by the Rehab A system and aggressively marketed through strong media coverage, civic activities, and systemwide educational opportunities. Initially, the staff included one full-time occupational therapist responsible for developing, implementing, and managing the program; two volunteers; and one horse. The facilities consisted of a public indoor arena that had a makeshift outdoor arena; the program had exclusive use of the facilities during weekdays.

In the beginning, a surge of referrals occurred for physical, occupational, and speech therapy using hippotherapy intervention strategies. The program expanded quickly over the first year. The staff added a full-time director, a physical therapist, and an occupational therapist, as well as a part-time speech–language pathologist. The herd grew to four horses, and the program moved to a private facility with therapy rooms, offices, and handicapped-accessible restroom facilities and parking. The program continued to flourish over a 2-year span until drastic changes occurred in 2000, again because of U.S. health care reform. Unfortunately, the Rehab A system became faced with fiscal challenges secondary to reimbursement changes and issues of corporate compliance. The hippotherapy program joined a long list of programs that were not considered "core" services for the organization during this financially challenging time. The program managed to survive the initial cuts, but challenges persisted.

The next challenge to overcome was the loss of a steady referral base. New productivity and accountability measures caused a shift in the program's patient referral base. Traditionally, patients were referred to hippotherapy from inpatient and outpatient rehabilitation services within the system. Because of stringent productivity conditions, therapists could not refer rehabilitation patients to the program and still meet daily requirements. Therefore, a business plan was constructed to address the challenge and alter the marketing approach to target patients in the local community instead of the traditional referral base. This approach was successful and yielded an 80% increase in the clientele, all of whom represented "new" reimbursement sources (i.e., clients who had not previously sought services from Rehab A).

Further challenges were encountered. A corporate compliance committee was established systemwide in an effort to oversee billing and compliance with U.S. Medicare rules and regulations. Hippotherapy was one of the first programs up for review. Diligent networking, pooling of information, and sharing of resources from other hippotherapy centers helped establish a strong case to allow billing of therapy services using the horse as a treatment strategy. Once again, the hippotherapy program persevered.

The final battle was too substantial for the program to overcome. Most patients seen by the program were pediatric and without insurance but Medicaid eligible. When the program started, Medicaid paid for any services the child needed. Under U.S. health care reform, private insurance organizations would be paid to manage services for Medicaid patients in an attempt to regulate health care spending. In Rehab A's state, Medicaid recipients could enroll in one of three programs. Unfortunately, Rehab A had a contract as a service provider with only one of the three companies and would not pursue contracting with others for reasons larger than the hippotherapy program.

The number of patients that could access hippotherapy services dropped by two-thirds. Given the decrease of referrals from within the system and the inability of many Medicaid patients to access the hippotherapy program, the Rehab A system was forced to evaluate the need for the program.

Strategic planning became more important than ever at this point. The options for sustaining the program included operating the program on a part-time basis, adding therapeutic riding services, soliciting mental health clients, and collaborating with another health care organization to provide the service. Unfortunately, those options did not come to fruition before the organization was forced to close the program.

Upon closure of the facility, one patient's family contacted a local news channel in one last effort to rescue the program. Although the outpouring of community support was encouraging, it was not enough to maintain the program under the auspices of the health care organization. It was, however, enough to purchase the equipment and supplies from the hospital and begin a new nonprofit therapeutic riding and hippotherapy program under a new name and independent organizational structure.

Summary

Strategic planning began again, establishing the program's mission, goals, and approach to meeting those goals. A business plan laid out the new organizational structure, the intended client population, and services to be provided. The plan included financial planning and marketing strategies to establish a strong foundation for the new program. A new facility was sought, horses and volunteers were trained, and within 4 months, the program was up and running. As of 2004, the program serves a client base of 75 children free of charge because of a strong volunteer base and community support.

References

Bryson, J. M. (1995). *Strategic planning for public and nonprofit organizations: A guide to strengthening and sustaining organizational achievement* (rev. ed.). San Francisco: Jossey-Bass.

Cleveland, H. (1993). *Birth of the new world: An open monument for international leadership.* San Francisco: Jossey-Bass.

Kaplan, R. S., & Norton, D. P. (2001). *The strategy-focused organization.* Boston: Harvard Business School.

Mintzberg, H. (1994). *The rise and fall of strategic planning: Reconceiving roles for planning, plans, and planners.* New York: Free Press.

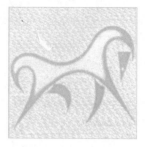

*A man on a horse is spiritually,
as well as physically,
bigger than a man on foot.*
—*John Steinbeck*

CHAPTER 37

Structured Occupational Therapy Internship

Kathy Splinter-Watkins, MOT, OTR/L, FAOTA, HPCS

Many aspiring occupational therapists discovered their calling by volunteering in a therapeutic riding or hippotherapy setting. Is it any wonder, then, that many of today's occupational therapy students wish to do at least one of their required fieldwork experiences in the field of hippotherapy? The educational needs of occupational therapy students and occupational therapy assistants and their desire to be involved with a therapeutic equine environment can be met in several different ways, as described in this chapter.

Brandenburger-Shasby and colleagues (1998) described *fieldwork* as the link between education and practice. Within occupational therapy is a need for occupation-based fieldwork to complement academic programs (Cohn & Crist, 1995). The *Occupational Therapy Practice Framework* (American Occupational Therapy Association [AOTA], 2002) defines the many different levels of practice that can apply to the world of equine-assisted therapy and hippotherapy. Both Level I and Level II fieldwork can be enhanced by participation in settings that offer hippotherapy or equine-assisted therapy. Working with horses can be occupation in the most basic sense, and it brings home the meaning of purposeful, occupation-based practice. Not only does the multidimensional movement of the horse affect client mobility and function, but this type of practice meets the client in a natural environment where tasks, occupations, and connections can be significantly adapted. Moreover, horse care and management can provide creative and realistic alternatives to the regular clinic environment.

Types of Fieldwork Experiences

Practitioners need to make decisions about the type of fieldwork experiences possible. The fieldwork will depend on the student's experience with horses and abilities in horsemanship, the other educational experiences that are needed to round out the student's fieldwork requirements, and the opportunities that are available. Interest in hippotherapy or equine-assisted therapy usually seems to stem from a lifelong passion for horses. Some occupational therapy students, however, discover the magic of horses later in life and are intrigued with the varied uses and dramatic results of equine-assisted therapy. Such students need to develop basic horsemanship skills to further understand safety issues and fully intertwine occupational therapy and equine experiences.

Hippotherapy is defined as "a physical, occupational, and speech therapy treatment strategy that utilizes equine movement" (American Hippotherapy Association, 2004). Within physical therapy and occupational therapy practice, hippotherapy is considered primarily for clients with physical disabilities. Indeed, hippotherapy may be used to facilitate balance, posture, mobility, and function. Occupational therapy, however, can be involved in many different equine-assisted therapy settings in institutional, community, or even camp settings for clients with mental, emotional, cognitive, behavioral, sensory-integrative, or developmental disabilities (Splinter-Watkins, 2004). A student with a mental health focus may want a fieldwork experience with an equine-facilitated mental health program. Equine-assisted therapy programs across the nation deal with juvenile delinquency, eating disorders, abuse and neglect, and depression or substance abuse. Prevocational skills, vocational rehabilitation, and back-to-work programs involving horses also can be areas for occupational therapy fieldwork experiences.

LaGrossa (2004) discussed the world of jockeys in thoroughbred racing. What are the occupational therapy implications for this group? For budding occupational therapists, both hippotherapy and equine-assisted therapy settings can be innovative educational, experiential, and career opportunities.

Requirements for Level I and Level II Fieldwork

According to the Accreditation Council for Occupational Therapy Education (ACOTE®) standards (AOTA, 2006), the goal of Level I fieldwork is "to introduce students to the fieldwork experience, and develop a basic comfort level with and understanding of the needs of clients" (p. 60). Along with enriching didactic coursework by providing experience with those with disabilities, fieldwork introduces the student to the variety of practice settings possible for occupational therapy. Having a full-time supervising occupational therapist is not required for Level I Fieldwork, and each academic program has the prerogative to meet the Level I standards in the way it feels is best. If a therapeutic riding center is used for Level I Fieldwork, however, an occupational or physical therapist should work in consultation with the therapeutic riding instructor (or the instructor may be dually credentialed as an occupational therapist). This arrangement allows the student to gain educationally relevant information and perspective. If the setting is hippotherapy practice, then the primary therapist can engage the student in provocative discussions and processing during and after the hippotherapy sessions.

In contrast, ACOTE standards (AOTA, 2006) state that the goal for Level II Fieldwork is to develop competent, entry-level, generalist occupational therapists or occupational therapy assistants. Level II fieldwork offers in-depth experience in delivering occupational therapy services. It focuses on the application of purposeful and meaningful occupation or research, administration, and management. An occupational therapist using hippotherapy or equine-assisted therapy in practice can illustrate a true merger of all these elements.

The ACOTE standards (AOTA, 2006) require inclusion of a variety of clients across the life span and a variety of settings (both traditional and emerging). Fieldwork may include 1 to 4 settings over the equivalent of 24 weeks. The flexibility of this standard allows for a variety of ways to meet this guideline. It is in the student's best learning interest to participate in a traditional fieldwork setting first and then to do a second fieldwork experience at a setting that includes hippotherapy. Alternatively, an additional 4 to 12 weeks in a setting with hippotherapy may be used as a specialty fieldwork after the required 24 weeks have been completed.

Considerations for Developing a Level II Hippotherapy Fieldwork Experience

A practitioner who takes on a Level I or II fieldwork occupational therapy student must attend to everything from terminology to safety to developing knowledge and skills. Because being a fieldwork educator requires preparation, the following sections outline some considerations for setting up a Level II fieldwork program as an example.

Time Frame

A first consideration is the time frame of the program. Is the program full-time and 5 days per week, or is it part-time, seasonal, contracted when appropriate, or connected with the school system? For Level I students, a part-time program could be perfectly adequate for observation and introduction to the world of hippotherapy or equine-assisted therapy. For Level II fieldwork, three-quarter or full-time work is preferred, or a combination of different practice settings may be possible. Often, an occupational therapist only uses hippotherapy as appropriate in his or her practice or only uses it part-time. Students in such settings could assist in other settings in the therapist's practice. Alternatively, a student may combine hours from 2 or 3 programs or settings. As long as communication lines are kept open and expectations are clear, students may be able to balance a couple of different settings and supervisors. Doing so, in fact, can enhance the fieldwork experience.

Clientele

What types of individuals or groups are served within the program? Is the caseload primarily pediatric clients or clients of a variety of ages? Does the program serve clients with physical disabilities, mental or behavioral challenges, or a mixture of the types? Is the practice defined as equine-facilitated mental health, equine-assisted therapy, or hippotherapy? Does it also offer driving, sport and competition for riders, or experiential and group therapy? Is the practice a family-comprehensive one, or does it focus primarily on the client? This information should be conveyed to the academic fieldwork coordinator at the university to best match students' learning needs to the practice.

Theoretical Framework

The practice's theoretical framework is a consideration. Do the therapists practice from a neurodevelopmental, psychosocial, cognitive behavioral, or sensory integrative framework? How does this match with what is taught in the university providing the fieldwork students? Programs hoping to sponsor students should request information about the academic program and curriculum. Coordinating the fieldwork experience with the curriculum at the university is important for consistency in education and practice.

Supervision

Who will supervise the students? Is the practice that of a sole practitioner? Are other disciplines involved in the practice? The members of the occupational therapy team make a difference when students are added into the mix. They should be supportive of having students and willing to teach students about their field of practice, share their perspective, and direct the student when the supervising therapist is unavailable.

University Support

How accessible is the university program for assistance in setting up the fieldwork program and providing ongoing support, problem-solving, and consultation? Will the program provide make onsite visits? University support is beneficial for everything from paperwork to program development to creative scheduling to problem solving.

Once a decision is made to become a fieldwork educator, it is time to talk with the academic fieldwork coordinator at a particular university occupational therapy program. Outline what the hippotherapy or equine-assisted therapy program has to offer, inquire as to the university's fieldwork needs, and find out what support is offered for program development. Send any required information, and ask for a contract. Contracts may take up to 6 months, or even a year, to negotiate, so plenty of time is available for program development.

Technology

Does the hippotherapy or equine-assisted therapy program have distance-learning or videotaping capabilities? Technology can enhance educational offerings and create another avenue for analyzing scenarios and solving problems involving treatment.

Legal and Ethical Considerations

Establishing a fieldwork program involves many legal and ethical considerations. What contracts are needed? Usually, a contract is required between the fieldwork program and the university, and administrative paperwork is a necessity. Contracts generally are either year-to-year or renew every 3 or 5 years.

Liability is an issue. What liability insurance does the fieldwork program have, and what does it cover?

Does the university provide any coverage? The student, either through the school or through an individual policy, must obtain liability insurance. Who might be liable in case of any accidents? If the program rents space at a local barn or riding facility, then it must have liability insurance. The board of directors and staff at a facility also may need liability coverage.

Fieldwork programs should be accredited. North American Riding for the Handicapped Association accreditation is the standard in the United States for therapeutic riding programs with a hippotherapy component. Fieldwork sponsors in private practice must follow state regulations (usually licensure).

Fieldwork programs must have a confidentiality statement. Health Insurance Portability and Accountability Act guidelines (Costa, 2004) must be followed. A document explaining the guidelines and specifying confidentiality expectations must be understood and signed by the student.

Program Content

Setting up a student program can be fun. Steps to creating a program can be found on the AOTA Web site (www.aota.org). Keys to a successful student program include developing a thorough orientation, setting up the structure or framework, evaluating the student fairly, and developing effective learning experiences (Splinter-Watkins, 2002a).

An orientation should include a notebook containing policies and procedures for the setting or program. It should include emergency procedures; safety guidelines; samples of documentation, including evaluation forms, progress notes, and discharge forms; location of tack and barn equipment; name, location, and idiosyncrasies of each horse; lists of staff and volunteers; and organizational configuration, including the program director and board of directors, as appropriate. The student should participate in formal orientation sessions with the volunteers and staff.

The structure or framework for the student program is important for clarifying expectations for the student and supervisor (see AOTA, 2000a; Costa, 2004; Splinter-Watkins, 2002b). The program objectives are probably most important from the academic point of view because they affect how the student is evaluated throughout the internship. Objectives need to be developed to match the Fieldwork Performance Evaluation form (FWPE; see Costa, 2004), which is the student evaluation tool. Several universities have developed helpful templates for developing objectives. Assistance with understanding the FWPE and writing objectives can be found on the AOTA Web site and in the manual (AOTA, 2000b). Also included in the structure should be a timeline and weekly expectations, because they provide the student with clear directions for performance.

Different assignments and projects may enhance the student's experience. Ideas include developing new adaptive equipment, reflective journals, guided observation, provocative questioning and discussion, and developing a new form or treatment protocol. Research on a certain diagnosis or a case study and following a specific client throughout the 12-week fieldwork assignment is a beneficial learning tool.

During the 12 weeks, the supervisor should provide regular feedback. Most fieldwork settings establish daily and weekly informal feedback sessions and formal midterm (6-week) and final (12-week) evaluations. The Fieldwork Experience Assessment Tool (Costa, 2004) can assist with connecting the student, supervisor, and environment; encouraging discussion of the fieldwork experience; and solving any problems that arise.

Space Considerations

What is needed to prepare for a student to be at the facility? Considerations may include housing, desk space, access to library and records, phone access, resources, other personnel, and financial assistance. Students, of course, love anything that can make their life conducive to learning, but a site does not have to offer anything but a good learning experience.

Student Considerations

What type of student can program staff best work with? How comfortable must the student be around horses? What level of horsemanship must he or she have attained? What are the student's motivation, personal goals, interpersonal skills, problem-solving abilities, and grasp of therapeutic concepts? Has the student completed a previous Level II fieldwork assignment? Interview the student either over the phone or, preferably, in person. This is someone with whom the program will be working for 3 months. Consider how to assess the student's level of responsibility and horsemanship skills in the interview. What will you accept? Not everyone needs to be a dressage expert, but a working knowledge of horses should be expected.

Conclusion

Providing an educational opportunity for occupational therapy students can be a tremendous experience and can evolve into mutually rewarding professional connections. Students can bring updated information to you in your practice and can provide the extra hands and brain power to puzzle over treatment challenges. It can be a joy to see them grow and develop into entry-level therapists and peers. By educating students in hippotherapy or other equine-assisted therapy, one not only shares one's enthusiasm for this area of practice but also presents students with creative occupation-based interventions and alternatives to traditional clinical practice.

References

American Hippotherapy Association. (2004). *What is hippotherapy?* Retrieved January 4, 2004, from www.americanhippotherapyassociation.org/aha_hpot.htm.

American Occupational Therapy Association. (2000a). *Steps to starting a fieldwork program.* Bethesda, MD: Author.

American Occupational Therapy Association. (2000b). *Strategies for creative fieldwork opportunities.* Bethesda, MD: Author.

American Occupational Therapy Association. (2002). Occupational therapy practice framework: Domain and process. *American Journal of Occupational Therapy, 56,* 609–639.

American Occupational Therapy Association. (2006). *The reference manual of the official documents of the American Occupational Therapy Association, Inc* (11th ed.). Bethesda, MD: AOTA Press.

Brandenburger-Shasby, S., Hills, L., Huie, C., Jansen, K., Johnson, L., Josey-Lamont, A., et al. (1998). Fieldwork: The critical link. *Education Special Interest Section Quarterly, 8*(3), 1–3.

Cohn, E. S., & Crist, P. (1995). Nationally Speaking—Back to the future: New approaches to fieldwork education. *American Journal of Occupational Therapy, 49,* 103–106.

Costa, D. (Ed.). (2004). *The essential guide to occupational therapy fieldwork education: Resources for today's educators and practitioners.* Bethesda, MD: AOTA Press.

LaGrossa, J. (2004). Racing for the glory. *Advance for Occupational Therapy Practitioners, 20*(15), 16–19.

Splinter-Watkins, K. L. (2002a). Choosing the right fieldwork sites. In K. Sladyk (Ed.), *The successful occupational therapy fieldwork student* (pp. 53–62). Thorofare, NJ: Slack.

Splinter-Watkins, K. L. (2002b). Creating the new fieldwork experience. *OT Practice, 7,* 11–15.

Splinter-Watkins, K. L. (2004). Equine-assisted therapy for adults with developmental disabilities. In M. Ross & S. Bachner (Eds.), *Adults with developmental disabilities: Current approaches in occupational therapy* (rev. ed., pp. 153–165). Bethesda, MD: AOTA Press.

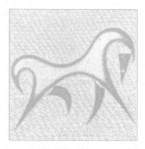

Horsemanship is "one."
—Jean-Claude Racinet

CHAPTER 38

Reimbursement for Occupational Therapy Services Using Hippotherapy as a Strategy

Amy Taylor Johnson, MS, OT

In an attempt to make reimbursement for therapy as easy as possible for occupational therapists in the United States, the following is a list of steps that therapists may use to increase the likelihood of obtaining insurance reimbursement. Following these steps does not guarantee payment by an insurance company but may assist clients in obtaining coverage.

Obtaining Coverage

1. Contact the physician to request an order for occupational therapy, physical therapy, or speech–language pathology (depending upon the professional providing service). Do not request orders for "hippotherapy."
2. Contact the insurance company to determine whether the requested therapy is a covered benefit.
3. If therapy is covered, determine whether the company will reimburse for private, out-client therapy or when it is paid out of pocket.
4. Ask the insurance company if it will reimburse for services furnished by a therapist who is not on the insurance company's list of providers.
5. Determine any limits on the number of therapy visits, deductibles, or co-pays.
6. Determine whether preauthorization is needed.
7. Determine whether recertification is needed, and if so, after how many treatment sessions.
8. If the client currently receives occupational therapy services from another provider, determine whether additional services will be covered.

Documentation

1. An evaluation by a credentialed therapist must be completed.
2. Functional goals should be written to emphasize functional gains off the horse.
3. Progress must be documented according to professional standards of practice and professional guidelines for documentation.
4. Terminology:

Avoid Using	Use Instead
Moving horse	Dynamic base of support
Halt–walk transitions	Stop–start transitions

Billing

1. Bill using *Current Procedural Terminology (CPT)* codes. Typical codes are as follows (but always check the latest version for the proper codes):
   a. 97110 B: therapeutic procedure/exercise
   b. 97112 B: neuromuscular reeducation
   c. 97530 B: therapeutic activities
   d. 97533: sensory integrative techniques
   e. 97532: development of cognitive skills
2. Typical charges may be $25 to $50 per *CPT* code. Establishing charges will depend on reasonable and customary charges in particular regions of the country and may increase or decrease.

*Movement is the expression
of the entire personality of
an individual.*
—Susan von Dietze

CHAPTER 39

Business Forms for a Hippotherapy Practice

Rebecca Cook, OTR, HPCS

When occupational therapists step into the world of hippotherapy, most are generally entering the realm of an autonomous or private practice, which carries with it a standard of professionalism beyond hippotherapy treatment proficiency. Basic business and organizational skills are essential.

The forms included in this chapter (Figures 39.1–39.7) were created for The Right Step, a therapy practice in Michigan. Although a lawyer has reviewed the liability releases of the forms, other states and countries may have different legal and wording requirements. It is the responsibility of anyone choosing to use or adapt these forms to acquire legal assistance to ensure adherence to their own state and national requirements. These forms are constantly evolving to include new information, legal updates, or changes in therapy practice. The forms in this book may differ from those currently in use at The Right Step.

Employee, Volunteer, Student Registration and Emergency Treatment

Date _____

No individual can be accepted as an employee, volunteer, or student at *The Right Step Therapy Services LLC* ("*TRS*") until this form has been completed by the individual if he/she is a legally competent adult age 18 or over or by his/her parent(s) or guardian. Therapy instructions will be under strict supervision, and although every effort will be made to avoid any accident, no liability can be accepted by any of the individuals or organizations concerned or by *TRS,* its personnel, or affiliates. Completion of this form constitutes (parent/guardian if applicable) permission for the named individual to participate as an employee, volunteer, or student in the program.

Name _____

Date of birth _____

Address _____

City_____ State _____ Zip_____

Home phone _____ Cell phone _____ Work phone _____

E-mail _____

Previous experience with horses _____

Parent/guardian name (if under 18 years) _____

Phone contact _____

Address_____

City_____ State _____ Zip_____

Physician's name _____

Phone contact _____

Address _____

City_____ State _____ Zip_____

Is there a medical condition requiring special precaution or treatment?   Yes ☐   No ☐

If yes, please describe _____

Medications being used?   Yes ☐   No ☐   If yes, please list dosage and description _____

Person who should be notified in case of emergency in absence of parent or guardian:

Emergency contact name _____ Phone_____ Relationship _____

References

1)_____ 2)_____ 3)_____

Relationship/Phone #

1)_____ 2)_____ 3)_____

Figure 39.1. Employee, Volunteer, Student Registration, and Emergency Treatment.

Authorization for Purpose of Providing Medical Treatment

You are being asked to complete this form to give an appropriate medical facility permission to treat _____ (employee, volunteer, or student's name) for minor injury or medical problems. In the event of serious injury or illness, the parent/guardian or person listed above will be contacted; treatment will proceed before contacting them only if the situation is urgent and does not permit delay.

Preferred medical facility _____

In case of medical emergency, the undersigned authorizes *TRS* and/or its affiliate to seek any medical and/or surgical treatment necessary for the care of _____, who is participating as an employee, volunteer, or student in *TRS* treatment program with parent/guardian permission if under 18 years.

I understand that NO LIABILITY can be accepted by any individual or organization concerned with this program in the event of any accident which may occur.

Health Insurance
Name of policyholder _____

Name of insurance company _____

Policy number(s) _____

If you have HMO or PHP insurance, please list the emergency phone number for treatment authorization _____

Name of policyholder's employer _____

The above designated person(s) is (are) hereby authorized to incur medical costs necessary to provide medical treatment for said participant for which we the undersigned shall be fully responsible. We also authorize the medical facility to release any and all information required to complete insurance claims and also authorize insurance payments directly to the medical facility.

Signature _____ Date _____

Printed Name _____
Parent/Guardian/Adult (circle appropriate title)

Witness _____

Figure 39.2. Authorization for Purpose of Providing Medical Treatment.

Informed Consent and Release of Liability Agreement

No individual can be accepted as an employee, volunteer, or student into *The Right Step Therapy Services LLC* ("*TRS*") until this form has been completed by the individual if he/she is a legally competent adult age 18 or over or by his/her parent(s)/guardian.

It is mutually understood that the liability release contained in this agreement shall constitute a waiver of liability beyond the provisions of the Michigan Equine Activity Liability Act, 1994 P.A. 351.

WARNING
Under the Michigan Equine Activity Liability Act [1994 P.A. 351], an equine professional is not liable for an injury to or the death of a participant in an equine activity resulting from an inherent risk of the equine activity.

I/we assume the risks and accept the consequences involved in the participation of _____ (employee, volunteer, or student's name) at *TRS* and its affiliates.

I/we are hereby informed of the possible dangers to me/my child/my ward that may result from participation in the program, including soft tissue (including skin and muscle) injury, ligament and tendon injury, bone/joint injury, and exacerbation of chronic conditions.

I/we recognize that the above listing may not be complete and that a fuller explanation of the possible consequences is available upon request. However, I/we do not wish further explanation.

I/we accept the responsibility for complying fully with all safety rules, regulations, and practices and I/we will consult with an authorized representative of *TRS* for advice in circumstances where safe practices are in doubt.

I/we hereby release *The Right Step Therapy Services LLC,* its owners, staff, students, volunteers, affiliates, and any other individuals and/or organizations involved from any liability for injury that may result from participation in the program and activities.

I/we do not have any type of criminal background and give permission for completion of a background check.

I/we have read and fully understand this document.

Signature _____

Parent/Guardian/Adult (circle appropriate title)

Date _____

Witness _____

Date _____ Time _____

Figure 39.3. Informed Consent and Release of Liability Agreement.

Video, Film, and Photography Release*

I authorize *TRS* to record and photograph my image and/or voice and/or that of the subject named below for use by *TRS* or its assignees in research, educational, and promotional programs. I understand and agree that these audio, video, film, and/or print images may be edited, duplicated, distributed with or without charge, reproduced, broadcast, and/or reformatted in any form and manner without payment of fees, in perpetuity.

Name of subject, employee, volunteer, student _____

Signature _____

Printed name _____

Parent/Guardian/Adult (circle appropriate title)

Address _____

Phone _____ E-mail _____

*Participation in *TRS* treatment activities is not contingent on the completion of this section.

Figure 39.4. Video, Film, and Photography Release.

Horse Handler, Assistant Instructor, and Instructor
Contractual Performance Outcomes

Evaluation for _____

1) All staff registration paperwork completed in full.

_____

2) Passed Horse Knowledge Quiz.

_____

3) Able to complete sessions that are 2 consecutive hours.

_____

4) Able to complete two or more of these sessions each date.

_____

5) Completes safety precheck for equipment.

_____

6) Completes soundness precheck for horse.

_____

7) Reports safety or soundness issues to therapist or instructor in charge.

_____

8) Follows rules and client confidentiality procedures.

_____

9) Comes at scheduled times.

_____

10) Demonstrates safe handling and instructing skills during sessions.

_____

Signature of Evaluator _____ Date _____

Signature of Contractor _____ Date _____

Comments

_____
_____
_____
_____
_____
_____
_____
_____

> For use of The Right Step only—
> YES___ NO___ Contract renewed as written or as revised below
>
> _____
> _____
> _____

Figure 39.5. Horse Handler, Assistant Instructor, and Instructor Contractual Performance Outcomes.

Horse Donation Form Letter

On behalf of the Therapeutic Riding Center and the hospital, we would like to thank you for considering donating your horse to our program. The Therapeutic Riding Center opened its doors in August of 1993 and has served the needs of children and adults from the community ever since. This would not be possible without our horses—they are the keys to our success!

Our program serves individuals of all ages with special needs, including physical, cognitive or emotional diagnoses. Our staff consists of occupational therapists and equestrian techs with considerable knowledge in the care and training of horses. Their skills combine several years of experience with breeding, training, and showing horses of various breeds in disciplines including Western, English, competitive trail riding, as well as therapeutic riding and hippotherapy.

After being contacted, the staff of the Therapeutic Riding Center will mail you a donation application and schedule a visit to conduct an initial screening of your horse. This screening in no way obligates either party to the donation of the horse. You will receive a copy of the results of the screening by mail. You are encouraged to call if you have questions.

Horses are selected on disposition, quality of movement, and conformation. Other factors considered are special training, age, vices, and conditions warranting special care. A negative Coggins test is required for the initial screening, although a new test may be necessary.

After the screening, if the staff determines your horse may be suitable for the program, they will contact you to schedule a 30-day trial period for the horse to be further screened at the Therapeutic Riding Center. A staff member will contact you after 2 weeks to give you a progress report. During this time, the hospital will be responsible for veterinary care if needed. You will be notified immediately if veterinary care is required.

Horses at our facility are provided with daily turnouts as well as their own 12×12 stall. They are fed twice a day with a 48-hour turnout on weekends. They are used 2 to 4 times daily during the week for 20 to 30 minutes during each treatment session. Horses are used in no more than two consecutive sessions.

Horses are vaccinated annually. Routine and emergency veterinary care is scheduled as needed. They are wormed rotationally and supplemented as directed by the veterinarian. All horses are trimmed or shod every 6 weeks. They are groomed daily and bathed once a week during the summer. Horses receive hoof treatments for conditioning and prevention of thrush each week.

During the trial period, the staff will further evaluate the horse in all areas listed on the initial screening, as well as in specific activities related to hippotherapy and therapeutic riding. Responses to natural horsemanship methods are also assessed. An additional 2 weeks of evaluation may be requested. Following the trial period, you will be contacted about your horse's performance. You will be given a copy of the final evaluation as well. If your horse is determined suitable for the program, you will receive your tax donation receipt within 2 weeks of the completion of the trial period.

Occasionally, some horses must be retired from the program due to age-related changes or the development of behavioral vices that are unsafe for our clients. If this occurs, you will be notified to determine your wishes. If you do not want to resume ownership, the staff will determine the most suitable home for your horse. The horse may be donated or sold through private treaty or a consignment sale. Absolutely will no horse be sold through public auction.

Thank you for your consideration.

Sincerely,

Figure 39.6. Horse Donation Form Letter.

Natural Horsemanship Handling Methods

Head down cue _____   Comment _____

Hindquarter yield _____   Comment _____

Friendly game _____   Comment _____

Back up _____   Comment _____

Come to _____   Comment _____

Desire to please _____   Comment _____

Rate of learning _____   Comment _____

Overall impression _____

_____

_____

_____

_____

Additional comments_____

_____

_____

_____   _____

Signature   Date

_____   _____

Signature   Date

_____   _____

Signature   Date

Figure 39.7. Final Horse Screening.

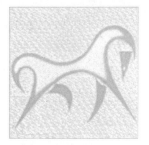

Yet when all the books have been read and reread, it boils down to the horse, his human companion, and what goes on between them.
—Walter Farley

CHAPTER 40

Insuring Equine-Assisted Occupational Therapy Practice

Debi DeTurk-Peloso, CPCU

Equine-assisted occupational therapy expands the treatment options available to those whose goal is increased function. Adding the horse to occupational therapy practice is helping many clients progress beyond their experiences with classical methods of occupational therapy.

Through riding and other associated equine activities, the treatment team of occupational therapist, equine professional, and the horse promotes increased function in a clearly defined therapeutic space and setting. Obtaining the proper insurance for these activities requires good communication between the practice and the insurer.

General Liability Insurance

Operations offering occupational therapy need general liability insurance protecting against bodily injury and property damage claims. A practice must be sure that the liability insurance it purchases insures the types of therapeutic activities it provides. The insurer must have a clear understanding of the practice to provide proper general liability coverage.

The ethical practice of occupational therapy requires a formal agreement between the client and the therapist prior to treatment. The therapist must be able to articulate the needs of the client and treatment plans and goals and be able to measure the treatment's effectiveness. A clearly defined treatment program will be able to purchase proper general liability insurance much easier than an unstructured, poorly defined operation.

The horse is an integral part of the treatment team. A general liability insurer who understands equine liability exposures may be the best choice when insuring equine-assisted occupational therapy practice.

Professional Liability for Therapists

While general liability coverage protects against suits alleging bodily injury or property damage, professional liability protects occupational therapy professionals against suits that allege they performed improperly. All practicing therapists must be sure they are covered by professional liability insurance whenever they provide professional services.

General liability would cover a lawsuit alleging a client received a bodily injury from falling while entering the treatment area. Professional liability coverage would respond to a lawsuit alleging that a client's condition deteriorated because of the therapist's prescribed treatment. It is possible that some suits might trigger both types of coverage.

Professionals who practice occupational therapy offer many treatment options. Manner of work and type of therapy is as diverse as types of licensing and credentials. Each professional is responsible for obtaining the correct credentials to practice and the correct professional liability coverage. Professional liability insurance for therapists may vary state to state, just like licensing requirements.

Providing Special Opportunities for People With Special Needs

The use of equine-assisted occupational therapy practice can make dramatic changes in people's lives. The introduction of a horse to the treatment team changes the therapeutic dynamic, usually in a positive way. Properly insuring your occupational therapy operation is an important part of a risk management plan to ensure your facility will continue providing exciting treatment opportunities for the many clients whose goal is improved function.

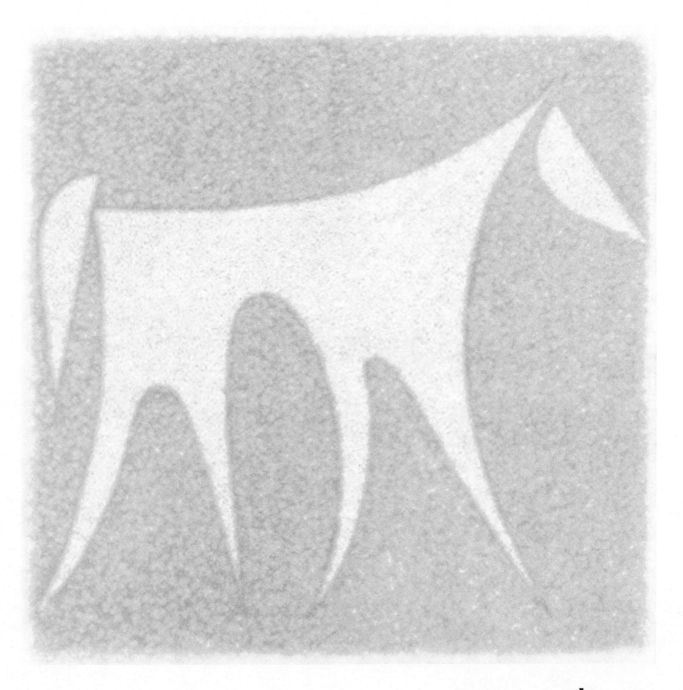

Appendixes

To be loved by a horse, or any animal,
should fill us with awe—for we have not deserved it.
—Marion Garretty

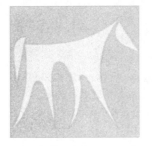

Because research adds to the knowledge base and therefore the value of the profession, obtaining grants and conducting research should not just be the job of academicians. It should be the job of both academicians and clinicians to research practice issues that help provide evidence on the effectiveness of occupational therapy services.
—Patricia Bowyer

APPENDIX A

How to Write a Journal Article for Publication

Joyce R. MacKinnon, PhD, OT(C), OTR

Some researchers are of the mistaken opinion that if they simply express their ideas, an editor will do the rest. This could not be further from the truth. A journal article must carefully follow the guidelines of the journal to which it will be submitted. Researchers who publish frequently will generate anywhere from three to eight drafts of a complete paper; each iteration improves upon the details of the document.

The typical sections of an article include the abstract, introduction, literature review, purpose of the study, research hypothesis or question, methods, results, discussion, conclusion, references, and acknowledgments.

The objective of this appendix is to give the novice hippotherapy researcher some guidance in preparing an article for publication. After describing each of the components of a research paper, the appendix concludes with practical tips to remember when writing a paper for publication.

Abstract

An *abstract,* often included at the beginning of a journal article, thesis, or report, is a short, comprehensive summary of the paper that is accurate, self-contained and concise. Weiss-Lambrou (1989) stated that an abstract must be a clear, succinct description of what the paper will examine; it should not use direct quotations, reference citations, or abbreviations not first written in full within the abstract. An abstract should contain the following elements:

- The purpose of the research
- The hypothesis or research question
- A description of the research design

- The rationale for the design
- Particulars of the methods and procedures, including special equipment, subject selection, and number of participants
- Data analyses (Hasselkus, 2001).

An abstract is one of the most important parts of a publication because readers use it to decide whether to read the entire article. It should be an interesting, brief reflection of the original work because it may be the only representation of the entire paper that readers see (Ballinger et al., 1996).

The content of the abstract depends on the type of abstract (as well as each journal's individual requirements); Day (1998) differentiates two types. An *informational abstract* addresses the issues examined, the methods used, and the results of the investigation and summarizes the conclusions. The *indicative abstract* serves as a narrative table of contents of the paper. This type of abstract can assist in determining whether the article will be useful to readers, but it does not substitute for reading the entire article. The differences in abstracts, as described by Day (1998) and Hasselkus (2001), follow methodological lines: The informational abstract is typically written for a quantitative paper, whereas the indicative abstract generally appears with qualitative research.

When Do You Write the Abstract?

Typically, an abstract is written after the entire work has been written (Ballinger et al., 1996; Weiss-Lambrou, 1989).

How Long Should the Abstract Be?

Journals generally provide guidelines. Some editors are very strict about the exact word count. Weiss-Lambrou (1989) indicated that, in her experience, abstracts range

Adapted with permission by the Federation of Riding for the Disabled. Original version of appendix appeared in the *Scientific and Educational Journal of Therapeutic Riding* (2005), pp. 40–49.

from 150 to 200 words, whereas Williams (2002) suggested that most journals permit 200 to 250 words. Whatever the word count, it is important to follow that guideline. An abstract is concise and focused!

After the abstract comes the introduction to the article.

Introduction

The introduction specifies the problem under study, presents relevant literature, and describes the research strategy. Some publications do not use the label "introduction" (American Psychological Association [APA], 2001). State the problem, then describe the approach to solving the problem (APA, 2001). Day (1998) recommended including the principal results of the study and the conclusions suggested by the results in the introduction. Typically, the last few sentences in the introduction define the variables under study and the hypothesis to be tested or research questions to be answered (APA, 2001; Day, 1998; Weiss-Lambrou, 1989).

Literature Review

The purpose of the literature review is to accomplish four major objectives, according to DePoy and Gitlin (1994):
• Summarize the previous research on the topic.
• Describe the level of theory and knowledge development.
• Describe the relevance of the current knowledge base to the problem area.
• Provide a rationale for the research strategy. (p. 47).

It is important to know what has already been researched on a given topic, how that research has been done, and whether it successfully answered the research questions posed. It also is important to determine whether the studies were well conceived and competently implemented. Additionally, when reporting studies' findings, it is critical to determine the level of knowledge within the field the study shows, how the study was generated, and what the limitations were. Once an understanding of the current state of knowledge on the topic is, the next step is to describe how it is relevant to the research questions posed by the paper. The final step is to clearly identify a rationale for the research strategy so that readers can see that the study follows on a logical continuum with other similar studies. Many of the ideas suggested by DePoy and Gitlin (1998) are reiterated by Weiss-Lambrou (1989).

How Long Should It Be?

The purpose and the type of research often dictate the length of the literature review. For example, if the research uses quantitative methods, it may be brief. If the work in question is a review article, the entire article will consist of the literature review. Unlike a research paper, a review paper is one in which no new research is undertaken, but the author critically examines research already published.

Despite these variations, the important aspect is not the length of the literature review but the thoroughness with which it is undertaken. It should cover the four major objectives specified by DePoy and Gitlin (1994). The rub here is how to balance thoroughness with eliminating nonessential information. Once researchers become involved in the process, they have great difficulty sorting relevant from irrelevant information. As Weiss-Lambrou (1989) stated, an exhaustive search must be completed before reporting that no other literature exists.

How Does One Conduct a Literature Review?

Developing a literature review is a stimulating process because many talents are brought into focus and used. It involves a search for information on the topic, sorting and analyzing the relevant literature, and summarizing the information. DePoy and Gitlin (1998) provided the following checklist:
• Determine when to conduct a search.
• Set parameters of what is searched.
• Access databases for periodicals, books, and documents.
• Organize the information.
• Critically evaluate the literature.
• Write the literature review. (p. 51)

Uses of a literature review vary, depending on whether it is for quantitative research or naturalistic inquiry (qualitative research). For the most part, however, review of the literature is done prior to undertaking the research. In quantitative research, it is always done prior to research, but with naturalistic inquiry, it may be reviewed at different points in time throughout the research (DePoy & Gitlin, 1994, 1998). Before launching into a review, the researcher needs to set parameters for what will be included and excluded. This process is mainly a function of the amount of material available on the topic. The most efficient way to search a topic is to access it from an online database that permits searching for material by topic, author, or title. Typically, resource personnel in the libraries can help researchers use the databases most effectively.

Many useful databases can help you find material in general, but when seeking information in a lesser-known area, such as hippotherapy, the search is much more time consuming. It will mean searching many databases to find a few references.

Once the material is collected, it will need to be sorted by topic or thematic area. Next, it is critiqued on several dimensions:

• Is it research based?
• Is the purpose of the paper clearly described?
• Does the purpose of the paper fit with the literature review and analyses?
• Does the author use up-to-date and quality references to support his or her opinions and ideas?
• Is there a valid conclusion (that is, does the conclusion relate back to the purpose and the literature review and follow from the results)?
• What is the theory underlying the paper?
• Is the paper clearly written and correctly documented?

What Format Should Be Used?

Authors must follow the format (also known as *editorial style*) specified by the journal or book to which the article or chapter is being submitted. Many mainstream occupational therapy journals, such as the *Canadian Journal of Occupational Therapy, American Journal of Occupational Therapy,* and *Occupational Therapy Journal of Research,* use the format of the *Publication Manual of the American Psychological Association* (APA, 2001), typically referred to as the "APA style manual." There are exceptions: The *Journal of Occupational Science* uses the Vancouver Style of the Committee of Medical Journal Editors. Although it accepts other styles, the *Scientific and Educational Journal of Therapeutic Riding* prefers APA format.

Editorial style provides specific directions regarding which headings to include, how to format references in the body of the publication and in the reference list, and requirements for tables and figures. This work is mechanical, but if your article does not follow these requirements to the letter, its chances to be accepted for publication may be hurt. Similarly, proofread the article for grammar and punctuation errors before submitting it.

Once a paper is rejected, typically it will not be reconsidered by that journal. It is a painful lesson, because it requires seeking another journal in which to publish the work.

Documentation

Evidence from published works should accompany every assertion put forward in the manuscript. Statistics, statements by other authors, and points of fact must be supported with references to the source of the information. References in a journal article provide the context for the paper and show how it builds on previous published works (Oermann, Mason, & Wilmes, 2002). They also assist readers in developing their understanding of a subject by giving them the information needed to locate related works on the subject (French, 1993; Oermann et al., 2002). Full reference information is a requirement for all mainstream journals. However, Day (1998) emphasized the importance of including only significant references that have been published. Authors who have not found support for an idea after an extensive literature search should not include it in the literature review of the paper because it is not supported or found in the literature. The idea may be proposed in the discussion section of the article.

Ideally, references should consist of primary sources—original research articles and books, for example. Secondary sources—references that come from one author who has referenced another author, such as articles in the popular press and previous literature reviews—are considered weak. Too many of them will undermine the credibility of the writer. It is always best to cite the original source. In some instances, however, it is not possible to access the original source (e.g., it is out of print); in such cases, use of a secondary source may be unavoidable. Before submitting an article for publication and again at the proof stage after acceptance, re-check every item within the reference list, as this is the one section of a manuscript that is most likely to contain errors (Day, 1998; Oermann et al., 2002).

Plagiarism

Plagiarism is taking someone else's work and passing it off as your own original idea. This offense is a serious one that has serious consequences for many parties, including the author of the original material, the scientific community, and the person who plagiarizes, including legal repercussions and loss of reputation (Oermann et al., 2002). For a university student, plagiarism can result in expulsion from the school. It is important to document the source of ideas, particularly those that are not universally accepted or that can be attributed to multiple writers (Cormack, 1994).

Paraphrasing is reporting the ideas of another author by using your own words and referencing the source. When an author's exact words are used, they must be put in quotation marks to indicate that they are the author's words. Keep in mind that direct quotes should be used sparingly and that it is generally preferable to paraphrase where possible (Williams, 2002). Too many direct quotes fragment the article, interrupt the flow of ideas, and make the manuscript difficult to read.

Where Should the Literature Review Take Readers?

The literature review should help readers and the writer understand the need for the study. It should demonstrate that the present study is not duplicating previous research or that if it is, why it is necessary to do so. It also provides a context for readers to understand the results of the study (Oermann et al., 2002; Weiss-Lambrou, 1989). In addition, the literature review should provide the framework and the theoretical background for the study (Weiss-Lambrou, 1989).

Where Do the Purpose of the Study and Research Questions Fit?

The rationale for reviewing the literature is to help readers understand the purpose of the study. The purpose should be clearly specified in the introduction section. The literature review justifies the study; the research questions or hypothesis should follow it. Typically these consist of three or four objectives, which may be stated as questions that the writer plans to address in the article.

Traditional research papers typically specify *hypotheses,* which are research questions asked in a specific form; they state a predicted outcome, in a particular direction. For example, a hypothesis might state that children with cerebral palsy will not make greater gains in hippotherapy than children with acquired head injuries. Another hypothesis could state that children with cerebral palsy would show greater gains in self-esteem when engaged in hippotherapy than when they are in a traditional therapy program. Hypotheses often suggest the methodology.

For qualitative research, the researcher may pose research questions, then interview the participants to find the answers to the questions. In such research, the emphasis is on exploring an area without imposing preconceived theories on the investigation (Cook, 2001). Occasionally, in qualitative research or naturalistic inquiry, questions are not posed at the beginning of the study (see DePoy & Gitlin, 1994, 1998).

Summary

- Sort the literature into subtopics or themes.
- Perform an exhaustive search of the literature.
- Reference all assertions.
- Do not plagiarize, but do paraphrase.
- Use primary sources.
- Limit quotations to avoid fragmenting the flow of ideas.
- Include the purpose of the study and research questions.

Method

The "Method" section describes the research design and how the data were analyzed.

Design

In hippotherapy, a variety of designs have been used throughout the literature; researchers suggest that qualitative designs may be more appropriate for hippotherapy than quantitative designs (Buck, 2001; Pauw, 1999). Reasons include the lack of homogeneity of hippotherapy treatment populations; the inability of standardized tools to measure clinically meaningful change; the dearth of reliable, valid instruments with which to measure horseback riding skills; the variability of skills within the population with a specific diagnosis; and the influence of environmental factors.

Ottenbacher and York (1986) discussed the single-subject design and offered useful information on its advantages and disadvantages. They stated that single-subject design is the preferred method for evaluating change in human services environments because it is clinically based and clinician oriented, so that a clinician can monitor progress and adjust the intervention as a result of the data produced. This is not possible with traditional quantitative data (Ottenbacher & York, 1986). It is tempting to apply the research results of a single-case design to another case, but doing so can be problematic because of the many unknown factors involved in a given outcome. Consequently, Ottenbacher and York suggested that single-case research results be related back to theory rather than directly to practice. "Therapeutic practice based on a synthesis of theory and research provides a firm foundation for clinical intervention that is removed from trial and error intuition" (p. 117).

The Method section should describe the following aspects of the study: participants, equipment, variables, assessment and interview instruments, and procedures (APA, 2001; Weiss-Lambrou, 1989). The participants must be described in sufficient detail that readers know how they were selected and, if applicable, randomized. The article should describe the extent to which the participants are representative of the larger population (Weiss-Lambrou, 1989; see also Oermann et al., 2002). If special equipment was used, it must be described in enough detail that another researcher can obtain the equipment and replicate the study. The variables tested in the study must be specified and described. Similarly, all measurement instruments must have their properties described (i.e., their reliability and validity). In addition, this section should outline the necessary credentials and the training for the person doing the testing.

If interviews or focus groups were used in the research, the article should include an outline of the interview and a description of how it captures the variables the researcher is examining. A subsection on procedures should include information on the instructions to participants, any experimental manipulation, and whether randomization or counterbalancing took place and how it was managed. If another language is involved, indicate how the translations were obtained.

In summary, the Method section should tell readers what was done in enough detail that the study can be replicated.

Results

The "Results" section often poses problems for new researchers. Writing the results section is a mechanical process that does not include any interpretation of the data. The writer is simply reporting the findings.

The type of analysis used to arrive at the results is the first piece of information your readers need to know. Researchers should always consult with a statistician (or invite one to sit in on the project) before embarking on any research. Statisticians are invaluable in helping determine sample size and designing the study to allow valid statistical analysis of the results.

The goal of the results section is to report the primary findings of the study, including both positive and negative outcomes (Weiss-Lambrou, 1989). It is important to stick to the facts, be concise, and report exactly what the data say without any interpretation. Tell the audience what is important for them to know rather than what is simply "nice to know" (Weiss-Lambrou, 1989). Be sure to disclose even those findings that contradict what was originally predicted (Oermann et al., 2002).

Tables and graphs are efficient ways to summarize the great quantity of information coming from most studies. The inclusion of tables depends on the data.

When comparing groups and looking for group differences using numeric data, then tables undeniably help consolidate the information. If the study primarily generated narrative data from interviews or focus groups, then tables generally will not be helpful, unless the narrative data are somehow consolidated and described quantitatively (e.g., the number of times different topics arose). Tables and figures should be as simple as possible (Weiss-Lambrou, 1989). Because their function is to support the text, they should not merely duplicate what has already been said in the text (Oermann et al., 2002).

Summary

- Simply report the findings, without comment.
- Report the primary findings.
- Consult with a statistician or qualitative researcher before beginning the study and again when summarizing results.

Discussion

The "Discussion" section is the most creative and exciting, but it also is the most challenging to write. The Discussion is where the author can let his or her creative juices flow. The author is no longer bogged down by documentation but can build arguments and interpretations of the findings that are based on the literature review, research, and experience.

The Discussion section relates the findings back to the literature and tries to make sense of unexpected results. The author is using his or her reasoning skills to uncover the real meaning of the results. Again, all quotations or statistics should be documented. This section should include recommendations for future research that would either improve on the current work or that would be important to have before additional research can be undertaken in the area of the current study.

Conclusion

The "Conclusion" section might include the theoretical or clinical implications of the study, recommendations for further study, and an indication of the significance of the work (Oermann et al., 2002; Weiss-Lambrou, 1989). If appropriate, the writer may encourage clinician readers to modify their current practice on the basis of the study's findings (Oermann et al., 2002).

Other Sections

An "Acknowledgments" section should follow the Conclusion, unless the journal has other requirements.

Briefly thank the sources of support, the participants (including riders, parents, technicians, and therapists), consultants (e.g., statisticians), and the riding centers involved in the research. All illustrations or photographs of horses or riders used in the research should have artist or photographer credit, as appropriate. The "References" section should follow the acknowledgments, and the tables and figures should be included last. Follow all journal requirements for art submission (art includes photographs, illustrations, tables, and figures—anything that is not text).

References

American Psychological Association. (2001). *Publication manual of the American Psychological Association* (5th ed.). Washington, DC: Author.

Ballinger, C., Curtin, M., Eakin, P., Hollis, V., Nicol, M., & Telford, R. (1996). Writing an abstract. *British Journal of Occupational Therapy, 59,* 33–35.

Buck, W. (2001). Therapeutic riding for children with emotional or behavioral disorders: Recommendations for research. *Scientific and Educational Journal of Therapeutic Riding, 7,* 76–90.

Cook, J. (2001). Qualitative research in occupational therapy. In J. Cook (Ed.), *Qualitative research in occupational therapy* (pp. 3–9). Albany, NY: Delmar.

Cormack, D. (1994). *Writing for health care professions.* Oxford: Blackwell Scientific.

Day, R. A. (1998). *How to write and publish a scientific paper* (5th ed.). Phoenix, AZ: Oryx Press.

DePoy, E., & Gitlin, L. N. (1994). *Introduction to research: Multiple strategies for health and human services.* Toronto: Mosby.

DePoy, E., & Gitlin, L. N. (1998). *Introduction to research: Understanding and applying multiple strategies.* Toronto: Mosby.

French, S. (1993). *Practical research: A guide for therapists.* Oxford: Butterworth-Heinemann.

Hasselkus, B. (2001). Writing the abstract: The most important part of the manuscript? *American Journal of Occupational Therapy, 55,* 127–128.

Oermann, M., Mason, N., & Wilmes, N. (2002). Accuracy of references in general readership nursing journals. *Nurse Educator, 27,* 260–264.

Ottenbacher, K., & York, J. (1986). Strategies for evaluating clinical change: Implications for practice and research. In K. Ottenbacher & B. Bonder (Eds.), *Scientific inquiry: Design and analysis issues in occupational therapy* (pp. 110–121). Rockville, MD: American Occupational Therapy Association.

Pauw, J. (1999). Data analytical problems experienced in therapeutic riding research and a statistical explanation to some of the problems. *Scientific and Educational Journal of Therapeutic Riding, 5,* 65–70.

Weiss-Lambrou, R. (1989). *The health professional's guide to writing for publication.* Springfield, IL: Charles C Thomas.

Williams, D. (2002). *Writing skills in practice: A practical guide for health professionals.* London: Jessica Kingsley.

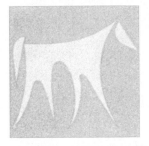

*He doth nothing
but talk of his horse.*
—*William Shakespeare*

APPENDIX B

How to Write a Research Proposal

Joyce R. MacKinnon, PhD, OT(C), OTR

Many clinicians will need to write a research proposal at some point during their careers. It may be for an employer who must accommodate a reduced workload to account for the research, for an ethics review board that must approve the project, for sites where the clinician hopes to recruit participants, or for funding agencies that may offer financial support (Cormack, 1994). From my experience sitting on national and provincial granting agencies, it appears that the success rate of funding requests for research proposals is about 30 percent; therefore, it is important that novice researchers be knowledgeable of the major factors that need to be considered when deciding to write a grant proposal for funding. Frequently, the granting agency rejects the proposal because some portion was neglected or the agency's guidelines were not followed. Missing the submission deadline may automatically bring a rejection.

The purpose, then, of this appendix is to provide readers with issues (modified from those presented by Portney and Watkins, 2000) to consider in creating a research proposal. The appendix is divided into three major areas: the research plan, budget support for the research, and other important topics.

Research Plan

The research plan should include the title, an abstract, a table of contents (if needed), a statement of the research problem, the purpose of the study, a literature review, the research methodology, a reference list, and documen-

tation of informed consent and institutional review board approval.

Title

The title must tell readers what the study is about in sufficient detail to be both informative and concise (Portney & Watkins, 2000). Miller and Salkind (2002) recommended providing a title page that includes the following information:
- Name of agency to which proposal is being submitted
- Name and address of institution submitting proposal
- Title of proposed project
- Name, title, phone number, e-mail address, and mailing address of project director
- Period of time over which the proposed research is to take place
- Requested amount of funds
- Date of proposal
- Endorsements.
Some funders require such a title page.

Table of Contents

This section is necessary only if the proposal is especially long and if including a table of contents will make it easier for readers to follow the proposal (Miller & Salkind, 2002).

Abstract

The abstract should "highlight the purpose and the importance of the proposed project" (Portney & Watkins, 2000, p. 635). Cormack (1994) suggested that the abstract be approximately 200 words (different funders have different requirements). Write the abstract after the entire proposal has been written to summarize most effectively the objectives of the proposal and the procedures (Miller & Salkind, 2002).

Adapted with permission by the Federation of Riding for the Disabled. Original version of appendix appeared in the *Scientific and Educational Journal of Therapeutic Riding* (2005), pp. 50–64.

Statement of the Research Problem

The statement of the research problem is the core of the study and the reason for undertaking the research (Bailey, 1991). This statement establishes the purpose of the study: its aims, objectives, hypotheses, and research questions. It also answers the question, What will the study achieve for one's clients, one's program, or one's profession (Bailey, 1991)? French (1993) suggested five sequential stages to move through when writing the statement of the research problem: identify a general problem area; connect the problem with existing theory; narrow the focus to clarify what concepts are being studied; decide how to measure those concepts; then, finally, state the hypotheses or research questions. The process moves the writer from the general to the specific. The results of the literature review should help narrow the research questions.

Literature Review

The literature review informs readers about what is known and unknown about the topic. According to French (1993), a literature search has many purposes: to understand the area of interest, suggest new ideas or clarify research questions, prevent duplication and avoid making others' mistakes, identify measurement instruments that might be valuable in the research, identify a study worth doing, and define terminology. Nolinske (1996) stated that a review of the literature justifies and supports the design of a project. It also provides a rationale and potential significance of the current project by putting it into context.

Two important and overarching principles guiding any literature review are to refute or confirm common beliefs regarding the topic of interest and to provide the theoretical basis to ground the study (French, 1993; Portney & Watkins, 2000; Stein & Cutler, 2000). Opinion is not appropriate in this section, unless it is supported with evidence (e.g., preferring one theory over another, rejecting the conclusions of previous research). For the literature review to have the necessary impact on readers, it needs to include the most recent and well-known literature in the field and strengthen the case for the proposed study (Tarling & Crofts, 2002).

Krathwohl (1998) outlined tips for the process of working through literature, which can be summarized as (1) read material, (2) organize it, and (3) talk—even daydream—about it. Krathwohl emphasized that one must read and become familiar with material related to, as well as specific to, the topic; "read actively," attempting to predict the writer's next thought; look for incon-sistencies in the material; and attempt to challenge conclusions using previous research results. It is important to mentally organize the material to find interrelationships between concepts. Krathwohl recommended that the researcher also talk with specialists in the area to gain new perspectives or to consolidate those already found. Before finishing the task, daydreaming and other methods of distraction allow for the release of creative energies and thoughts.

Research Methodology

The research methodology establishes the specific purpose of your study—its aims, objectives and research questions, and hypotheses. It answers the question, What does the author want to achieve for his or her clients, program, or profession (Bailey, 1991)? The results of the literature review should help narrow the research questions. From there, French (1993) suggested five sequential stages:

1. Identify a general problem area.
2. Connect the problem with existing theory.
3. Narrow the focus of the questions so it becomes clearer what concepts are being studied.
4. Decide how to measure the concepts being studied, and be specific about that.
5. State the hypotheses or research questions.

In essence, this process involves moving from the general to the specific.

Most or all sources should come from scholarly journals; avoid merely listing different authors, followed by their findings. Grouping authors by common themes is more logical and reader friendly. Keep investigating literature until the same references begin to appear repeatedly, and report only sources that have a direct relationship to the research question (see Appendix A in this book). A recent article by Coster and Vergara (2004) offered some practical suggestions for people who are conducting literature searches away from university campuses.

Portney and Watkins (2000) stated that the "method section is probably the most important part of the proposal, and should be both clear and concise" (p. 637). Exhibit B.1 outlines some of the issues relating to methodology that may be of assistance to beginning researchers.

Participants and Sample Size

This section specifies the sampling methods, number of participants, plans for recruitment, inclusion and exclusion criteria, and specific characteristics (e.g., age,

Exhibit B.1.
Research Methodology—Qualitative (Naturalistic Inquiry) or Quantitative?

Occupational therapists often seem confused as to whether they should use qualitative or quantitative research methodology. The setting in which the researcher operates may introduce biases of its own. Some employers and health authorities provide guidelines on how to conduct research, and their forms for creating proposals often are biased toward quantitative research using a medical model (Morton-Cooper, 2000).

When should a researcher use each type of research? This exhibit offers some advice on when to use each type of research.

Qualitative Methodology

Although qualitative design yields much richer data, it is labor intensive. Qualitative researchers often are more interested in the process than in predicting the outcome (Cook, 2001). Cook stated that in practical terms, this means that qualitative researchers focus on understanding the problem rather than testing predetermined solutions. Krathwohl (1998) offered help when he suggested that qualitative methods may be appropriate in the following situations:

- A lack of research exists.
- The emphasis is on exploration of the topic rather than supporting a particular hypothesis.
- The topic involves complex interactions.
- The focus is on the inherent qualities of a phenomenon, rather than its effects.
- The focus is on details and diversity within a phenomenon, rather than comparing those elements to standard measures.
- Standardized measures would be inappropriate, intrusive, or impossible to conduct.
- No standardized measures are available, and it would be impractical to develop one for the study.
- Fresh perspectives are sought (e.g., when research progress has plateaued).
- There is reason to believe participants' perspectives differ from observers in a way that might explain their behavior.
- Unanticipated side effects could be an important issue.

Quantitative Methodology

Qualitative methods are not appropriate for all situations. Seale and Barnard (1998) suggested that the following situations warrant a quantitative approach:
- Effectiveness of a particular therapeutic procedure is important to establish.
- A procedure must be demonstrated to be valid with particular clients in a certain clinical environment.
- Measurements must be quantified, rather than guessed or approximated.

Traynor, Rafferty, and Spragg (2003) reported that proposals are most likely to receive funding when they integrate both qualitative and quantitative methods.

sex, disability) of the population to be studied (Portney & Watkins, 2000). Nolinske (1996) stated that a sample should describe the population at large, if generalization of results is a goal of the study.

The way people are selected for research participation depends on the purpose of the study (see DePoy & Gitlin, 1998; Tarling & Crofts, 2002). Approaches can be divided into six categories:

1. *Maximum variation:* Participants are extreme in their contrasts along a particular dimension.
2. *Homogeneous selection:* Participants have similar experiences.
3. *Theory-based selection:* Participants exhibit a particular construct under study (e.g., loneliness).
4. *Confirming and disconfirming cases:* Researcher expands understanding of a particular phenomenon as a means of developing theory or interpretations.
5. *Extreme or variant cases:* Participants are extreme cases of the phenomenon.
6. *Typical cases:* Participants are average on the particular dimension.

The next question to be addressed involves the number of participants be recruited. According to DePoy and Gitlin (1998, p. 174), determining sample size involves four primary considerations:

1. Data analytic procedures to be used
2. Statistical significance (usually chosen at $p = .05$ or .01)
3. Statistical power (.80 acceptable)
4. Effect size.

It is recommended that the researcher solicit the help of a seasoned statistician to help with this aspect of research design.

According to Sommer and Sommer (1997), the researcher should decide on a sample size before beginning the research; otherwise, the research may appear to be biased (e.g., a researcher may add participants until he or she obtains the desired results). French (1993) advised researchers to consider the following issues:

- *Practical matters:* What are the availability of participants and the costs involved?
- *Representation and generalization:* Other things being equal, large sample sizes provide better reliability and representation than do small samples (Sommer & Sommer, 1997).
- *Variability of results:* If expected results (or characteristics of the population) are highly variable, a larger sample size is needed.
- *Purpose of the study:* Is the goal to test out a research design (pilot study) or to determine characteristics of the population?

- *Size of the population:* If the population is small, a smaller sample size may be adequately representative.
- *Commitment of participants:* Recruit enough participants to accommodate dropouts.
- *Ethical considerations:* Consider any discomfort, inconvenience, or disadvantage to be endured by participants.

In qualitative research, no specific rules exist regarding the numbers of people needed in a study, because this type of research focuses on in-depth observation or interviewing (see DePoy & Gitlin, 1998). If the intent is to examine a phenomenon that is a shared experience, a homogeneous population should be used to reduce the variance; a small number, such as 5 to 10 participants, is probably adequate. DePoy and Gitlin suggested that to maximize the variation in experiences, the researcher may need 20 to 50 participants.

Unfortunately, quantitative research strategies for selecting participants are not appropriate for hippotherapy, because hippotherapy involves such small numbers of participants and, therefore, small sample sizes. French (1993) is a good source for information on types of sampling. Additional information on this topic can be found in Exhibit B.2.

Types of sampling include probability and nonprobability sampling. Nonprobability sampling, according to French (1993), involves the researcher's subjective judgment in selecting the sample. This method is less reliable but may be adequate for the study's purpose, and it is easier to implement than probability sampling. The various types of nonprobability sampling, as presented by French are as follows:

- *Purposive sampling:* The sample is "hand picked."
- *Snowball sampling:* The sample is recruited via word of mouth.
- *Quota sampling:* The sample is chosen as in stratified random sampling (where the sampling frame is divided into non-overlapping groups), but the process is performed in a nonrandom way (in a particular place, for example).

Materials

The proposal should specify any equipment, materials, or assessment instruments that are intended to be used (Portney & Watkins, 2000)

Procedures

The procedures section should explain the research plan from the beginning of the project to its completion. A timetable is helpful; it should include milestones for training, subject recruitment, assignment, assessment, treatment, reassessment, and final report to the funding agency.

Qualitative Research Design

Qualitative approaches to research include the following (see DePoy & Gitlin, 1998; Llewellyn, Cutler, & Stein, 2000):

- *Case study (prospective or retrospective):* In-depth data collection of a person, organization, or event from multiple sources
- *Grounded theory* or *heuristic study:* Method for generating theory during the data collection.
- *Phenomenological:* Universal meanings are generated from individual descriptions.
- *Ethnography* or *field study:* Using participant observation to examine a culture or social group.
- *Biography:* Study of an individual through life histories, profiles, journals, case studies, or autobiographies.

Cook (2001), an occupational therapist, provided an abbreviated list of qualitative methods that includes participant action research, in-depth interviewing, and participant observation. She also provided several chapters on what she calls "personal journeys," which are written by a number of occupational therapy graduate students regarding their experience as they undertake their qualitative research.

Exhibit B.2.
Probability Sampling

Probability sampling involves randomly selecting from the population to be studied in an effort to gain a sample that is generalizable to the larger population. Following are some examples of types of probability sampling (see French, 1993):

- *Simple random sampling:* A completely random sample (e.g., a raffle).
- *Systematic sampling (quasi-random):* Selection of every *n*th person on a list.
- *Stratified random sampling:* A sample meant to mirror the population in some predetermined way (e.g. gender proportion).
- *Multistage sampling:* A random selection of groups is selected, then a random selection within those groups is made (e.g., the researcher randomly selects certain hospitals, then randomly selects patients within these hospitals).
- *Cluster sampling:* Random selection of subjects by group membership (homogeneity of clusters is crucial to be able to make statements about populations as a whole).

Quantitative Approaches

DePoy and Gitlin (1998) described the following experimental or quantitative approaches:
- True experimental design
- Variations of experimental design
- Quasi-experimental design
- Pre-experimental designs
- Nonexperimental designs.

Data Analysis

Data analysis outlines how data will be recorded, stored, and analyzed. Qualitative and quantitative approaches use different methods of data analysis.

At the start of qualitative analysis, the researcher will be thinking about the processes, then developing categories and taxonomies and discovering underlying themes (DePoy & Gitlin, 1998; Tarling & Crofts, 2002). During the next phase, the researcher will examine the accuracy and rigor in the analysis (DePoy & Gitlin, 1998) by using the following techniques:
- *Triangulation:* The study of one phenomenon using more than one strategy (e.g., interviewing and direct observation)
- *Saturation:* Occurs when additional information does not lead to new insights
- *Member checks:* Confirming assumptions with another participant (e.g., checking with the rider to see if your impressions are accurate)
- *Reflexivity:* A process of self-examination by the researcher to determine what has been learned (e.g., the researcher does not know what it is like to be a rider with disabilities and so changes perceptions of and assumptions about riders with disabilities as the research progresses)
- *Audit trail:* The researcher keeps notes in detail so that another researcher can follow them; the researcher should be able not only to report but also to explain the results
- *Peer debriefing:* The researcher shares results with another researcher and seeks agreement.

Quantitative analysis always involves numbers and statistics. Statistics can be categorized into three categories (see, e.g., DePoy & Gitlin, 1998):
- *Descriptive statistics:* Data analysis using measures of central tendency, measures of variability, and bivariate descriptive statistics.
- *Inferential statistics:* Analysis based on inferences from the data; it includes parametric and nonparametric statistics.

- *Association and relationship:* Analysis that attempts to determine causality by examining correlations; it includes multivariate analysis (e.g., multiple regression, discriminate analysis, path analysis).

Reference List

The sources of literature cited in the proposal should be included in a reference list.

Ethics Approval and Informed Consent

Before a research proposal can be sent to a granting agency, the researchers must show evidence of having the proposal approved by an ethics board for human subjects (typically, these boards are referred to as institutional review boards [IRBs], and all hospitals, universities, and treatment centers have one). All aspects of the proposal must be vetted by an IRB.

The researcher may be required to seek approval not only from a hospital or treatment center, but also the university with which he or she is affiliated. This task can be time intensive, particularly because many IRBs review proposals on a fixed schedule, usually once per month. Once a decision is rendered, then the researcher will be contacted as to whether revisions are required or whether he or she may proceed with the study. Should more than one level of approval be required, the process can be stressful and time consuming for the researcher.

Many boards have two types of review: (1) *full review,* which requires the entire board's approval, and (2) *expedited review,* which consists of a subgroup of the board, who may grant approval to proposals that do not involve invasive procedures or high risk to participants. For the most part, research involving vulnerable participants, such as children, people with disabilities, or people deemed incompetent, would require a full review.

You will need IRB approval prior to submission of the proposal (Portney & Watkins, 2000). A copy of the informed consent should be included with the proposal. It is a good idea to build IRB approval into your research timetable.

Budget Support for Research

In addition to the plan of research, the granting agency will need information on the budget for the research project, which should include personnel, travel, equipment, supplies, and equipment rental. Most agencies will fund only for a specific project and will not grant funds for operating costs (Camarena, 2000). Project-specific costs include supplies, insurance, and training and staffing needs (be sure to specify the type of staff and the number of hours per week needed). Some funders will cover construction costs. If your project will receive revenue from clients, indicate how that will be applied to research expenses. (See Kirk-Smith, 1996; Nolinske, 1996; Tarling & Crofts, 2002; and Turner, 1996 for more information on budgeting.) A narrative budget justification section that addresses each line item of the budget is helpful, even if the funder does not request it, because it demonstrates accountability.

Conclusion

In summary, it is very important to follow a research plan. If the proposal is being written for a granting agency, all information requested must be completed. Should information on the application form be unclear or not understood, then the researchers need to contact the granting agency and clarify. The application form also should be complete. If the question on the form does not apply, then indicate it. Proposals must satisfy granting agency staff guidelines (e.g., meeting the deadline date) or it will rejected before it even has the opportunity of being considered for funding. Outside reviewers, for the most part, are researchers who volunteer their time and have other full time jobs; therefore, they might reject an otherwise excellent proposal simply because of missing information or some aspect of the proposal that is not presented clearly. In addition, researchers should be clear about their research methodology, providing sufficient details and the rationale for using it. All budget details need to be included, because researchers have only one chance to request funding; important omissions can adversely affect the outcome of the proposed research.

The best advice is to prepare the research proposal well ahead of time, plan the methodology carefully, and submit a budget with precision, accuracy, and attention to details. Finally, it reflects positively on researchers to submit a proposal that is esthetically pleasing, following the guidelines of the granting agency.

References

Bailey, D. (1991). *Research for the health professional: A practical guide*. Philadelphia: F. A. Davis.

Camarena, J. (2000). A wealth of information on foundations and the grant seeking process. *Computers in Libraries, 20*(5), 26–31.

Cook, J. (2001). Qualitative research in occupational therapy. In J. Cook (Ed.), *Qualitative research in occupational therapy* (pp. 3–9). Albany, NY: Delmar.

Cormack, D. (1994). *Writing for health care professions*. Oxford: Blackwell Scientific.

Coster W., & Vergara, E. (2004, March). Finding resources to support EBP: What to do when the university isn't next door. *OT Practice*, pp. 10–15.

DePoy, E., & Gitlin, L. N. (1998). *Introduction to research: Understanding and applying multiple strategies*. Toronto: Mosby.

French, S. (1993). *Practical research: A guide for therapists*. Oxford: Butterworth-Heinemann.

Kirk-Smith, M. (1996). Winning ways with research proposals and reports. *Nursing Times, 92*(11), 36–38.

Krathwohl, D. (1998). *Methods of educational and social science research: An integrated approach*. New York: Longman.

Llewellyn, G., Cutler, S. K., & Stein, F. (2000). Qualitative research models. In F. Stein & S. K. Cutler (Eds.), *Clinical research in occupational therapy*. New York: Singular Thompson Learning.

Miller, D., & Salkind, N. (Eds.). (2002). *Handbook of research design and social measurement*. Thousand Oaks, CA: Sage.

Morton-Cooper, A. (2000). *Action research in health care*. Oxford: Blackwell Science.

Nolinske, T. (1996). Research forum: Writing a research proposal. *Journal of Prosthetics and Orthotics, 8,* 132–137.

Portney, L. G., & Watkins, M. P. (2000). *Foundations of clinical research: Applications to practice*. Toronto: Prentice Hall.

Seale, J., & Barnard, S. (1998). *Therapy research: Processes and practicalities*. Oxford: Butterworth-Heinemann.

Sommer, R., & Sommer, B. (1997). *A practical guide to behavioural research* (4th ed.). Oxford: Oxford University Press.

Stein, F., & Cutler, S. K. (2000). *Clinical research in occupational therapy*. New York: Singular Thompson Learning.

Tarling, M., & Crofts, L. (2002). Writing a proposal. In M. Tarling & L. Crofts (Eds.), *The essential researcher's handbook for nurses and healthcare professionals* (2nd ed., pp. 82–89). Edinburgh, Scotland: Baillere Tindall.

Traynor, M., Rafferty, A., & Spragg, J. (2003). Decent proposals. *Nursing Standard, 17*(28), 112.

Turner, S. O. (1996). How to write a winning proposal. *American Journal of Nursing, 96*(7), 64–65.

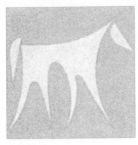

APPENDIX C

Recommended Reading for Hippotherapy

Bennet, D. (1988). *Principles of conformation analysis* (Vol. 1). Gaithersburg, MD: Fleet Street.

Harris, S. E. (1993). *Horse gaits, balance, and movement.* New York: Howell Book House/Macmillan.

Henriquet, M. (2004). *Henriquet on dressage.* North Pomfret, VT: Trafalgar Square.

Reide, D. (1988). *Physiotherapy on the horse.* Riderwood, MD: Therapeutic Riding Services & The Delta Society.

Russell, M., & Steele, A. W. (2004). *Lessons in lightness: The art of educating the horse.* Gilford CT: Lynons.

Schusdziarra, H., & Schusdziarra, V. (1978). *An anatomy of riding.* Briarcliff, NY: Breakthrough.

Stewart, D. (2004). *Riding right.* North Pomfret, VT: Trafalgar Square.

Strauss, I. (1995). *Hippotherapy: Neurological therapy on the horse.* Ontario: Ontario Therapeutic Riding Association.

Swift, S. (2002). *Centered riding 2; further exploration.* North Pomfret, VT: Trafalgar Square.

Von Dietz, S. (2005). *Balance in movement: How to achieve the perfect seat.* North Pomfret, VT: Trafalgar Square.

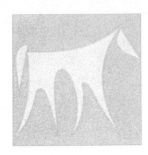

Index

NOTE: Page numbers followed by *f* indicate a figure will be found on that page. Page numbers followed by *t* indicate a table will be found on that page.

A

acceleration transducer, 57
accelerometry, 65
acknowledgment skills, 204
Acredolo, L., 223, 226
activities
    equine-assisted, 4
    occupation-based, 32
activities of daily living, 232
adaptation, 143
adaptive responses, 220
adaptive riding. *See* riding
adductor spasticity, 54
AHA. *See* American Hippotherapy Association
Allan, D. E., 58–59
Allen, A. S., 187
Allen, Claudia K., 26
Allori, P., 63
American Hippotherapy Association (AHA)
    on the benefits of hippotherapy, 11–12
    development of hippotherapy, 3
    German–Swiss–Austrian model, 4
    hippotherapy, definition of, 8
    integration of hippotherapy into mainstream therapy, 180–181
American Occupational Therapy Association (AOTA)
    activity analysis process, 185–191
    Practice Framework, 30–31
    The Scope of Practice, 202
    Web site, 264
analysis of covariance (ANCOVA), 59
anatomical directions of development, 196
Andrade, C. K., 61
ANOVA summary table, 96*t*

AOTA. *See* American Occupational Therapy Association; *Occupational Therapy Practice Framework*
appropriate adaptive responses, 220
apraxia, 21
Armstrong, C. A., 56
arsenic, 100
The Art of Horsemanship (Xenophon), 36
Ary, D., 84
assessments, 231
asymmetrical weight bearing, 200*f*
athetoid cerebral palsy, 9
atresia. *See* CHARGE syndrome
auditory system, 212–213, 216
autism, 59, 103–110, 107*t*–109*t*, 119–125, 242
autonomy, 17
Avaliani, I. A., 62–63, 65–66
avoidance and psychological fleeing response, 230
Ayalon, A., 56
Ayres, Jean
    discriminatory system, 212
    integrative frame of reference, 103
    reticular formation, definition of, 211
    sensory integration, 192–193, 220
    sensory therapy, 42–43
    work of, 21–22

B

back pain, 62
backriding, 40–41
Baker, E. A., 57–58, 87
balance, 38–39, 56, 64–65, 144–145
Bar, D., 56
Barbour, R. S., 170
Baucher, François, 36–37
Baum, Carolyn M., 7, 25
Baumann, J. U., 47–48, 53, 93
BCOPD. *see* body center of pressure dispersion area

Let Me Teach You

When you are tense, let me teach you to relax.
When you are short tempered, let me teach you to be patient.
When you are short sighted, let me teach you to see.
When you are quick to react, let me teach you to be thoughtful.
When you are angry, let me teach you to be serene.
When you feel superior, let me teach you to be respectful.
When you are self-absorbed, let me teach you to think of greater things.
When you are arrogant, let me teach you humility.
When you are lonely, let me be your companion.
When you are tired, let me carry your load.
When you need to learn, let me teach you.

After all, I am your horse.

—*Willis Lamm*
(Reprinted with permission)